HORIZONS IN CANCER RESEARCH

HORIZONS IN CANCER RESEARCH

VOLUME 54

HORIZONS IN CANCER RESEARCH

Additional books in this series can be found on Nova's website
under the Series tab.

Additional e-books in this series can be found on Nova's website
under the e-book tab.

HORIZONS IN CANCER RESEARCH

VOLUME 54

HIROTO S. WATANABE
EDITOR

Nova Biomedical

New York

For permission to use material from this book please contact us:
Telephone 631-231-7269; Fax 631-231-8175
Web Site: http://www.novapublishers.com

Library of Congress Cataloging-in-Publication Data

ISSN: 2159-1326

ISBN: 978-1-63321-389-0

Published by Nova Science Publishers, Inc. † New York

Contents

Preface

This book presents original research results on the leading edge of cancer. Topics discussed include the risk factors, diagnosis and treatment options for glioblastoma; the biology of the interleukin-2 (il-2)-based immunotherapies in cancer and autoimmune disease; rna interference (rnai)/rna activation (rnaa) for cancer therapeutics; melanoma progression to metastatic disease; proteins, polysaccharide-peptide complexes and polysaccharides with antiproliferative and anticancer activities of mushrooms; low-molecular-weight compounds with anticancer activity of mushroom origin; lifestyle and cancer prevention; and the pathology and pathogenesis of Hodgkin's lymphoma.

Chapter 1 - Glioblastoma (GBM), also known as glioblastoma *multiforme*, is the most common and lethal primary brain tumor which exhibits clinical, radiological and pathological heterogeneity. Based on the fact that the incidence has been documented to be constant in various reports, genetic variation is more likely to play a major role in developing GBM than environmental, geographical and nutritional factors. MRI with contrast enhancement is the most commonly used method in the initial evaluation and follow-up after treatment. The typical finding of GBM is ring enhanced white matter lesion with central necrosis and perilesional edema on MRI. Microvascular proliferation and necrosis have been used as the most critical factor in pathological confirmation. Recently, some biomarkers such as O^6-methylguanine-DNA methyltransferase (MGMT) methylation, BRAF fusions, and IDH1 mutations have been suggested as possible prognostic and grading factors. Standard therapy includes microsurgical resection and a multimodal treatment of concomitant radiotherapy and chemotherapy, followed by adjuvant chemotherapy with temozolomide. In addition to functional or diffusion tensor MRI with navigation system or intraoperative MRI, fluorescence-guided resection helps surgeons to increase safety and accuracy in GBM surgery. MR spectroscopy and positron-emission tomography (PET) scans may provide useful information in differential diagnosis and making treatment plans. Anti-angiogenic therapy with antivascular endothelial growth factor antibodies (bevacizumab) is on its way into clinical practice. In this article, the authors discuss and highlight the advances in diagnosis and treatment of GBM with relevant reviews.

Chapter 2 - Interleukin-2 (IL-2) is an important T cell growth factor with the capacity to promote T cell expansion. Consistent with this idea, IL-2 is used clinically to enhance T cell responses to viral and tumor antigens in both preclinical models and patients. However, the role of IL-2 in immune responses is far more complex than initially expected. In addition to its ability to promote immune responses, IL-2 signaling is essential for the differentiation of regulatory T cells (Tregs), which suppress immune responses. Thus, IL-2 signaling can both promote and inhibit immune responses depending on the context, the dose, and the nature of the IL-2/IL-2 receptor interactions. As a result, IL-2 therapies that selectively target Tregs may be useful for treating autoimmune diseases, whereas IL-2 therapies that selectively target effector T cells may improve cancer immunotherapy. In this chapter the authors summarize their current understanding of the biology of IL-2-based immunotherapies for cancer and autoimmune disease.

Chapter 3 - Small double-stranded RNAs (dsRNAs) have emerged as main key regulators of gene expression. The small RNA molecules which suppress their target gene expression have been termed RNA interference (RNAi). The ability of transcriptional upregulation has been referred to RNA activation (RNAa). New evidences have shown that silencing hyperactive genes or activating genes targeted against the specific promoter region induce significant tumor responses. The recent preclinical animal model studies show strong evidence that dsRNA can be effective in treating liver cancer. The advanced technologies of nucleic acid therapeutics make small dsRNAs promising cancer therapeutics. The authors describe here strategies to turn genes off or on with small RNAs along with their tumor-specific delivery for the treatment of cancer. Given the potential of RNAs as druggable therapeutics, dsRNAs-based drugs can be exploited in fast growing therapeutic market.

Chapter 4 - Worldwide, melanoma has the most rapidly rising incidence rate of any human cancer. It arises from the malignant transformation of the melanocyte cells of the skin. Due to the inefficacy of present chemotherapeutic regimens and the resistance of melanocyte cells to radiotherapy, 95% of stage IV metastatic melanoma patients die within five years of diagnosis. Metastasis, the spread of a cancer from the site of the primary tumour to distant sites of the body, makes melanoma very hard to treat. Risk factors associated with malignant melanoma include excessive sun exposure and associated mutations in specific genes and deregulation of signal transduction pathways.

Malignant melanoma is characterized by frequent metastasis; however, specific changes that cause this malignancy are yet to be characterized. Several oncogenes, tumour suppressor genes, and pathways are implicated in melanoma; for example, NRAS, which activates RAF kinases in response to growth factors is overactive in 15–20% of melanomas. P16 (INK4A) tumour suppressor expression is lost by mutation, deletion, or transcriptional silencing of the CDKN2A locus in many melanomas. BRAF mutations are often found alongside P16 mutations. Phosphatase and tensin homolog (PTEN) mutations and deletions are also present in a significant number of melanomas, coinciding with BRAF mutations. Since these two mutations often occur together PTEN loss reflects the importance of two RAS-effector pathways in melanoma. Another genomic aberration associated with melanoma is the amplification of microphthalmia-associated transcription factor (MITF).

The occurrence of several different mutations implies that several signal transduction pathways are perturbed in melanoma. Of particular interest to this review are mutations in the Wnt/β-catenin pathway as well as the PI3K pathway. Elevated levels of nuclear β-catenin are observed in ~30% of human melanomas. In fact, melanoma is one of the first cancer types associated with β-catenin/Wnt signaling mutations. Mutations in the Wnt signaling pathway that result in over-activation of β-catenin signaling are readily observed in melanomas, but the functional implications of these mutations in melanoma progression remain unclear.

The PI3K pathway is likely the most frequently deregulated pathway in melanoma, although the mechanism underlying the over-activation in most cases remains largely elusive.

Growth factor stimulation of receptor tyrosine kinases (RTK) and/or non-RTKs results in the activation of PI3K and the conversion of phosphatidylinositol-bis-phosphate (PIP2) to phosphatidylinositol-tri- phosphate (PIP3). The presence of PIP3 mediates the phosphorylation and activation of Akt/PKB by PDK1/PDK2 at Threonine 308 (T308) and Serine 473 (S473). Activated Akt (phosphorylated Akt [P-Akt]) is the central effector of many downstream signaling pathways regulating protein synthesis, cell cycle, cell death, cell growth, and cell survival. In Melanoma, the loss of the tumour suppressor protein and negative regulator of the PI3K/Akt pathway, PTEN, is a common event leading to the constitutive activation of PI3K/Akt signaling. The consitutive activation of this pathway with PTEN loss and the resulting elevation of the P-AKT signaling axis may be a method for promoting/sustaining melanoma progression. This includes modes of regulation between PI3K/Akt and other pathways such as 1) cross-talk with the Wnt/GSK3β/β- catenin pathway, 2) cross-talk with FOXO family of transcription factors and 3) mammalian target of rapamycin (mTOR).

This review will discuss the current evidence available for PI3K/PTEN/Akt and Wnt- β-catenin mediated signaling in melanoma progression.

Chapter 5 - Proteins with antiproliferative activity toward cancer cells *in vitro* and/or anticancer activity *in vivo* are discussed in this review. Lectins, fungal immunomodulatory proteins, ribonucleases, ribosome-inactivating proteins, polysaccharide-peptide complexes, laccases, a hemolysin, a ubiquitin-like peptide, a protease, and a translation inhibiting protein are included in the discussion. The lectins comprise those from *Agaricus bisporus*, *Clitocybe nebularis*, *Cordyceps militaris*, *Flammulina velutipes*, *Ganoderma capense*, *Hericium erinaceum, Lactarius flavidulus, Pholiota adiposa, Pleurotus eous, Polyporus adusta, Russula delica, R.lepida, Schizophyllum commune, Tricholoma mongolicum, Xerocomus chrysenteron, Xylaria hypoxylon* and *Volvariella volvacea.* The fungal immunomodulatory proteins encompass those from *Flammulina velutipes, Ganoderma lucidum,* and *G. tsugae.* The ribonucleases comprise those from *Hypsizigus marmoreus, Pleurotus ostreatus, P. sajor-caju, Russula delica* and *Tuber indicum.* Ribosome-inactivating proteins include hypsin and marmorin, both from *Hypsizigus marmoreus.* The polysaccharide-peptide complexes include those from *Agaricus blazei*, *Coriolus versicolor*, *Grifola frondosa, Pleurotus abalones* and *P.pulmonarius.* The polysaccharides comprise those from *Armillaria mellea, Grifola frondosa, Lentinula edodes, Pleurotus abalones* and *P. nebrodensis. Pleurotus eryngii* hemolysin, *Agaricus placomyces* laccase, *Agrocybe cylindracea* laccase, *Agrocybe cylindracea* ubiquitin-like peptide, *Amanita farinosa* protease, and *Calvatia caelata* translation-inhibiting protein also display antiproliferative activity.

Chapter 6 - The following low-molecular-weight compounds of mushroom origins exhibit anticancer activity toward various cancer cells. The list of compounds include active hexose correlated compound, gamma-L-glutaminyl-4-hydroxybenzene derivatives from *Agaricus bisporus, Albatrellus confluens* grifolin, *Antrodia camphorata* ubiquinone derivative (antroquinonol), *Antrodia camphorata* sesquiterpene lactone (antrocin), *Astraeus odoratus* lanostane triterpenes (astraodoric acids A-D), *Boletus pseudocalopus* grifolin derivatives and phenolic compounds, *Chondrostereum sp.* hirsutane sesquiterpenoid (hirsutanol A), *Coprinus plicatilis* guanacastane-type diterpenoids, *Coprinus radians* diterpenoid (radianspene C), *Daedalea gibbosa* oleylamine-carbonyl-valinol, *Epicoccum sp* glycosylated tetramic acid derivative (epicoccamide D), ergosterol peroxide, *Fomitopsis nigra* lanostane triterpene glycoside (fomitoside-K), *Ganoderma lucidum* lanostanoid triterpene (ganodermanontriol), *Ganoderma lucidum* triterpene, *Ganoderma lucidum* ganoderic acids, *Ganoderma lucidum* ergosta-7,22-diene-2β,3α,9α-triol, *Hypholoma sublateritium* clavaric acid, *Inonotus obliquus* ergosterol peroxide and trametenolic acid, *Lentinus connatus* hirsutane sesquiterpenes (dihydrohypnophilin, panepoxydione, and panepoxydone), *Leucopaxillus gentianeus* cucurbitane triterpenoid (cucurbitacin B), L-glutamic acid dihydroxyanilide, *Naematoloma fasciculare* lanostane derivatives, *Naematoloma fasciculare* lanostane triterpenoids, *Omphalotus* illudin S derivative (Irofulven) and droxymethylacylfulvene, *Phellinus igniarius* phenolic (hispolon), *Phellinus linteus* phenolic (hispidin), *Poria cocos* triterpenes, *Thelephora aurantiotincta* thelephantin O and vialinin A, *Tomophagus cattienensis* steroids (cattienoids A-C), and *Tomophagus cattienensis* steroids (cattienoids A-C).

Chapter 7 - The burden of modern lifestyle diseases is enormous and the true unifying factor for most cancers seems to be lifestyle. The intervention with the modification of lifestyle factors seems to be a physiological and safe approach for the prevention and management of modern lifestyle diseases including cancer. Defining the precise role of diet and other lifestyle factors in cancer may require the elucidation of genetic susceptibility and genetic-environmental interactions. The modifications in the diet along with secondary prevention measures may have a major impact on reducing the mortality from cancer. Lifestyle modifications offer an important strategy for cancer prevention. However, a change in only one lifestyle factor is unlikely to reduce the risk of cancer or other diseases. Environmental exposures by themselves do not cause cancer. Cancer is complex and involves many gene-gene interactions that occur inside you and are not well understood. Over your lifetime, random gene changes are passed along as your body cells grow and divide, so they accumulate. The unique patterns that evolve over time may make some people more likely than others to increase their risk for cancer after exposure to a particular chemical or after choosing a particular behavior. Whether a future obesity-related cancer burden is realized will depend greatly on competing risks and survival from other affected chronic diseases—cardiovascular disease and diabetes in particular. Similarly for alcohol, multiple competing risks of mortality from, for instance, accidents and violence, alcohol poisoning, and acute ischemic heart disease will affect whether individuals survive to be at risk for cancer.

Chapter 8 - The histopathological and fine-needle aspiration (FNA) cytologic diagnosis of Hodgkin's lymphoma (HL) is based on demonstration of the so called pathognomonic mononucleated Hodgkin's and bi- to multinucleated Reed-Sternberg (HRS) cells among reactive cellular component composed of lymphocytes, benign histiocytes, neutrophils and eosinophils. Hodgkin's lymphoma (HL) is one of the most common lymphomas in the developed world with an incidence of approximately three per 100,000 person-years but it is uncommon in the Far-East countries as compared to rest of the world and relatively uncommon in Sub-Saharan African countries**.** When the reported frequency in the Far-East countries was compared with the rest of the world, it exceeded 20% in none of the reports from the Far-East countries, as opposed to 15 (68.2%) from rest of the world ($p=0.00002$). When Sub-Saharan African countries were compared with rest of the non-Far-East countries of the world, it was observed that the frequency of HL exceeded 20% in 2 (28.6%) of the Sub-Saharan African countries and in13 (86.7%) of the 15 other counties ($p=0.01355$). Nearly five decades ago Hodgkin's lymphoma, then known as Hodgkin's disease (HD) was categorized under Rye classification into lymphocytic predominant (LP), nodular sclerosis

(NS), mixed cellularity (MC) and lymphocytic depletion (LD) sub-types. Analysis of 33 reports on Rye classification from various countries revealed that the median percentages for LP, NS, MC and LD subtypes were 10.0%, 58.5%, 26.0% and 2.6%, respectively, from the developed economies and the corresponding figures from the developing countries were 9.5%, 29.4%, 44.1% and 8.9%, respectively. In NS subtype, the frequency exceeded 50% in significantly higher number of reports from the developed (9 of 13, 69.2%) than developing countries (3 of 20, 15.0%, p= 0.00281). A reverse trend was observed in MC subtype wherein frequency exceeding 30% of cases were compared (23.1% of the reports in developed vs. 90.0% in the developing world, p=0.00016). However, there was no significant difference between the developed and developing countries in respect of LP and LD subtypes when the number of reports with frequency exceeding 10% were compared (p=1.0000, and =0.70059, respectively).

The sub-classification of HL into LP, MC, and LD in histology as well as cytology depends on relative proportion of neoplastic HRS cells and reactive cellular components. In nodular sclerosis type of HL, islands of neoplastic cells including a special type of R-S cells called lacunar cells and reactive cell components are surrounded by collagenous bands, which are not appreciated in cytologic preparations leading to limitation of cytology in the diagnosis of NS subtype. HL is an unusual malignancy in which the malignant cells are much less (about 1% cells in tumor tissue) compared to reactive cell components. In the past, various possibilities put forth regarding nature of Hodgkin's disease were inflammatory, neoplastic, autoimmune reaction and an intermediate stage between inflammatory & neoplastic lesions. HRS cells were traditionally believed to be abnormal reticulum cells. With the advent of immunological markers in 1970s, three candidates emerged as possible sources of HRS cells: T-lymphocytes, B-lymphocytes and macrophages; interdigitating reticulm cells and early progenitor myeloid cells subsequently joined the membership club of progenitor cells. Based on observation of R-S cell and T-lymphocyte interaction, and stepwise cytolysis of R-S cells in scanning electron microscopic study, it was proposed that Hodgkin's disease was a war between T-lymphocytes and transformed macrophages; the various histological subtypes depended upon the outcome of this war. During this period, the understanding of nature of cells in the formation of non-Hodgkin's lymphoma (NHL) led to the emergence of a number of classifications and wide range of controversies was associated with it. Unlike non-Hodgkin's lymphoma, the fortress of Hodgkin's lymphoma seemed invincible in seventies through eighties into early nineties. But gradually notes of dissent started to appear. In earlier reports, Reed-Sternberg-like cells were reported not only in benign lymphoproliferative conditions like reactive lymphoid hyperplasia and infectious mononucleosis, but some of nonHodgkin lymphoma subtypes, e.g., chronic lymphocytic leukemia, mycosis fungoides, Burkitt's lymphoma, lymphoepithelioid lymphoma and immunoblastic lymphoma, and non-lymphoid malignancies like metastatic carcinoma, melanoma, sarcomas and germ cell tumors revealed presence of RS-like cells. It was subsequently found that some subtypes of non-Hodgkin lymphoma like anaplastic large cell lymphoma (ALCL), T-cell-histiocytic-rich B-cell lymphoma (TCHRBCL), and pleomorphic peripheral T-cell lymphoma were most commonly misdiagnosed as Hodgkin's disease. The immunocytochemical markers like CD15, CD30, CD45, CD3 and CD20 were of help in differentiating these entities. The immunocytochemical markers for HL were CD15+, CD30+, CD45-, B-, T-, and EMA-. ALCL were CD15-, CD30+, CD45+, B±, T±, EMA± and Alk1 ±; later B+ cases were excluded from ALCL pool. The neoplastic cells in TCHRBCL were CD15-, CD30-, CD45+,

CD3-, CD20+, EMA-; the accompanying rich lymphoid cell population was CD3+ and histiocytes were CD68+. With the separation of these entities, the empire of Hodgkin's disease started disintegrating. New immunohistochemical and molecular studies proved that the neoplastic cells in Hodgkin's disease was of B-cell origin and it was renamed as Hodgkin's lymphoma. In the WHO classification of Tumors of Hematopoietic and Lymphoid Tissue, Hodgkin's lymphoma was classified as nodular lymphocytic predominant HL and classical HL which was in turn classified into lymphocyte-rich, mixed cellular, lymphocytic depleted and nodular sclerosis subtypes. At present there is compelling evidence that HRS cells are clonal B-cells that have lost their B-cell phenotype. Whereas, classical HL is associated with crippling mutation of immunoglobulin genes, which prevents the production of a functional immunoglobulin molecule, the nodular lymphocytic predominance HL is associated with ongoing immunoglobulin gene hypermutation but absence of crippling mutation in their immunoglobulin genes. Mature B-cells lacking B-cell receptors would normally die by apoptosis. The rescue of Hodgkin cells and R-S cells from apoptosis is a key event in HL pathogenesis. Hodgkin cells and R-S cells express a number of receptors (at least six receptors that belong to TNF receptor family) that regulate tumor cell survival. Epstein-Barr virus (EBV), which was initially implicated in the pathogenesis of Burkitt's lymphoma, was found to be associated with other nonlymphoid malignancies (e.g., nasoparyngeal carcinoma and gastric carcinoma) and lymphoid neoplasms (B- and T-cell NHL). HL in varying proportions (ranged 26.1%to 93.8%, with a median 46.8%) was found to be associated with EBV in different studies. The escape from apoptosis and transcriptional reprogramming of HRS cells are interlinked and appear central to pathogenesis of HL. It is likely that EBV plays a role in reprogramming and survival through dysregulation of several signaling networks and transcription factors. As regards the reactive cellular infiltrate in HL, there is increased number of T-cells (CD4 and NKT subsets), decreased B-cells, and increased regulatory T-cells in comparision with reactive hyperplasia of lymph node; the tumor associated macrophages in HL are of prognostic importance. As it stands today, most of the cases of NHL and HL cases can be diagnosed based on cyto/histomorphology, immunocytochemistry, cytogenetic and molecular studies. However, there were some grey zone lymphomas, which do not exactly fall into either HL or NHL sub-types like ALCL and TCHRBCL. It appears that Hodgkin lymphoma and its pathogenesis is still in a stage of evolution and only future will tell when this turbulent phase will settle down.

In: Horizons in Cancer Research. Volume 54
Editor: Hiroto S. Watanabe
ISBN: 978-1-63321-389-0

Chapter 1

Glioblastoma: Risk Factors, Diagnosis and Treatment Options

Kyung-Sub Moon and Maciej S. Lesniak*
The Brain Tumor Center, The University of Chicago Medical Center, Chicago, IL, US

Abstract

Glioblastoma (GBM), also known as glioblastoma *multiforme*, is the most common and lethal primary brain tumor which exhibits clinical, radiological and pathological heterogeneity. Based on the fact that the incidence has been documented to be constant in various reports, genetic variation is more likely to play a major role in developing GBM than environmental, geographical and nutritional factors. MRI with contrast enhancement is the most commonly used method in the initial evaluation and follow-up after treatment. The typical finding of GBM is ring enhanced white matter lesion with central necrosis and perilesional edema on MRI. Microvascular proliferation and necrosis have been used as the most critical factor in pathological confirmation. Recently, some biomarkers such as O^6-methylguanine-DNA methyltransferase (MGMT) methylation, BRAF fusions, and IDH1 mutations have been suggested as possible prognostic and grading factors. Standard therapy includes microsurgical resection and a multimodal treatment of concomitant radiotherapy and chemotherapy, followed by adjuvant chemotherapy with temozolomide. In addition to functional or diffusion tensor MRI with navigation system or intraoperative MRI, fluorescence-guided resection helps surgeons to increase safety and accuracy in GBM surgery. MR spectroscopy and positron-emission tomography (PET) scans may provide useful information in differential diagnosis and making treatment plans. Anti-angiogenic therapy with antivascular endothelial growth factor antibodies (bevacizumab) is on its way into clinical practice. In this article, the authors discuss and highlight the advances in diagnosis and treatment of GBM with relevant reviews.

Keywords: Diagnosis, glioblastoma, glioma, risk factors, treatment options

* Correspondence to: Maciej S. Lesniak, MD, University of Chicago Brain Tumor Center, 5841 S Maryland Ave, MC 3026, Chicago, IL 60637. E-mail: mlesniak@surgery.bsd.uchicago.edu

Introduction

Glioblastoma (GBM) is the most malignant glioma (World Health Organization [WHO] grade IV) with an average life expectancy of 14 months after diagnosis, despite the best standard of care. This dismal disease entity represents various radiological and pathological features. Although majority of the diagnosed patients follow the poor clinical course with rapid recurrence and infiltration into deeper portions of the central nervous system, a small fraction of the patients do much better than the expected. Furthermore, various new treatment strategies based on the tremendous discoveries in basic and translational research have been adopted in recent years. In this chapter, the authors review the recently published articles and discuss the advances in diagnosis and treatment of GBM.

Risk Factor

GBM accounts for 12-15% of all brain tumors and 60-75% of astrocytomas. The incidence of GBM is in the range of 3-4 new cases per 100,000 population per year but the poor prognosis makes it a considerable public health issue [1, 2]. The peak incidence is between 45 and 75 years, with a mean age of 61.3 years: more than 80% of patients are older than 50 years [3]. GBM is a relatively frequent intracranial neoplasm in adults (12–20% of all intracranial tumors) [4]. However, it is unusual in pediatric patients and constitutes 7–8.8% of all pediatric brain tumors [5].

Generally, the incidence of primary brain tumors (including gliomas) has been highly reported in developed countries including Western Europe, North America, and Australia [6]. In population-based studies, the incidence of GBM is fairly constant in United States and Europe [1, 2]. This result may lead one to conclude that environmental, geographical and nutritional factors probably do not play a major role in gliomagenesis, whereas genetics is more likely to tip the scale of etiology [6]. The lower incidence in developing countries can be partly explained by under-estimation, but ethnic differences as a possible factor in glioma development should be considered. According to the data of Central Brain Tumor Registry of the United States, blacks are relatively protected, as their incidence is lower than other ethnic groups such as whites, latinos and Asians [7, 8]. The incidence of GBM is approximately twice as common in whites as in blacks [6]. It is slightly more common in men, with a male to female ratio of 1.3:1 [1]. The reasons for this gender distribution have not been revealed. Some studies suggest a possible relationship between season of birth and risk of GBM. Based on these studies, GBM patients are generally born in winter, particularly in the month of February and January [9, 10]. Perinatal viral origin (infection with an unknown oncovirus, integrating in the genome) has subsequently been put forward, but no hard evidence has yet been found to support it. The association with an oncogenic virus, SV40, remains controversial [11, 12]. Recent study suggests the involvement of host genetic factors in susceptibility to cytomegalovirus-induced GBM [13]. Although most GBMs originate in a sporadic fashion without any known genetic predisposition, several genetic disorders are associated with increased incidence, including tuberous sclerosis, neurofibromatosis type 1 and type 2, von Hippel Lindau disease, as well as some well-known hereditary tumor syndromes (Turcot's syndrome or Li–Fraumeni syndrome) [14, 15].

There is a proven association between GBM and exposure to ionizing radiation or polyvinyl chloride [16, 17]. A large-scale cohort study for childhood cancer patients demonstrated that radiation exposure was associated with increased risk of subsequent glioma and meningioma. Considering the higher risk of subsequent glioma in children irradiated at a very young age, the developing brain may be more susceptible to radiation. Even low-dose therapeutic radiation may result in subsequent development of brain tumors [18]. Long-term exposure to polyvinyl chloride has been reported to cause hepatic angiosarcoma. Moreover, it may also carry a slightly enhanced risk of developing GBM [17]. Polycyclic aromatic hydrocarbons and non-arsenical insecticides were suggested as possible occupational carcinogens associated with an excess risk of brain tumors [19]. Some studies have shown a significant inverse correlation between glioma and allergic conditions such as asthma, eczema and atopy [20, 21]. Based on the observation that total immunoglobulin E levels were lower in glioma patients than control subjects [22] and partly explained by interleukin-13 polymorphism [23], immunological factors may influence glioma development. No definitive links have been found between GBM and smoking, diet, cellular phones or electromagnetic fields [6]. However, recent meta-analysis studies came down on the side of suggesting that there may a possible role of cellular phone use in gliomagenesis [24, 25]. Additionally, a recent study provides evidence of an association between alcohol consumption and risk of GBM. This study also postulates whether the increased risk of GBM associated with alcohol consumption is modified by cigarette smoking, folate intake, or genetic variants in the alcohol-dehydrogenase and acetaldehyde dehydrogenase genes [26].

Diagnosis

Contrast–enhanced multiplanar MRI is the standard assessment technique for GBM, particularly useful in evaluating anatomical location, extension, and characteristics. The mass usually demonstrates low-signal intensity, as a hypodense necrotic central area surrounded by thick, irregularly-enhanced rim, corresponding to the central necrosis with the peripheral cellular vascularized wall, on T_1-weighted images. It conversely appears as high-signal intensity mass on T_2–weighted images. The lesion seems to be much broader and less well defined, overlapping with the perilesional edema. Although it is sometimes difficult to distinguish the lesion from surrounding edema, T_2–weighted images are the best to reveal the surrounding vasogenic edema. GBM generally shows marked and somewhat heterogenous gadolinium enhancement, indicating angiogenesis and vascular permeability. It frequently follows the ring-enhancement pattern, demonstrating enhancement along with the peripheral rim surrounding non-enhanced necrotic portion.

However, these conventional imaging sequences can not fully reflect the complicated biology of infiltrative gliomas [27] and have limited specificity in the identification of features necessary for glioma grading or aggressiveness [28-31]. Basically, GBMs typically show microvascular proliferation and necrosis, in addition to increased cellularity and pleomorphism. New blood vessel formation, essential to maintain high proliferative property, has somewhat different biological features. This disorganized vascular network consists of dilated, tortuous and hyperpermeable vessels induced by oversecretion of proangiogenic cytokines such as vascular endothelial growth factor [32]. It also leads to heterogeneity within tumor blood flow with some areas receiving high blood flow whereas others receiving very little [33]. Under normal conditions, the contrast agent can not leak into the brain across the blood-brain-barrier. However, tumor vasculature is abnormally hyperpermeable, thus gadolinium can leak into the area of the tumor. Although the size of the tumor can be identified by the extent of contrast leakage, this leakage is not consistent within patients and can vary from scan to scan depending on the amount of gadolinium used or the precision of the contrast injection. Some drugs used in glioma patients, such as dexamethasone and antiangiogenic agents can also affect the permeability of the blood-brain-barrier, causing a decrease in the leakage of gadolinium into the brain. However, this decrease in enhancement does not reflect a decrease in tumor cell density or apoptosis [34].

The introduction of physiology-based MRI sequences, such as diffusion and perfusion MRI, overcome the limitation of contrast leakage as a measure of tumor size and response to treatment. These techniques stress the angiogenic features and proliferative ability of tumor cells to distinguish the tumor from surrounding normal tissue [33, 35] and hold promise in the quantitative assessment of aggressiveness [30, 31, 36-41]. Diffusion MRI focuses on cell density and enables the acquisition of images of white matter tracts to evaluate vasogenic edema and tumor infiltration. Perfusion MRI evaluates hemodynamic properties of the tumor such as blood volume or blood flow, oxygenation, vessel size, and vascular permeability [33].

The measuring of the water diffusivity within brain tissue is a fundamental principal of diffusion-weighted imaging. The clinical application using this technique can be divided into apparent diffusion coefficient (ADC) maps for evaluation of cell density and fractional anisotropy maps (diffusion tensor imaging: DTI) for morphology of the white matter track. ADC is calculated to quantitatively measure relative degrees of hydrogen motion within the extracellular space [42]. Less water movement represents low ADC value (dark appearance) and has correlated with increased cellularity and proliferation in pathological studies of gliomas [43-45]. However, similar studies involving mixed-grade gliomas have yielded various results [42, 46-49]. In contrast to the cellular portion, water content can move freely in vasogenic edema, thus this increased movement appears bright on ADC. ADC can be used as a noninvasive biomarker for prediction of treatment response in glioma patients. Increase in tumor diffusion value, particularly in treated area, has been positively associated with subsequent volumetric tumor response and overall survival after treatment [50-52].

White matter tracts (DTI) can be visualized based on the fraction anisotropy value of water molecule in tissue. Isotropy theoretically means that all water molecules diffuse at the same speed and quantity. In nervous tissue, however, water diffusion is imparted in certain directions by white matter fiber bundle. This ‘diffusion anisotropy’ is significantly decreased when the tumor infiltration destroys white matter fibers [53]. Some studies showed that DTI enables the differentiation of tumor infiltration from purely vasogenic edema [54, 55]. Using this technique, restoration of white matter tracts was confirmed in the patients who responded to the pan-VEGF receptor tyrosine kinase inhibitor, leading to normalization of tumor vasculature and alleviation of vasogenic edema [35]. Serial DTI may thus show resolution of vasogenic edema and potentially the arrest of tumor growth along white matter tracts after GBM treatment. DTI can be successfully combined with neuronavigation for surgical planning and contributes to maximum resection when the tumor is in an eloquent area while minimizing postoperative deficits [56].

Perfusion-weighted MRI is used to quantitatively measure cerebral hemodynamic characteristics [30]. Cerebral blood volume, peak height, and percentage of signal intensity recovery are three imaging measurements previously shown to be clinically useful in predicting glioma histopathologic grade and distinguishing recurrent brain tumors from radiation necrosis [30, 36-38, 41]. Currently, dynamic susceptibility contrast (DSC) MRI has been most widely used to determine cerebral blood volume and flow. It measures the amount of gadolinium that enters into and flushes out from each voxel and this amount is proportional to the cerebral blood volume in the particular region of the brain [33]. The strong correlation between the maximum cerebral blood volume measured in a tumor and the histologic tumor grade has been generally accepted [39, 57]. Regional cerebral blood volume has also been correlated with microvessel density in glioma model and human sample [40, 58, 59]. However, DSC measurements are not considered a valid biomarker of GBM angiogenesis because a direct comparison with tissue specimens obtained through image-guided biopsy has yet to be extensively reported [39, 40, 60, 61].

Although conventional MRI provides the structural information, MR spectroscopy (MRS) provides a qualitative analysis of a number of metabolites within the brain, and a quantitative analysis if a reference of known concentration is used. The principal peaks observed in the brain tumors at 1.5T include branch chain amino acid (0.9-1.0 ppm), lipid (0.9-1.5 ppm), lactate (1.3 ppm), alanine (1.5 ppm), *N*-acetyl aspartate (NAA; 2.0 ppm), choline (3.2 ppm), creatine (3.0 and 3.9 ppm), and myoinositol (3.6 ppm) [62, 63]. Each metabolite represents the status of neuronal integrity, cell membrane proliferation or degradation, energy metabolism or necrotic transformation of brain or tumor tissue. Through the summation of these spectra data, colorful metabolite map depicting the spatial distribution of the different heights, areas, or peak ratio can be produced. Although the main data assessed from the spectral graphs can limit the clinical diagnostic value, MRS provides information about a number of disease processes and adds another dimension to imaging diagnosis [62]. The typical pattern of glioma spectra is well defined as high choline (metabolism of cell membrane) and low or absent NAA peaks (viable neuron), with lipid and lactate peaks (necrosis) often seen in GBM [31, 63]. However, numerous investigations have failed to prove the definitive role of MRS in differential diagnosis of tumor types or of tumor from non-neoplastic processes such as demyelination, ischemia, and gliosis [64-67]. The use of MRS for biopsies targeted to the areas with high Choline/NAA ratios has been reported to increase the accuracy of tumor biopsy. It can reduce the false negative rate by targeting metabolically active areas within heterogeneous glioma [68-70].

Conventional MRI has a major limitation to differentiate tumor recurrence from radiation necrosis after GBM treatment. Both lesions generally show various enhancement patterns and degrees possibly with mass effect. Ideally, progressive decrease in NAA and choline peaks and lactate/lipid peaks can suggest necrosis. Significant increase in choline with decrease in NAA can be an indicator of tumor recurrence. However, in most clinical settings, recurrent tumor and necrosis may occur concomitantly and this mixture can make MRS patterns less definitive. In addition to different acquisition on voxel placement or technique, spatial variation of important peaks in individual tumor can be augmented over serial scan time. Some studies stress the Choline/Creatin ratio in mixed tumor recurrence and necrosis [71-73]. A ratio greater than specific value (2.23) with enlargement indicates the predominance of recurrence [71]. This discrimination ability of MRS can be enhanced by the combination with diffusion and/or perfusion MRI [72, 73]. Serial changes in MRS findings of gliomas after treatment have shown encouraging results. Increased Choline/Creatinin ratio was checked in lesions before a subsequent contrast enhancement [74].56 E.E. Graves, S.J. Nelson and D.B.

Vigneron et al., Serial proton MR spectroscopic imaging of recurrent malignant gliomas after gamma knife radio surgery, AJNR Am J Neuroradiol 22 (2001), pp. 613–624. View Record in Scopus | Cited By in Scopus (87) Incorporation of spatial information from MRS guaranteed more accurate planning and prolonged survival in stereotactic radiosurgery for GBM [75].

PET with ^{18}F-fluorodeoxyglucose (FDG) has been widely used in diagnosis and treatment of systemic cancer. However, because there are some problematic obstacles as an imaging tool for brain [76], new PET tracers, such as ^{18}F-fluoro-L-thymidine (FLT) and ^{18}F-fluoromisonidazole (FMISO), ^{11}C-methionine (MET), and 3,4-dihydroxy-6-18F-fluoro-L-phenylalanine (FDOPA) have been developed and introduced to the clinics [33, 77]. FLT is the most extensively investigated tracer to image cell proliferation. FLT is a thymidine analogue and is correlated with expression of thymidine kinase-1 activity, an enzyme important in DNA synthesis. Thus, it can provide a measure of DNA synthesis and tumor cell proliferation [78]. With some limitations in correlation with Ki-67 labeling, FLT tracer uptake is essential for the in vivo assessment of tumor proliferation in high-grade gliomas [79, 80]. FLT-PET can be used as an imaging biomarker in assessing proliferation and serve as a predictive tool in overall survival for GBM, especially in the treatment with anti-angiogenic agents or with cytostatic therapy possibly leading to unreliable results on conventional MRI [81]. FMISO, as a tracer for determining tumor hypoxia, binds selectively to hypoxic cells [82]. In glioma patients, elevated FMISO uptake representing hypoxic area has been associated with cell proliferation and patient outcome after treatment [83, 84]. MET readily cross the intact blood-blood-barrier using specific amino acid transporters and incorporates into the active proliferative area. Elevated MET uptake correlates with grades, proliferation, accurate extension and biological aggressiveness in gliomas [85-87].

Treatment

In addition to the definitive antitumor therapy, the management of GBM patients involves providing effective supportive care. The most common problems include seizure, peritumoral edema, venous thromboembolism, gastrointestinal disturbance, osteoporosis, cognitive dysfunction, infection and mood disturbance [88].

It remains controversial to use prophylactic antiepileptic drugs (AEDs) in patients with malignant gliomas who have never had a seizure. However, given the potential for adverse effects and the lack of clear evidence that AEDs reduce the incidence of new-onset seizures, routine prophylactic AED therapy in brain tumor patients is probably unnecessary [89]. Patients with brain tumors who present with seizures should be treated with standard AED. Because some AEDs, such as phenytoin or carbamazepine, induce cytochrome P450 to increase the metabolism for chemotherapeutic agents, AED without induction of cytochrome P450, such as levetiracetam, are preferred [88].

To treat the peritumoral edema, the use of corticosteroid such as dexamethasone is indispensable. Glucose intolerance, Cushing's syndrome, steroid myopathy, and peptic ulceration may occur in prolonged treatment with high doses of corticosteroids. The use of moderate to high doses of corticosteroid can result in clinically significant suppression of the immune system and vulnerability to opportunistic infections. Among these infectious diseases, *Pneumocystis jiroveci (previously known as carinii)* can cause life-threatening pneumonitis. Although the clinical features of *Pneumocystis jiroveci* pneumonitis are usually those of an acute pneumonia, the presentation can be subtle and non-specific in immunocompromised state. Thus, physicians should maintain a high index of suspicion for this diagnosis in any patient developing respiratory symptoms. The use of prophylactic antibiotic therapy against this infection can be considered for brain tumor patients receiving prolonged corticosteroid treatment. However, its benefit is still controversial [88, 90]. As new treatment modalities improve survival rate of malignant glioma, long-term steroid complications previously unrecognized, including osteoporosis, compression fractures, and neuropsychiatric disturbance, are becoming more problematic. Vitamin D, calcium supplements, and bisphosphonates should be considered as the preventive measures [88].

Venous thromboembolism is the common cause of perioperative morbidity and mortality in malignant gliomas, with the incidence of 20 to 30% [91]. Old age (>60 years), large sized tumor and paralytic leg can be regarded as risk factors [92]. Patients with malignant gliomas are often suppose to have increased risk of intracranial hemorrhage after anticoagulation therapy because of the increased vascularity of the tumors. According to a previous report, however, only 2% of intratumoral hemorrhage was complicated by anticoagulation therapy for venous thromboembolism. This complication rate was similar to that of the non-treated group [93]. Currently, it is generally accepted to use low-molecular weight heparin for venous thromboembolism, except in cases with intracerebral hemorrhage or other complications [94]. During and just after the surgery and chemoradiotherapy, patients with malignant gliomas frequently complain of profound fatigue. It is possibly associated with anemia, adverse effect of AED or steroid, and other various factors. Modafinil or methylphenidate may be useful in reducing the fatigue in this situation [95]. Donepezil may improve the decreased cognitive function including attention, mood and verbal memory after radiation treatment [96]. Neuropsychiatric problems can be overlooked in patients with malignant gliomas, and antidepressants and psychiatric support are often invaluable [97].

Although the mainstay of therapy for GBM consists of surgery, radiation and chemotherapy, several make GBM treatment notoriously difficult, including the intrinsic resistance of these lesions to conventional therapy, limited capacity of the brain to repair itself, infiltrative feature of the tumor cells into brain parenchyma, the variably disrupted blood–brain-barrier complicating drug delivery [98]. Current standard treatment is composed of maximal surgical resection and involved-field RT (60 Gy administered in 5 times weekly fractions over 6 weeks) with concurrent TMZ (75 mg/m^2/d). After 4 weeks of rest, patients receive 6-12 cycles of adjuvant TMZ (150 mg/m^2/d for 5 days at the beginning of the first 28-day cycle, followed by 200 mg/m^2/d for 5 days at the beginning of the each subsequent 28-day cycle) [99, 100].

Surgery

Surgical treatment for GBM remains critical for confirming the diagnosis, alleviating symptoms of mass effect and ICP, and reducing tumor volume [101].

There have been a lot of technical advances focusing on maximizing resection while minimizing injury to surrounding normal tissue. In addition, tissue obtained during the procedure can eventually be used for design of targeted therapies through the individualized analysis of the molecular signature [102]. The extent of surgical resection depends on location and eloquence of the brain areas involved.

However, surgery is always an incomplete debulking, since GBM is a highly infiltrating tumor and cannot be resected completely. Some advantages of radical resection include good relief of intracranial pressure, reversal of some neurologic deficits, lowering of seizure incidence, a definitive pathological diagnosis, and ultimately improved survival.

Although the value of radical microsurgical resection in GBM remains controversial, recent studies suggest that extent of resection is associated with better survival of the patients with GBM [103-106]. Especially, according to the most recent study, the extent of resection beyond critical threshold (eg, 78%), may impact patient survival [105].

To resect the tumor to the greatest extent, several technical advances should be accompanied simultaneously. New techniques for preoperative radiological evaluations (DTI combined with functional MRI), intraoperative MRI, three dimensional-image guidance or neuronavigation for tumor delineation, electrophysiological mapping for eloquent areas or 5-aminolevulinic acid (ALA) and, if needed, multimodal combined approach could be considered.

Neuronavigation, widely used for brain tumor surgery, has been assessed prospectively as to whether it improves resection or causes neurological deficits [107]. There was no benefit in terms of the extent of tumor resection and prognosis. This result may be closely related with brain shift and intraoperative distortion of anatomy, compared with that seen on preoperative imaging, mainly due to change of cerebrospinal fluid dynamics and tumor tissue volume [108-110].

Intraoperative collaboration with other techniques, however, has been attempted to overcome the limit of neuronavigation. In addition to integration with DTI, functional MRI, or PET [111-115], three dimensional ultrasonography [112, 114, 116, 117] and intraoperative neurophysiological monitoring [118-120] have been coupled with neuronavigation system.

Despite high cost, low quality of images, and limits of functional evaluation, intraoperative MRI also has been used in glioma surgery. It provides optimization of extent of resection in real time and can be coupled with other modalities, such as neuronavigation or electrophysiological studies [121-127].

The effects of a fluorescent tumor marker (5-ALA) on the degree of resection and survival in GBM surgery have also been recently analyzed [128-131]. The use of intraoperative 5-ALA and fluorescence-guided resection was shown to enhance the total resection rate and offer a survival benefit.

Basically, the non-fluorescent prodrug is metabolized to fluorescent protoporphyrin IX in tumor tissue through the heme biosynthesis pathway. The accumulation of protoporphyrin IX in malignant gliomas may be explained by higher 5-ALA uptake in tumor tissue or increased enzyme activity for hemoglobin biosynthesis in tumor cells. Higher 5-ALA uptake may be related to disrupted BBB, increased neovascularization, and the overexpression of membrane transporters in glioma tissue.

Because the protoporphyrin IX level induced by 5-ALA in normal brain tissue is very low, macroscopic visualization of the tumor under the specialized microscope may allow more reliability to neurosurgeons than neuronavigation or standard microscope [102].

Radiation Therapy

External beam radiotherapy (RT) has been used to treat malignant gliomas for decades. It destructs tumor cells through the damage of ionizing radiation in the DNA helix by electrons and free radicals. Although the type of radiation has not been changed substantially, technical advancements have improved significantly to minimize the radiation dose for surrounding normal tissue. The rationale of RT in malignant gliomas is based on the landmark report that showed prolonged survival in treated group compared with the supportive group [132]. RT is usually started within 4 to 6 weeks after surgery and performed with a standard fractionated dose over 6 to 7 weeks [133-135]. Because of the infiltrative nature of malignant gliomas, wide margins are usually included to the treatment plan. The standard dose of external beam RT is 60 Gy in single daily fractions of 1.7-2 Gy, 5 times a week. The decision of margin generally follows the ECORTC and RTOG guidelines [136]. For initial treated volume, the margin expands 2 cm around abnormal area on FLAIR T_2 (46 grays [Gy] at 2 Gy/day). It includes 2 cm around the enhancing tumor/tumor bed for the boost volume (14 Gy at 2 Gy/day, total 60 Gy). Prior to therapy, the regions at risk are mapped and a conformal treatment plan is generated that encompasses target volume. Current processes render the significant sparing of surrounding normal tissues while maintaining high dose to the targeted area [137].

Although radiation has a major role in the standard therapy for newly diagnosed malignant gliomas, reirradiation is strongly restricted for recurrent cases because of significant risk for the development of necrosis [138]. However, considering factors such as the patient's performance status, the volume of recurrence tumor, the proximity of the recurrence to previous treated lesion, and the length of time since previous irradiation, reirradiation could be a useful modality with other salvage treatment [139, 140]. In a view of limiting treatment volume and dose reduction, single-fraction stereotactic radiosurgery (SRS) is used to a focal area of small (<3-4 cm) recurrence [141, 142]. SRS has not been associated with benefit for newly diagnosed GBMs as a boost to a standard RT [143]. In recurrence cases, however, it may lengthen the time to disease progression [144, 145]. Another option is the stereotactic brachytherapy, using stereotactic technique for implanting or infusing the radioactive isotope (eg, ^{125}I, ^{192}Ir, ^{252}Californium) within the confined tumor cavity [146, 147]. It delivers an additional 50-65 Gy of radiation during 4-7 days, bringing the total dose of radiation up to 110-120 Gy [138]. As a primary treatment, it is mainly adopted for well-defined, unilateral supratentorial tumors less than 5 cm in diameter without involvement of corpus callosum, brain stem, or ependymal surface. Although both SRS and brachytherapy are performed in a single treatment session, they can cause radiation necrosis of the residual tumor and sometimes the surrounding brain, which can necessitate surgery for relief of mass effect [148]. Recent studies, however, provide evidence that stereotactic RT has therapeutic effect in recurrent malignant gliomas both in terms of survival duration and morbidity, compared with other treatment strategies [149-152]. According to the most recent study, more favorable prognosis was found in younger patients, patients with less-extensive areas of disease progression or a short time interval between initial diagnosis and progression [149]. Reirradiation by means of hypofractionated delivery might have particular appeal for patients who have recurrent tumors that are too large to be considered for single-fraction SRS. Further investigations should be performed about the possibility of combining radiation with conventional chemotherapy, molecularly targeted therapy, or immunotherapy at the time of progression [153].

Chemotherapy

Among many chemotherapeutics tested for treatment of GBM, alkylating agents have frequently been used in clinical setting. Alkylating agents (including the nitrosoureas, procarbazine and TMZ) work by alkylating cellular DNA, leading to DNA cross-links and cell death. Alkylation at the O^6 site on guanine is particularly important [99, 154]. These agents can be classified into methylating drugs like TMZ and procarbazine, and chloroethylating drugs like carmustine (bis-(2-cholorethyl)-nitrosourea, BCNU) and lomustine (1-(2-chloroethyl)-3-cyclohexyl-1-nitrosourea, CCNU), according to the alkyl group donated to O^6-guanine by O^6-alkylguanine DNA alkyltransferase (AGT) [154].

Nitrosourea compounds (BCNU and CCNU) act by forming O^6-chloroethylguanine lesions, converted to G-C interstrand crosslinks within 8-12 hours of formation [155], and these are very poorly repaired in mammalian cells. It is estimated that 2-5 crosslinks can kill a cell whereas over 5000 O^6-methylguanine lesions are required to do the same [156]. However, an aggressive regimen with these agents causes considerable side effects, leading to dose reductions and corresponding decreases in therapeutic efficacy [157]. Because of lipid solubility and ability to cross the blood-brain-barrier, nitrosoureas have been used for early randomized clinical trials as a adjuvant chemotherapy for malignant gliomas [158, 159]. In addition to the positive result from these studies, meta-analyses confirm that chemotherapy offers a modest survival benefit (a 6%–10% increase in 1-year survival) for patients with malignant glioma [160, 161]. Based on this data, the most commonly used regimens are BCNU or PCV (combination of procarbazine, CCNU, and vincristine). However, prospective randomized trials using these regimens have failed to demonstrate a survival benefit [162].

TMZ, an oral alkylating agent, can reach maximum plasma concentration 30 to 90 minutes after intake with the plasma half-life of 2 hours [163]. Methylation of the O^6 site on guanine, the biologically most pertinent site of DNA methylation by TMZ, will trigger activation of the mismatch repair process [164] to result in G2 checkpoint activation leading to G2/M cell cycle arrest and eventually to induction of apoptosis [165-167]. Severe or life-threatening toxicity is rare. Common mild to moderate adverse effects are nausea and vomiting, constipation, and some fatigue. Noncumulative myelosuppression, particularly thrombocytopenia occurring 3 to 4 weeks after treatment start, is the most serious and dose-limiting toxicity, observed in less than 10% of patients [168-170].

A new standard of treatment for GBM emerged in 2005 [134]. A large, randomized, multicenter, phase III trial included 573 newly diagnosed GBM patients. The patients who were surgical candidates underwent maximal feasible resection. Then, all patients consecutively received standard RT (60 Gy over 6 weeks) and were randomly assigned to receive TMZ chemotherapy or no chemotherapy. In the chemotherapy arm, patients received radiotherapy with concurrent TMZ at a dose of 75 $mg/m^2/d$ for 6 weeks. After a 4-week break, patients received 6 cycles of adjuvant TMZ (150 to 200 $mg/m^2/d$ for 5 days during each 28-day cycle). Median survival in chemotherapy group improved to 14.6 months (*vs* 12.1 mos in non-chemotherapy group). More strikingly, the 2-year survival rate improved with TMZ therapy, from 10.4% to 26.5% ($P < 0.001$). The trial tumor specimens were evaluated for O^6-methylguanine-DNA methyltransferase (MGMT) gene silencing [133]. Previous studies hypothesized that DNA methylation of the MGMT gene promoter region is an epigenetic modification that can reduce DNA repair activity and increase susceptibility to chemotherapy [171-173]. Among TMZ treated patients with MGMT promoter methylation, median survival was 21.7 months, and 2-year survival was a remarkable 46%. In contrast, temozolomide-treated patients without MGMT promoter methylation had a significantly shorter median survival of only 12.7 months, and a 2-year survival of 13.8%. This study provided evidence that MGMT promoter methylation was associated with better outcome in the RT and TMZ group, suggesting that it may be a predictive marker for sensitivity to alkylating chemotherapy. Several investigational approaches to suppress MGMT activity include dose intense TMZ regimens [174, 175] and combination therapy with O^6-benzylguanine or other MGMT inhibitors [176]. In addition to MGMT, the DNA repair enzyme poly(ADP-ribose) polymerase (PARP) may promote chemotherapy resistance in patients with malignant gliomas. PARP inhibitors such as BSI-201, ABT-888, and several others may be effective when combined with RT and TMZ [177, 178].

However, more than 50% of patients with GBM retain MGMT expression and demonstrate less sensitivity to TMZ, presumably because MGMT repairs the TMZ-induced DNA damage. These unmethylated patients who received TMZ had an approximate 10%–15% actuarial overall survival time at the 2-year survival point, compared with 0% in those who did not receive TMZ. Recent study showed that MGMT methylation is a predictive marker of radiation response, independently of TMZ treatment and may be a general surrogate marker of favorable prognosis in GBM [179]. This observation indicates that MGMT methylation status is not the sole predictor of GBM response to TMZ and this drug of choice, as the standard of care, should not be withheld from any GBM patient.

Gliadel wafer, an interstitial chemotherapy drug implanted within the tumor resection cavity, contains the BCNU and biodegradable polyanhydride copolymer. The advantages of this approach include achieving high concentrations of chemotherapeutic agent at the local resection site with minimal systemic toxicity and eliminating the problem of brain-blood-barrier penetration. Techniques that have been used include up to 8 Gliadel wafers that are placed in the resection cavity and designed to release BCNU slowly over a period of 2-3 weeks. Clinical trials results have shown that Gliadel prolonged survival in a statistically albeit modest manner in newly diagnosed patients [180]. The patients enrolled in this study received either conventional therapy (surgery followed by RT) with placement of a BCNU wafer or conventional therapy with placement of an identical placebo wafer. The median survival was increased for the BCNU wafer group (13.9 months) compared with the placebo wafer group (11.6 months), with 1-year survival rates of 59.2% and 49.6%, respectively (P=0.03), a 28% reduction in the risk of death and significant sustaining in neuroperformance status. This survival advantage was maintained at 2 and 3 years [181]. Although there have been reports that use of Gliadel wafer was not associated with an increase in perioperative morbidity after surgical treatment of malignant glioma, its use may have side-effects including seizure, brain edema, wound healing problems, intracranial infection, and delay in the administration of other drugs [180, 182]. Combination of both treatment strategies, local chemotherapy with Gliadel wafer and the standard concomitant radiochemotherapy, appears attractive in aggressive multimodal treatment schedules [183]. However, questionable survival benefit and possible increased toxicity warrant further evaluation [184, 185].

Although second line cytotoxic agents including carboplatin, etoposide, oxaliplatin, and irinotecan can be considered for the patients who do not respond to standard TMZ therapy, they produce low response rates and no significant survival benefit [101].

Target Therapy

Various potential therapeutic targets have been developed based on the understanding of molecular mechanism and pathogenesis of glioma development and recognition of differences explaining various clinical courses among tumors with similar morphology. Molecular profiling of glioma has presented signaling pathways driving the malignant behavior of tumors and induction of cell migration and tumor invasiveness [186-188]. These pathways are activated by amplification of receptor tyrosine kinases such as the epidermal growth factor receptor (EGFR), platelet-derived growth factor receptor (PDGFR), insulin-like growth factor receptor (IGFR), and others that lead to activation of downstream mediators if unopposed by tumor suppressors such as PTEN (phosphatase and tensin homolog on chromosome 10). PTEN, frequently inactivated in malignant glioma, is a negative regulator of phosphatidylinositol-3 kinase (PI3K), through several pathways linked with tumor-promoting function (eg, protein kinase C and the activated ras pathway) [99, 189]. Main targets have focused on receptor tyrosine kinases inhibitors such as EGFR and PDGFR, as well as on signal-transduction inhibitors targeting mTOR, farnesyltransferase, and PI3K [35, 190-193]. However, single agent therapies have been disappointing in malignant gliomas, with response rates of 10-15% or less and no prolongation of survival [100, 194, 195]. These results can be explained by some factors.

Malignant gliomas have coactivation of multiple tyrosine kinases [196], including redundant signaling pathway, and limit the activity of single agent. In addition, many of these agents have poor penetration ability through the blood-brain-barrier. Current developing strategies to increase the effectiveness of targeted molecular therapies include the use of a single agent targeted against several kinases, combinations of targeted agents, and targeted agents combined with radiotherapy and chemotherapy [194, 195, 197].

Vascular endothelial growth factor (VEGF) and its receptors (VEGFR) have emerged as other therapeutic targets. Because malignant gliomas are the most vascular among human tumors, VEGF is a critical stimulatory factor in tumor angiogenesis, as well as in the production of peritumoral edema [32, 198].

After bevacizumab (Avastin, humanized monoclonal antibody against VEGF) was approved by FDA for colon cancer, this agent had been introduced into neurooncological field for recurrent malignant gliomas often in combination with irinotecan.

According to the early clinical data, its response rate has been reported from 25% to 74%, with 6-month progression-free survival (PFS6) rate of 32% to 64% [199-205].

These results are superior to the 5-8% response rate and 21% PFS6 rate reported for TMZ [206]. The first trial randomly assigned 167 patients with recurrent GBM to bevacizumab therapy (10mg/kg IV every 2 weeks) with or without irinotecan (340 mg/m^2 IV with enzyme-inducing antiepileptic drug or 125 mg/m^2 without antiepileptic drug) [207]. Objective response rates were reported to be between 28% and 38%, and PFS6 rates ranged from 43% to 50%. In addition to hemorrhagic and thromboembolic complications, common toxicities observed in these studies included hypertension, proteinuria, fatigue, and wound-healing complications.

In another trial, bevacizumab monotherapy was tested in 48 heavily pretreated patients with recurrent GBM [208]. The radiological response rate was 35%, and the PFS6 rate was 29%. Phase III studies are ongoing for evaluation of the combination of bevacizumab with standard TMZ and RT. Preliminary results report that the addition of bevacizumab with standard TMZ and RT was found to be associated with minimal toxicity in patients newly diagnosed with GM [209].

Recently, a phase II trial for the combination of bevacizumab and irinotecan with standard TMZ and RT reported moderate toxicity and possible efficacy compared with the standard therapy [210].

Median overall survival was 21.2 months, and 65% of the patients were alive at 16 months. The median progression-free survival was 14.2 months. Combination of bevacizumab and other chemotherapeutics and targeted molecular drugs is also currently in clinical trial.

Recurrent GBM

Recurrence is generally found as an increase in tumor size (≥25%) associated with increased edema and mass effect on MRI (or newly developed mass with a variable free interval, after complete removal documented on postoperative MRI) or unequivocal neurological deterioration. The Macdonald criteria, which rely on consecutive contrast-enhanced T1-weighted MRI or CT scans, use the enhancing tumor area as the primary parameter [211]. In addition to the difficulty of measuring the irregular-shaped glioma, however, recent observations have revealed the fundamental limitations to this approach [27, 212, 213]. These limitations include variable differences in different observers, the lack of assessment of non-enhancing component, the lack of the guidance for multifocal tumors, and the difficulty in measuring enhancing lesions in the wall of cystic or surgical cavities. Currently, it has been recommended to use the updated response assessment in Neuro-Oncology (RANO) criteria for radiological evaluation in malignant glioma treatment [214]. Although this criteria is also based on the maximal cross-sectional enhancing diameter to determine the size of the contrast-enhancing lesion (>5 mm increase in maximal diameter or ≥25% increase in sum of the products of perpendicular diameters of enhancing lesions), it includes evaluation of non-enhancing MRI (T2-weighted or FLAIR images) for volume changes of tumor. The RANO criteria also modify the definition of measurable disease and introduce the clear definition for pseudoprogression. Tumor cyst, surgical cavity and nodular enhanced (< 10 mm) should not be measured in determining response. The neurological deterioration, based on the KPS, is defined as a decline to 70 or less from 90 or 100, a decline of at least 20 from 80 or less, or a decline to 50 or less without comorbid events or changes in steroid dose.

Pseudoprogression can be defined as radiological progression after adjuvant chemoradiotherapy, which stabilizes or improves with the same treatment or no further therapy [215]. Among the radiological aggravation after concurrent RT and TMZ, 20-50% of the cases were diagnosed with pseudoprogression [216-218]. According to the recent published data [219], median survival was significantly prolonged in pseudoprogression group compared with that of the patient with true progression (125 vs 36 weeks). This survival prolongation can be explained by the possible correlation of pseudoprogression with the status of MGMT promoter methylation [220]. Considering the difficulty in differentiating pseudoprogression from true progression in the first 3 months after concurrent chemoradiotherapy, adjuvant TMZ should be continued for a minimum of 3 cycles with close observation unless new enhanced lesion develops clearly outside the RT field [214, 215]. Although various kinds of imaging modalities, such as MRS, diffusion or perfusion MR, and PET scan, have been introduced to help the diagnosis of pseudoprogression [27], repeated imaging studies may ultimately distinguish the true progression from pseudoprogression.

The treatment approach can be influenced by several factors including patient age, performance status, histology, extent initial resection, response to initial therapy, time since diagnosis, and recurrence feature (local vs diffuse). Reoperation may be indicated in selected patients with a high KPS score and an easily accessible location [215]. Even though reirradiation or SRT has been shown to be beneficial, their usefulness remains controversial [138]. Medtromic TMZ, bevacizumab alone or in combination with irinotecan, nitrosourea-based regimens (BCNU, PCV), and various investigational therapies have been used for recurrent GBM.

References

[1] Kleihues P, Nakazato Y, Burger PC, Plate KH, Aldape KD, Giangaspero F, Brat DJ, von Deimling A, Biernat W, Ohgaki H et al.: Glioblastoma. In: *WHO Classification of Tumours of the Central Nervous System.* Edited by Louis DN, Ohgaki H, Wiestler OD, Cavenee WK. Lyon: IARC Press; 2007: 33-49.

[2] Ohgaki H, Kleihues P: Population-based studies on incidence, survival rates, and genetic alterations in astrocytic and oligodendroglial gliomas. *Journal of neuropathology and experimental neurology* 2005, 64(6):479-489.

[3] Ohgaki H, Dessen P, Jourde B, Horstmann S, Nishikawa T, Di Patre PL, Burkhard C, Schuler D, Probst-Hensch NM, Maiorka PC et al.: Genetic pathways to glioblastoma: a population-based study. Cancer research 2004, 64(19):6892-6899.

[4] Salcman M: Glioblastoma multiforme and anaplastic astrocytoma. In: *Brain tumors: an encyclopedic approach.* Edited by Kaye AH, Laws ER Jr. London: Churchill Livingstone; 2001: 494-523.

[5] Sanchez-Herrera F, Castro-Sierra E, Gordillo-Dominguez LF, Vaca-Ruiz MA, Santana-Montero B, Perezpena-Diazconti M, Gonzalez-Carranza V, Torres-Garcia S, Chico-Ponce de Leon F: Glioblastoma multiforme in children: experience at Hospital Infantil de Mexico Federico Gomez. *Childs Nerv. Syst.* 2009, 25(5):551-557.

[6] Ohgaki H: Epidemiology of brain tumors. *Methods in molecular biology* 2009, 472:323-342.

[7] Fan KJ, Pezeshkpour GH: Ethnic distribution of primary central nervous system tumors in Washington, DC, 1971 to 1985. *Journal of the National Medical Association* 1992, 84(10):858-863.

[8] McLendon RE, Robinson JS, Jr., Chambers DB, Grufferman S, Burger PC: The glioblastoma multiforme in Georgia, 1977-1981. *Cancer* 1985, 56(4):894-897.

[9] Koch HJ, Klinkhammer-Schalke M, Hofstadter F, Bogdahn U, Hau P: Seasonal patterns of birth in patients with glioblastoma. *Chronobiology international* 2006, 23(5):1047-1052.

[10] Brenner AV, Linet MS, Shapiro WR, Selker RG, Fine HA, Black PM, Inskip PD: Season of birth and risk of brain tumors in adults. *Neurology* 2004, 63(2):276-281.

[11] Ohgaki H, Huang H, Haltia M, Vainio H, Kleihues P: More about: cell and molecular biology of simian virus 40: implications for human infections and disease. *Journal of the National Cancer Institute* 2000, 92(6):495-497.

[12] Vilchez RA, Kozinetz CA, Arrington AS, Madden CR, Butel JS: Simian virus 40 in human cancers. *The American journal of medicine* 2003, 114(8):675-684.

[13] Pandey JP: Genetic and Viral Etiology of Glioblastoma--a Unifying Hypothesis. *Cancer Epidemiol Biomarkers Prev* 2011, 20(6):1061-1063.

[14] Farrell CJ, Plotkin SR: Genetic causes of brain tumors: neurofibromatosis, tuberous sclerosis, von Hippel-Lindau, and other syndromes. *Neurologic clinics* 2007, 25(4):925-946, viii.

[15] Tamber MS, Rutka JT: Pediatric supratentorial high-grade gliomas. *Neurosurgical focus* 2003, 14(2):e1.

[16] Fisher JL, Schwartzbaum JA, Wrensch M, Wiemels JL: Epidemiology of brain tumors. *Neurologic clinics* 2007, 25(4):867-890, vii.

[17] Moss AR: Occupational exposure and brain tumors. *Journal of toxicology and environmental health* 1985, 16(5):703-711.

[18] Ron E, Modan B, Boice JD, Jr., Alfandary E, Stovall M, Chetrit A, Katz L: Tumors of the brain and nervous system after radiotherapy in childhood. *The New England journal of medicine* 1988, 319(16):1033-1039.

[19] Siemiatycki J, Richardson L, Straif K, Latreille B, Lakhani R, Campbell S, Rousseau MC, Boffetta P: Listing occupational carcinogens. *Environmental health perspectives* 2004, 112(15):1447-1459.

[20] Linos E, Raine T, Alonso A, Michaud D: Atopy and risk of brain tumors: a meta-analysis. *Journal of the National Cancer Institute* 2007, 99(20):1544-1550.

[21] Schoemaker MJ, Swerdlow AJ, Hepworth SJ, McKinney PA, van Tongeren M, Muir KR: History of allergies and risk of glioma in adults. *International journal of cancer* 2006, 119(9):2165-2172.

[22] Wiemels JL, Wiencke JK, Patoka J, Moghadassi M, Chew T, McMillan A, Miike R, Barger G, Wrensch M: Reduced immunoglobulin E and allergy among adults with glioma compared with controls. *Cancer research* 2004, 64(22):8468-8473.

[23] Wiemels JL, Wiencke JK, Kelsey KT, Moghadassi M, Rice T, Urayama KY, Miike R, Wrensch M: Allergy-related polymorphisms influence glioma status and serum IgE levels. *Cancer Epidemiol Biomarkers Prev* 2007, 16(6):1229-1235.

[24] Khurana VG, Teo C, Kundi M, Hardell L, Carlberg M: Cell phones and brain tumors: a review including the long-term epidemiologic data. *Surgical neurology* 2009, 72(3):205-214.

[25] Myung SK, Ju W, McDonnell DD, Lee YJ, Kazinets G, Cheng CT, Moskowitz JM: Mobile phone use and risk of tumors: a meta-analysis. *J. Clin. Oncol* 2009, 27(33):5565-5572.

[26] Baglietto L, Giles GG, English DR, Karahalios A, Hopper JL, Severi G: Alcohol consumption and risk of glioblastoma; evidence from the Melbourne Collaborative Cohort Study. *International journal of cancer*, 128(8):1929-1934.

[27] Sorensen AG, Batchelor TT, Wen PY, Zhang WT, Jain RK: Response criteria for glioma. *Nature clinical practice* 2008, 5(11):634-644.

[28] Jackson A, Kassner A, Annesley-Williams D, Reid H, Zhu XP, Li KL: Abnormalities in the recirculation phase of contrast agent bolus passage in cerebral gliomas: comparison with relative blood volume and tumor grade. *Ajnr.* 2002, 23(1):7-14.

[29] Law M, Oh S, Johnson G, Babb JS, Zagzag D, Golfinos J, Kelly PJ: Perfusion magnetic resonance imaging predicts patient outcome as an adjunct to histopathology: a second reference standard in the surgical and nonsurgical treatment of low-grade gliomas. *Neurosurgery* 2006, 58(6):1099-1107.

[30] Lev MH, Rosen BR: Clinical applications of intracranial perfusion MR imaging. *Neuroimaging clinics of North America* 1999, 9(2):309-331.

[31] Cha S: Update on brain tumor imaging: from anatomy to physiology. *Ajnr* 2006, 27(3):475-487.

[32] Jain RK, di Tomaso E, Duda DG, Loeffler JS, Sorensen AG, Batchelor TT: Angiogenesis in brain tumours. *Nature reviews* 2007, 8(8):610-622.

[33] Gerstner ER, Sorensen AG, Jain RK, Batchelor TT: Advances in neuroimaging techniques for the evaluation of tumor growth, vascular permeability, and angiogenesis in gliomas. *Current opinion in neurology* 2008, 21(6):728-735.

[34] Claes A, Wesseling P, Jeuken J, Maass C, Heerschap A, Leenders WP: Antiangiogenic compounds interfere with chemotherapy of brain tumors due to vessel normalization. *Molecular cancer therapeutics* 2008, 7(1):71-78.

[35] Batchelor TT, Sorensen AG, di Tomaso E, Zhang WT, Duda DG, Cohen KS, Kozak KR, Cahill DP, Chen PJ, Zhu M et al.: AZD2171, a pan-VEGF receptor tyrosine kinase inhibitor, normalizes tumor vasculature and alleviates edema in glioblastoma patients. *Cancer cell* 2007, 11(1):83-95.

[36] Barajas RF, Jr., Chang JS, Segal MR, Parsa AT, McDermott MW, Berger MS, Cha S: Differentiation of recurrent glioblastoma multiforme from radiation necrosis after external beam radiation therapy with dynamic susceptibility-weighted contrast-enhanced perfusion MR imaging. *Radiology* 2009, 253(2):486-496.

[37] Henry RG, Vigneron DB, Fischbein NJ, Grant PE, Day MR, Noworolski SM, Star-Lack JM, Wald LL, Dillon WP, Chang SM et al.: Comparison of relative cerebral blood volume and proton spectroscopy in patients with treated gliomas. *Ajnr.* 2000, 21(2):357-366.

[38] Lupo JM, Cha S, Chang SM, Nelson SJ: Dynamic susceptibility-weighted perfusion imaging of high-grade gliomas: characterization of spatial heterogeneity. *Ajnr.* 2005, 26(6):1446-1454.

[39] Maia AC, Jr., Malheiros SM, da Rocha AJ, da Silva CJ, Gabbai AA, Ferraz FA, Stavale JN: MR cerebral blood volume maps correlated with vascular endothelial growth factor expression and tumor grade in nonenhancing gliomas. *Ajnr.* 2005, 26(4):777-783.

[40] Sadeghi N, D'Haene N, Decaestecker C, Levivier M, Metens T, Maris C, Wikler D, Baleriaux D, Salmon I, Goldman S: Apparent diffusion coefficient and cerebral blood volume in brain gliomas: relation to tumor cell density and tumor microvessel density based on stereotactic biopsies. *Ajnr.* 2008, 29(3):476-482.

[41] Sugahara T, Korogi Y, Kochi M, Ikushima I, Hirai T, Okuda T, Shigematsu Y, Liang L, Ge Y, Ushio Y et al.: Correlation of MR imaging-determined cerebral blood volume maps with histologic and angiographic determination of vascularity of gliomas. *Ajnr.* 1998, 171(6):1479-1486.

[42] Le Bihan D, Breton E, Lallemand D, Grenier P, Cabanis E, Laval-Jeantet M: MR imaging of intravoxel incoherent motions: application to diffusion and perfusion in neurologic disorders. *Radiology* 1986, 161(2):401-407.

[43] Chenevert TL, Stegman LD, Taylor JM, Robertson PL, Greenberg HS, Rehemtulla A, Ross BD: Diffusion magnetic resonance imaging: an early surrogate marker of therapeutic efficacy in brain tumors. *Journal of the National Cancer Institute* 2000, 92(24):2029-2036.

[44] Higano S, Yun X, Kumabe T, Watanabe M, Mugikura S, Umetsu A, Sato A, Yamada T, Takahashi S: Malignant astrocytic tumors: clinical importance of apparent diffusion coefficient in prediction of grade and prognosis. *Radiology.* 2006, 241(3):839-846.

[45] Kitis O, Altay H, Calli C, Yunten N, Akalin T, Yurtseven T: Minimum apparent diffusion coefficients in the evaluation of brain tumors. *European journal of radiology.* 2005, 55(3):393-400.

[46] Sugahara T, Korogi Y, Kochi M, Ikushima I, Shigematu Y, Hirai T, Okuda T, Liang L, Ge Y, Komohara Y et al.: Usefulness of diffusion-weighted MRI with echo-planar technique in the evaluation of cellularity in gliomas. *J Magn Reson Imaging* 1999, 9(1):53-60.

[47] Guo AC, Cummings TJ, Dash RC, Provenzale JM: Lymphomas and high-grade astrocytomas: comparison of water diffusibility and histologic characteristics. *Radiology.* 2002, 224(1):177-183.

[48] Stadnik TW, Chaskis C, Michotte A, Shabana WM, van Rompaey K, Luypaert R, Budinsky L, Jellus V, Osteaux M: Diffusion-weighted MR imaging of intracerebral masses: comparison with conventional MR imaging and histologic findings. *Ajnr.* 2001, 22(5):969-976.

[49] Gupta RK, Cloughesy TF, Sinha U, Garakian J, Lazareff J, Rubino G, Rubino L, Becker DP, Vinters HV, Alger JR: Relationships between choline magnetic resonance spectroscopy, apparent diffusion coefficient and quantitative histopathology in human glioma. *Journal of neuro-oncology.* 2000, 50(3):215-226.

[50] Mardor Y, Pfeffer R, Spiegelmann R, Roth Y, Maier SE, Nissim O, Berger R, Glicksman A, Baram J, Orenstein A et al.: Early detection of response to radiation therapy in patients with brain malignancies using conventional and high b-value diffusion-weighted magnetic resonance imaging. *J. Clin. Oncol.* 2003, 21(6):1094-1100.

[51] Moffat BA, Chenevert TL, Lawrence TS, Meyer CR, Johnson TD, Dong Q, Tsien C, Mukherji S, Quint DJ, Gebarski SS et al.: Functional diffusion map: a noninvasive MRI biomarker for early stratification of clinical brain tumor response. *Proceedings of the National Academy of Sciences of the United States of America.* 2005, 102(15):5524-5529.

[52] Hamstra DA, Galban CJ, Meyer CR, Johnson TD, Sundgren PC, Tsien C, Lawrence TS, Junck L, Ross DJ, Rehemtulla A et al.: Functional diffusion map as an early imaging biomarker for high-grade glioma: correlation with conventional radiologic response and overall survival. *J. Clin. Oncol.* 2008, 26(20):3387-3394.

[53] Basser PJ, Pajevic S, Pierpaoli C, Duda J, Aldroubi A: In vivo fiber tractography using DT-MRI data. *Magn Reson Med* 2000, 44(4):625-632.

[54] Morita K, Matsuzawa H, Fujii Y, Tanaka R, Kwee IL, Nakada T: Diffusion tensor analysis of peritumoral edema using lambda chart analysis indicative of the heterogeneity of the microstructure within edema. *Journal of neurosurgery.* 2005, 102(2):336-341.

[55] Lu S, Ahn D, Johnson G, Law M, Zagzag D, Grossman RI: Diffusion-tensor MR imaging of intracranial neoplasia and associated peritumoral edema: introduction of the tumor infiltration index. *Radiology.* 2004, 232(1):221-228.

[56] Wu JS, Zhou LF, Tang WJ, Mao Y, Hu J, Song YY, Hong XN, Du GH: Clinical evaluation and follow-up outcome of diffusion tensor imaging-based functional neuronavigation: a prospective, controlled study in patients with gliomas involving pyramidal tracts. *Neurosurgery.* 2007, 61(5):935-948.

[57] Chaskis C, Stadnik T, Michotte A, Van Rompaey K, D'Haens J: Prognostic value of perfusion-weighted imaging in brain glioma: a prospective study. *Acta neurochirurgica.* 2006, 148(3):277-285.

[58] Pathak AP, Schmainda KM, Ward BD, Linderman JR, Rebro KJ, Greene AS: MR-derived cerebral blood volume maps: issues regarding histological validation and assessment of tumor angiogenesis. *Magn. Reson Med.* 2001, 46(4):735-747.

[59] Aronen HJ, Pardo FS, Kennedy DN, Belliveau JW, Packard SD, Hsu DW, Hochberg FH, Fischman AJ, Rosen BR: High microvascular blood volume is associated with high glucose uptake and tumor angiogenesis in human gliomas. *Clin. Cancer Res.* 2000, 6(6):2189-2200.

[60] Aronen HJ, Gazit IE, Louis DN, Buchbinder BR, Pardo FS, Weisskoff RM, Harsh GR, Cosgrove GR, Halpern EF, Hochberg FH et al.: Cerebral blood volume maps of gliomas: comparison with tumor grade and histologic findings. *Radiology.* 1994, 191(1):41-51.

[61] Cha S, Johnson G, Wadghiri YZ, Jin O, Babb J, Zagzag D, Turnbull DH: Dynamic, contrast-enhanced perfusion MRI in mouse gliomas: correlation with histopathology. *Magn. Reson. Med.* 2003, 49(5):848-855.

[62] Sibtain NA, Howe FA, Saunders DE: The clinical value of proton magnetic resonance spectroscopy in adult brain tumours. *Clinical radiology.* 2007, 62(2):109-119.

[63] Young GS: Advanced MRI of adult brain tumors. *Neurologic clinics* 2007, 25(4):947-973, viii.

[64] Gajewicz W, Papierz W, Szymczak W, Goraj B: The use of proton MRS in the differential diagnosis of brain tumors and tumor-like processes. *Med. Sci. Monit.* 2003, 9(9):MT97-105.

[65] Del Sole A, Falini A, Ravasi L, Ottobrini L, De Marchis D, Bombardieri E, Lucignani G: Anatomical and biochemical investigation of primary brain tumours. *European journal of nuclear medicine.* 2001, 28(12):1851-1872.

[66] Delorme S, Weber MA: Applications of MRS in the evaluation of focal malignant brain lesions. *Cancer Imaging.* 2006, 6:95-99.

[67] Nelson SJ, McKnight TR, Henry RG: Characterization of untreated gliomas by magnetic resonance spectroscopic imaging. *Neuroimaging clinics of North America.* 2002, 12(4):599-613.

[68] Dowling C, Bollen AW, Noworolski SM, McDermott MW, Barbaro NM, Day MR, Henry RG, Chang SM, Dillon WP, Nelson SJ et al.: Preoperative proton MR spectroscopic imaging of brain tumors: correlation with histopathologic analysis of resection specimens. *Ajnr.* 2001, 22(4):604-612.

[69] Nelson SJ: Multivoxel magnetic resonance spectroscopy of brain tumors. *Molecular cancer therapeutics.* 2003, 2(5):497-507.

[70] Pirzkall A, McKnight TR, Graves EE, Carol MP, Sneed PK, Wara WW, Nelson SJ, Verhey LJ, Larson DA: MR-spectroscopy guided target delineation for high-grade gliomas. *International journal of radiation oncology, biology, physics.* 2001, 50(4):915-928.

[71] Rock JP, Scarpace L, Hearshen D, Gutierrez J, Fisher JL, Rosenblum M, Mikkelsen T: Associations among magnetic resonance spectroscopy, apparent diffusion coefficients, and image-guided histopathology with special attention to radiation necrosis. *Neurosurgery.* 2004, 54(5):1111-1117.

[72] Matsusue E, Fink JR, Rockhill JK, Ogawa T, Maravilla KR: Distinction between glioma progression and post-radiation change by combined physiologic MR imaging. *Neuroradiology*, 52(4):297-306.

[73] Zeng QS, Li CF, Liu H, Zhen JH, Feng DC: Distinction between recurrent glioma and radiation injury using magnetic resonance spectroscopy in combination with diffusion-weighted imaging. *International journal of radiation oncology, biology, physics.* 2007, 68(1):151-158.

[74] Graves EE, Nelson SJ, Vigneron DB, Verhey L, McDermott M, Larson D, Chang S, Prados MD, Dillon WP: Serial proton MR spectroscopic imaging of recurrent malignant gliomas after gamma knife radiosurgery. *Ajnr* 2001, 22(4):613-624.

[75] Chan AA, Lau A, Pirzkall A, Chang SM, Verhey LJ, Larson D, McDermott MW, Dillon WP, Nelson SJ: Proton magnetic resonance spectroscopy imaging in the evaluation of patients undergoing gamma knife surgery for Grade IV glioma. *Journal of neurosurgery.* 2004, 101(3):467-475.

[76] Vallabhajosula S: (18)F-labeled positron emission tomographic radiopharmaceuticals in oncology: an overview of radiochemistry and mechanisms of tumor localization. *Seminars in nuclear medicine.* 2007, 37(6):400-419.

[77] Chen W: Clinical applications of PET in brain tumors. *J. Nucl. Med.* 2007, 48(9):1468-1481.

[78] Barwick T, Bencherif B, Mountz JM, Avril N: Molecular PET and PET/CT imaging of tumour cell proliferation using F-18 fluoro-L-thymidine: a comprehensive evaluation. *Nuclear medicine communications.* 2009, 30(12):908-917.

[79] Ullrich R, Backes H, Li H, Kracht L, Miletic H, Kesper K, Neumaier B, Heiss WD, Wienhard K, Jacobs AH: Glioma proliferation as assessed by 3'-fluoro-3'-deoxy-L-thymidine positron emission tomography in patients with newly diagnosed high-grade glioma. *Clin. Cancer Res.* 2008, 14(7):2049-2055.

[80] Chen W, Cloughesy T, Kamdar N, Satyamurthy N, Bergsneider M, Liau L, Mischel P, Czernin J, Phelps ME, Silverman DH: Imaging proliferation in brain tumors with 18F-FLT PET: comparison with 18F-FDG. *J. Nucl. Med..* 2005, 46(6):945-952.

[81] Chen W, Delaloye S, Silverman DH, Geist C, Czernin J, Sayre J, Satyamurthy N, Pope W, Lai A, Phelps ME et al.: Predicting treatment response of malignant gliomas to

bevacizumab and irinotecan by imaging proliferation with [18F] fluorothymidine positron emission tomography: a pilot study. *J. Clin. Oncol.* 2007, 25(30):4714-4721.

[82] Rasey JS, Grunbaum Z, Magee S, Nelson NJ, Olive PL, Durand RE, Krohn KA: Characterization of radiolabeled fluoromisonidazole as a probe for hypoxic cells. *Radiation research.* 1987, 111(2):292-304.

[83] Cher LM, Murone C, Lawrentschuk N, Ramdave S, Papenfuss A, Hannah A, O'Keefe GJ, Sachinidis JI, Berlangieri SU, Fabinyi G et al.: Correlation of hypoxic cell fraction and angiogenesis with glucose metabolic rate in gliomas using 18F-fluoromisonidazole, 18F-FDG PET, and immunohistochemical studies. *J. Nucl. Med.* 2006, 47(3):410-418.

[84] Spence AM, Muzi M, Swanson KR, O'Sullivan F, Rockhill JK, Rajendran JG, Adamsen TC, Link JM, Swanson PE, Yagle KJ et al.: Regional hypoxia in glioblastoma multiforme quantified with [18F]fluoromisonidazole positron emission tomography before radiotherapy: correlation with time to progression and survival. *Clin. Cancer Res.* 2008, 14(9):2623-2630.

[85] Kawai N, Maeda Y, Kudomi N, Miyake K, Okada M, Yamamoto Y, Nishiyama Y, Tamiya T: Correlation of biological aggressiveness assessed by 11C-methionine PET and hypoxic burden assessed by 18F-fluoromisonidazole PET in newly diagnosed glioblastoma. *European journal of nuclear medicine and molecular imaging*, 38(3):441-450.

[86] Hatakeyama T, Kawai N, Nishiyama Y, Yamamoto Y, Sasakawa Y, Ichikawa T, Tamiya T: 11C-methionine (MET) and 18F-fluorothymidine (FLT) PET in patients with newly diagnosed glioma. *European journal of nuclear medicine and molecular imaging.* 2008, 35(11):2009-2017.

[87] Miwa K, Shinoda J, Yano H, Okumura A, Iwama T, Nakashima T, Sakai N: Discrepancy between lesion distributions on methionine PET and MR images in patients with glioblastoma multiforme: insight from a PET and MR fusion image study. *Journal of neurology, neurosurgery, and psychiatry* 2004, 75(10):1457-1462.

[88] Wen PY, Schiff D, Kesari S, Drappatz J, Gigas DC, Doherty L: Medical management of patients with brain tumors. *Journal of neuro-oncology.* 2006, 80(3):313-332.

[89] Glantz MJ, Cole BF, Forsyth PA, Recht LD, Wen PY, Chamberlain MC, Grossman SA, Cairncross JG: Practice parameter: anticonvulsant prophylaxis in patients with newly diagnosed brain tumors. Report of the Quality Standards Subcommittee of the American Academy of Neurology. *Neurology.* 2000, 54(10):1886-1893.

[90] Green H, Paul M, Vidal L, Leibovici L: Prophylaxis of Pneumocystis pneumonia in immunocompromised non-HIV-infected patients: systematic review and meta-analysis of randomized controlled trials. *Mayo Clinic proceedings.* 2007, 82(9):1052-1059.

[91] Gerber DE, Grossman SA, Streiff MB: Management of venous thromboembolism in patients with primary and metastatic brain tumors. *J. Clin. Oncol.* 2006, 24(8):1310-1318.

[92] Pruitt AA: Medical management of patients with brain tumors. *Current treatment options in neurology*, 13(4):413-426.

[93] Ruff RL, Posner JB: Incidence and treatment of peripheral venous thrombosis in patients with glioma. *Annals. of neurology.* 1983, 13(3):334-336.

[94] Lee AY, Levine MN, Baker RI, Bowden C, Kakkar AK, Prins M, Rickles FR, Julian JA, Haley S, Kovacs MJ et al.: Low-molecular-weight heparin versus a coumarin for

the prevention of recurrent venous thromboembolism in patients with cancer. *The New England journal of medicine.* 2003, 349(2):146-153.
[95] Meyers CA, Weitzner MA, Valentine AD, Levin VA: Methylphenidate therapy improves cognition, mood, and function of brain tumor patients. *J. Clin. Oncol.* 1998, 16(7):2522-2527.
[96] Shaw EG, Rosdhal R, D'Agostino RB, Jr., Lovato J, Naughton MJ, Robbins ME, Rapp SR: Phase II study of donepezil in irradiated brain tumor patients: effect on cognitive function, mood, and quality of life. *J. Clin. Oncol.* 2006, 24(9):1415-1420.
[97] Litofsky NS, Farace E, Anderson F, Jr., Meyers CA, Huang W, Laws ER, Jr.: Depression in patients with high-grade glioma: results of the Glioma Outcomes Project. *Neurosurgery.* 2004, 54(2):358-366.
[98] Chamberlain MC: Treatment options for glioblastoma. *Neurosurgical focus* 2006, 20(4):E19.
[99] Norden AD, Wen PY: Glioma therapy in adults. *The neurologist.* 2006, 12(6):279-292.
[100] Wen PY, Kesari S: Malignant gliomas in adults. *The New England journal of medicine.* 2008, 359(5):492-507.
[101] Grossman SA, Batara JF: Current management of glioblastoma multiforme. *Seminars in oncology.* 2004, 31(5):635-644.
[102] Van Meir EG, Hadjipanayis CG, Norden AD, Shu HK, Wen PY, Olson JJ: Exciting new advances in neuro-oncology: the avenue to a cure for malignant glioma. *CA: a cancer journal for clinicians*, 60(3):166-193.
[103] Lacroix M, Abi-Said D, Fourney DR, Gokaslan ZL, Shi W, DeMonte F, Lang FF, McCutcheon IE, Hassenbusch SJ, Holland E et al.: A multivariate analysis of 416 patients with glioblastoma multiforme: prognosis, extent of resection, and survival. *Journal of neurosurgery.* 2001, 95(2):190-198.
[104] Sanai N, Berger MS: Glioma extent of resection and its impact on patient outcome. *Neurosurgery* 2008, 62(4):753-764.
[105] Sanai N, Polley MY, McDermott MW, Parsa AT, Berger MS: An extent of resection threshold for newly diagnosed glioblastomas. *Journal of neurosurgery.* 2011, 115(1):3-8.
[106] Vuorinen V, Hinkka S, Farkkila M, Jaaskelainen J: Debulking or biopsy of malignant glioma in elderly people - a randomised study. *Acta neurochirurgica.* 2003, 145(1):5-10.
[107] Willems PW, Taphoorn MJ, Burger H, Berkelbach van der Sprenkel JW, Tulleken CA: Effectiveness of neuronavigation in resecting solitary intracerebral contrast-enhancing tumors: a randomized controlled trial. *Journal of neurosurgery.* 2006, 104(3):360-368.
[108] Letteboer MM, Willems PW, Viergever MA, Niessen WJ: Brain shift estimation in image-guided neurosurgery using 3-D ultrasound. *IEEE transactions on bio-medical engineering.* 2005, 52(2):268-276.
[109] Trantakis C, Tittgemeyer M, Schneider JP, Lindner D, Winkler D, Strauss G, Meixensberger J: Investigation of time-dependency of intracranial brain shift and its relation to the extent of tumor removal using intra-operative MRI. *Neurological research.* 2003, 25(1):9-12.
[110] Nimsky C, Grummich P, Sorensen AG, Fahlbusch R, Ganslandt O: Visualization of the pyramidal tract in glioma surgery by integrating diffusion tensor imaging in functional neuronavigation. *Zentralblatt fur Neurochirurgie.* 2005, 66(3):133-141.

[111] Braun V, Dempf S, Tomczak R, Wunderlich A, Weller R, Richter HP: Multimodal cranial neuronavigation: direct integration of functional magnetic resonance imaging and positron emission tomography data: technical note. *Neurosurgery.* 2001, 48(5):1178-1181.

[112] Rasmussen IA, Jr., Lindseth F, Rygh OM, Berntsen EM, Selbekk T, Xu J, Nagelhus Hernes TA, Harg E, Haberg A, Unsgaard G: Functional neuronavigation combined with intra-operative 3D ultrasound: initial experiences during surgical resections close to eloquent brain areas and future directions in automatic brain shift compensation of preoperative data. *Acta neurochirurgica.* 2007, 149(4):365-378.

[113] Coenen VA, Krings T, Weidemann J, Hans FJ, Reinacher P, Gilsbach JM, Rohde V: Sequential visualization of brain and fiber tract deformation during intracranial surgery with three-dimensional ultrasound: an approach to evaluate the effect of brain shift. *Neurosurgery.* 2005, 56(1 Suppl):133-141.

[114] Berntsen EM, Gulati S, Solheim O, Kvistad KA, Torp SH, Selbekk T, Unsgard G, Haberg AK: Functional magnetic resonance imaging and diffusion tensor tractography incorporated into an intraoperative 3-dimensional ultrasound-based neuronavigation system: impact on therapeutic strategies, extent of resection, and clinical outcome. *Neurosurgery*, 67(2):251-264.

[115] Pirotte B, Goldman S, Dewitte O, Massager N, Wikler D, Lefranc F, Ben Taib NO, Rorive S, David P, Brotchi J et al.: Integrated positron emission tomography and magnetic resonance imaging-guided resection of brain tumors: a report of 103 consecutive procedures. *Journal of neurosurgery.* 2006, 104(2):238-253.

[116] Muns A, Meixensberger J, Arnold S, Schmitgen A, Arlt F, Chalopin C, Lindner D: Integration of a 3D ultrasound probe into neuronavigation. *Acta neurochirurgica*, 153(7):1529-1533.

[117] Schlaier JR, Warnat J, Dorenbeck U, Proescholdt M, Schebesch KM, Brawanski A: Image fusion of MR images and real-time ultrasonography: evaluation of fusion accuracy combining two commercial instruments, a neuronavigation system and a ultrasound system. *Acta neurochirurgica.* 2004, 146(3):271-276.

[118] Nossek E, Korn A, Shahar T, Kanner AA, Yaffe H, Marcovici D, Ben-Harosh C, Ben Ami H, Weinstein M, Shapira-Lichter I et al.: Intraoperative mapping and monitoring of the corticospinal tracts with neurophysiological assessment and 3-dimensional ultrasonography-based navigation. Clinical article. *Journal of neurosurgery*, 114(3):738-746.

[119] Gonzalez-Darder JM, Gonzalez-Lopez P, Talamantes F, Quilis V, Cortes V, Garcia-March G, Roldan P: Multimodal navigation in the functional microsurgical resection of intrinsic brain tumors located in eloquent motor areas: role of tractography. *Neurosurgical focus*, 28(2):E5.

[120] Shamov T, Spiriev T, Tzvetanov P, Petkov A: The combination of neuronavigation with transcranial magnetic stimulation for treatment of opercular gliomas of the dominant brain hemisphere. *Clinical neurology and neurosurgery*, 112(8):672-677.

[121] Senft C, Franz K, Ulrich CT, Bink A, Szelenyi A, Gasser T, Seifert V: Low field intraoperative MRI-guided surgery of gliomas: a single center experience. *Clinical neurology and neurosurgery*, 112(3):237-243.

[122] Muragaki Y, Iseki H, Maruyama T, Kawamata T, Yamane F, Nakamura R, Kubo O, Takakura K, Hori T: Usefulness of intraoperative magnetic resonance imaging for glioma surgery. *Acta. Neurochir. Suppl.* 2006, 98:67-75.

[123] Hatiboglu MA, Weinberg JS, Suki D, Rao G, Prabhu SS, Shah K, Jackson E, Sawaya R: Impact of intraoperative high-field magnetic resonance imaging guidance on glioma surgery: a prospective volumetric analysis. *Neurosurgery.* 2009, 64(6):1073-1081.

[124] Jankovski A, Francotte F, Vaz G, Fomekong E, Duprez T, Van Boven M, Docquier MA, Hermoye L, Cosnard G, Raftopoulos C: Intraoperative magnetic resonance imaging at 3-T using a dual independent operating room-magnetic resonance imaging suite: development, feasibility, safety, and preliminary experience. *Neurosurgery.* 2008, 63(3):412-424.

[125] Sun GC, Chen XL, Zhao Y, Wang F, Hou BK, Wang YB, Song ZJ, Wang D, Xu BN: Intraoperative High-Field Magnetic Resonance Imaging Combined With Fiber Tract Neuronavigation Guided Resection Of Cerebral Lesions Involving Optic Radiation. *Neurosurgery.* 2011, *Jun. 7.*

[126] Parney IF, Goerss SJ, McGee K, Huston J, 3rd, Perkins WJ, Meyer FB: Awake craniotomy, electrophysiologic mapping, and tumor resection with high-field intraoperative MRI. *World neurosurgery*, 73(5):547-551.

[127] Kuhnt D, Ganslandt O, Schlaffer SM, Buchfelder M, Nimsky C: Quantification of glioma removal by intraoperative high-field magnetic resonance imaging - an update. *Neurosurgery.* 2011, *May 26.*

[128] Pichlmeier U, Bink A, Schackert G, Stummer W: Resection and survival in glioblastoma multiforme: an RTOG recursive partitioning analysis of ALA study patients. *Neuro-oncology.* 2008, 10(6):1025-1034.

[129] Stummer W, Pichlmeier U, Meinel T, Wiestler OD, Zanella F, Reulen HJ: Fluorescence-guided surgery with 5-aminolevulinic acid for resection of malignant glioma: a randomised controlled multicentre phase III trial. *The lancet oncology.* 2006, 7(5):392-401.

[130] Stummer W, Reulen HJ, Meinel T, Pichlmeier U, Schumacher W, Tonn JC, Rohde V, Oppel F, Turowski B, Woiciechowsky C et al.: Extent of resection and survival in glioblastoma multiforme: identification of and adjustment for bias. *Neurosurgery.* 2008, 62(3):564-576.

[131] Tonn JC, Stummer W: Fluorescence-guided resection of malignant gliomas using 5-aminolevulinic acid: practical use, risks, and pitfalls. *Clinical neurosurgery.* 2008, 55:20-26.

[132] Walker MD, Strike TA, Sheline GE: An analysis of dose-effect relationship in the radiotherapy of malignant gliomas. *International journal of radiation oncology, biology, physics.* 1979, 5(10):1725-1731.

[133] Hegi ME, Diserens AC, Gorlia T, Hamou MF, de Tribolet N, Weller M, Kros JM, Hainfellner JA, Mason W, Mariani L et al.: MGMT gene silencing and benefit from temozolomide in glioblastoma. *The New England journal of medicine.* 2005, 352(10):997-1003.

[134] Stupp R, Mason WP, van den Bent MJ, Weller M, Fisher B, Taphoorn MJ, Belanger K, Brandes AA, Marosi C, Bogdahn U et al.: Radiotherapy plus concomitant and adjuvant temozolomide for glioblastoma. *The New England journal of medicine.* 2005, 352(10):987-996.

[135] Stupp R, van den Bent MJ, Hegi ME: Optimal role of temozolomide in the treatment of malignant gliomas. *Current neurology and neuroscience reports.* 2005, 5(3):198-206.
[136] Ataman F, Poortmans P, Stupp R, Fisher B, Mirimanoff RO: Quality assurance of the EORTC 26981/22981; NCIC CE3 intergroup trial on radiotherapy with or without temozolomide for newly-diagnosed glioblastoma multiforme: the individual case review. *Eur. J. Cancer* 2004, 40(11):1724-1730.
[137] Chan MF, Schupak K, Burman C, Chui CS, Ling CC: Comparison of intensity-modulated radiotherapy with three-dimensional conformal radiation therapy planning for glioblastoma multiforme. *Med. Dosim.* 2003, 28(4):261-265.
[138] Butowski NA, Sneed PK, Chang SM: Diagnosis and treatment of recurrent high-grade astrocytoma. *J. Clin. Oncol.* 2006, 24(8):1273-1280.
[139] Nieder C, Astner ST, Mehta MP, Grosu AL, Molls M: Improvement, clinical course, and quality of life after palliative radiotherapy for recurrent glioblastoma. *American journal of clinical oncology.* 2008, 31(3):300-305.
[140] Mayer R, Sminia P: Reirradiation tolerance of the human brain. *International journal of radiation oncology, biology, physics.* 2008, 70(5):1350-1360.
[141] Larson DA, Gutin PH, McDermott M, Lamborn K, Sneed PK, Wara WM, Flickinger JC, Kondziolka D, Lunsford LD, Hudgins WR et al.: Gamma knife for glioma: selection factors and survival. *International journal of radiation oncology, biology, physics.* 1996, 36(5):1045-1053.
[142] Kondziolka D, Flickinger JC, Bissonette DJ, Bozik M, Lunsford LD: Survival benefit of stereotactic radiosurgery for patients with malignant glial neoplasms. *Neurosurgery.* 1997, 41(4):776-783.
[143] Souhami L, Seiferheld W, Brachman D, Podgorsak EB, Werner-Wasik M, Lustig R, Schultz CJ, Sause W, Okunieff P, Buckner J et al.: Randomized comparison of stereotactic radiosurgery followed by conventional radiotherapy with carmustine to conventional radiotherapy with carmustine for patients with glioblastoma multiforme: report of Radiation Therapy Oncology Group 93-05 protocol. *International journal of radiation oncology, biology, physics.* 2004, 60(3):853-860.
[144] Larson DA, Prados M, Lamborn KR, Smith V, Sneed PK, Chang S, Nicholas KM, Wara WM, Devriendt D, Kunwar S et al.: Phase II study of high central dose Gamma Knife radiosurgery and marimastat in patients with recurrent malignant glioma. *International journal of radiation oncology, biology, physics.* 2002, 54(5):1397-1404.
[145] Combs SE, Widmer V, Thilmann C, Hof H, Debus J, Schulz-Ertner D: Stereotactic radiosurgery (SRS): treatment option for recurrent glioblastoma multiforme (GBM). *Cancer* 2005, 104(10):2168-2173.
[146] Bernstein M, Laperriere N, Glen J, Leung P, Thomason C, Landon AE: Brachytherapy for recurrent malignant astrocytoma. *International journal of radiation oncology, biology, physics.* 1994, 30(5):1213-1217.
[147] Gabayan AJ, Green SB, Sanan A, Jenrette J, Schultz C, Papagikos M, Tatter SP, Patel A, Amin P, Lustig R et al.: GliaSite brachytherapy for treatment of recurrent malignant gliomas: a retrospective multi-institutional analysis. *Neurosurgery.* 2006, 58(4):701-709.
[148] Quant EC, Drappatz J, Wen PY, Norden AD: Recurrent high-grade glioma. *Current treatment options in neurology*, 12(4):321-333.

[149] Fogh SE, Andrews DW, Glass J, Curran W, Glass C, Champ C, Evans JJ, Hyslop T, Pequignot E, Downes B et al.: Hypofractionated stereotactic radiation therapy: an effective therapy for recurrent high-grade gliomas. *J. Clin. Oncol*, 28(18):3048-3053.
[150] Fokas E, Wacker U, Gross MW, Henzel M, Encheva E, Engenhart-Cabillic R: Hypofractionated stereotactic reirradiation of recurrent glioblastomas : a beneficial treatment option after high-dose radiotherapy? *Strahlenther Onkol.* 2009, 185(4):235-240.
[151] Combs SE, Thilmann C, Edler L, Debus J, Schulz-Ertner D: Efficacy of fractionated stereotactic reirradiation in recurrent gliomas: long-term results in 172 patients treated in a single institution. *J. Clin. Oncol.* 2005, 23(34):8863-8869.
[152] Grosu AL, Weber WA, Franz M, Stark S, Piert M, Thamm R, Gumprecht H, Schwaiger M, Molls M, Nieder C: Reirradiation of recurrent high-grade gliomas using amino acid PET (SPECT)/CT/MRI image fusion to determine gross tumor volume for stereotactic fractionated radiotherapy. *International journal of radiation oncology, biology, physics.* 2005, 63(2):511-519.
[153] Pollack IF: Neuro-oncology: Therapeutic benefits of reirradiation for recurrent brain tumors. *Nat. Rev. Neurol*, 6(10):533-535.
[154] Gerson SL: MGMT: its role in cancer aetiology and cancer therapeutics. *Nat. Rev. Cancer* 2004, 4(4):296-307.
[155] Gonzaga PE, Brent TP: Affinity purification and characterization of human O6-alkylguanine-DNA alkyltransferase complexed with BCNU-treated, synthetic oligonucleotide. *Nucleic. acids research* 1989, 17(16):6581-6590.
[156] Day RS, 3rd, Ziolkowski CH, Scudiero DA, Meyer SA, Lubiniecki AS, Girardi AJ, Galloway SM, Bynum GD: Defective repair of alkylated DNA by human tumour and SV40-transformed human cell strains. *Nature.* 1980, 288(5792):724-727.
[157] Lonardi S, Tosoni A, Brandes AA: Adjuvant chemotherapy in the treatment of high grade gliomas. *Cancer treatment reviews.* 2005, 31(2):79-89.
[158] Hildebrand J, Sahmoud T, Mignolet F, Brucher JM, Afra D: Adjuvant therapy with dibromodulcitol and BCNU increases survival of adults with malignant gliomas. EORTC Brain Tumor Group. *Neurology.* 1994, 44(8):1479-1483.
[159] Walker MD, Green SB, Byar DP, Alexander E, Jr., Batzdorf U, Brooks WH, Hunt WE, MacCarty CS, Mahaley MS, Jr., Mealey J, Jr. et al.: Randomized comparisons of radiotherapy and nitrosoureas for the treatment of malignant glioma after surgery. *The New England journal of medicine.* 1980, 303(23):1323-1329.
[160] Fine HA, Dear KB, Loeffler JS, Black PM, Canellos GP: Meta-analysis of radiation therapy with and without adjuvant chemotherapy for malignant gliomas in adults. *Cancer.* 1993, 71(8):2585-2597.
[161] Stewart LA: Chemotherapy in adult high-grade glioma: a systematic review and meta-analysis of individual patient data from 12 randomised trials. *Lancet.* 2002, 359(9311):1011-1018.
[162] Randomized trial of procarbazine, lomustine, and vincristine in the adjuvant treatment of high-grade astrocytoma: a Medical Research Council trial. *J. Clin. Oncol.* 2001, 19(2):509-518.
[163] Brada M, Judson I, Beale P, Moore S, Reidenberg P, Statkevich P, Dugan M, Batra V, Cutler D: Phase I dose-escalation and pharmacokinetic study of temozolomide (SCH

52365) for refractory or relapsing malignancies. *British journal of cancer.* 1999, 81(6):1022-1030.

[164] Kaina B, Ziouta A, Ochs K, Coquerelle T: Chromosomal instability, reproductive cell death and apoptosis induced by O6-methylguanine in Mex-, Mex+ and methylation-tolerant mismatch repair compromised cells: facts and models. *Mutation research.* 1997, 381(2):227-241.

[165] Hirose Y, Berger MS, Pieper RO: p53 effects both the duration of G2/M arrest and the fate of temozolomide-treated human glioblastoma cells. *Cancer research.* 2001, 61(5):1957-1963.

[166] Hirose Y, Berger MS, Pieper RO: Abrogation of the Chk1-mediated G(2) checkpoint pathway potentiates temozolomide-induced toxicity in a p53-independent manner in human glioblastoma cells. *Cancer research.* 2001, 61(15):5843-5849.

[167] Hirose Y, Kreklau EL, Erickson LC, Berger MS, Pieper RO: Delayed repletion of O6-methylguanine-DNA methyltransferase resulting in failure to protect the human glioblastoma cell line SF767 from temozolomide-induced cytotoxicity. *Journal of neurosurgery.* 2003, 98(3):591-598.

[168] Newlands ES, Stevens MF, Wedge SR, Wheelhouse RT, Brock C: Temozolomide: a review of its discovery, chemical properties, pre-clinical development and clinical trials. *Cancer treatment reviews.* 1997, 23(1):35-61.

[169] Friedman HS, Kerby T, Calvert H: Temozolomide and treatment of malignant glioma. *Clin. Cancer. Res* 2000, 6(7):2585-2597.

[170] Mutter N, Stupp R: Temozolomide: a milestone in neuro-oncology and beyond? *Expert review of anticancer therapy.* 2006, 6(8):1187-1204.

[171] Hegi ME, Diserens AC, Godard S, Dietrich PY, Regli L, Ostermann S, Otten P, Van Melle G, de Tribolet N, Stupp R: Clinical trial substantiates the predictive value of O-6-methylguanine-DNA methyltransferase promoter methylation in glioblastoma patients treated with temozolomide. *Clin. Cancer Res.* 2004, 10(6):1871-1874.

[172] Esteller M, Garcia-Foncillas J, Andion E, Goodman SN, Hidalgo OF, Vanaclocha V, Baylin SB, Herman JG: Inactivation of the DNA-repair gene MGMT and the clinical response of gliomas to alkylating agents. *The New England journal of medicine.* 2000, 343(19):1350-1354.

[173] Paz MF, Yaya-Tur R, Rojas-Marcos I, Reynes G, Pollan M, Aguirre-Cruz L, Garcia-Lopez JL, Piquer J, Safont MJ, Balana C et al.: CpG island hypermethylation of the DNA repair enzyme methyltransferase predicts response to temozolomide in primary gliomas. *Clin. Cancer Res.* 2004, 10(15):4933-4938.

[174] Robinson CG, Palomo JM, Rahmathulla G, McGraw M, Donze J, Liu L, Vogelbaum MA: Effect of alternative temozolomide schedules on glioblastoma O(6)-methylguanine-DNA methyltransferase activity and survival. *British journal of cancer,* 103(4):498-504.

[175] Tolcher AW, Gerson SL, Denis L, Geyer C, Hammond LA, Patnaik A, Goetz AD, Schwartz G, Edwards T, Reyderman L et al.: Marked inactivation of O6-alkylguanine-DNA alkyltransferase activity with protracted temozolomide schedules. *British journal of cancer.* 2003, 88(7):1004-1011.

[176] Broniscer A, Gururangan S, MacDonald TJ, Goldman S, Packer RJ, Stewart CF, Wallace D, Danks MK, Friedman HS, Poussaint TY et al.: Phase I trial of single-dose temozolomide and continuous administration of o6-benzylguanine in children with

brain tumors: a pediatric brain tumor consortium report. *Clin. Cancer Res.* 2007, 13(22 Pt 1):6712-6718.

[177] Donawho CK, Luo Y, Luo Y, Penning TD, Bauch JL, Bouska JJ, Bontcheva-Diaz VD, Cox BF, DeWeese TL, Dillehay LE et al.: ABT-888, an orally active poly(ADP-ribose) polymerase inhibitor that potentiates DNA-damaging agents in preclinical tumor models. *Clin. Cancer Res.* 2007, 13(9):2728-2737.

[178] Clarke MJ, Mulligan EA, Grogan PT, Mladek AC, Carlson BL, Schroeder MA, Curtin NJ, Lou Z, Decker PA, Wu W et al.: Effective sensitization of temozolomide by ABT-888 is lost with development of temozolomide resistance in glioblastoma xenograft lines. *Molecular cancer therapeutics.* 2009, 8(2):407-414.

[179] Rivera AL, Pelloski CE, Gilbert MR, Colman H, De La Cruz C, Sulman EP, Bekele BN, Aldape KD: MGMT promoter methylation is predictive of response to radiotherapy and prognostic in the absence of adjuvant alkylating chemotherapy for glioblastoma. *Neuro-oncology*, 12(2):116-121.

[180] Westphal M, Hilt DC, Bortey E, Delavault P, Olivares R, Warnke PC, Whittle IR, Jaaskelainen J, Ram Z: A phase 3 trial of local chemotherapy with biodegradable carmustine (BCNU) wafers (Gliadel wafers) in patients with primary malignant glioma. *Neuro-oncology.* 2003, 5(2):79-88.

[181] Westphal M, Ram Z, Riddle V, Hilt D, Bortey E: Gliadel wafer in initial surgery for malignant glioma: long-term follow-up of a multicenter controlled trial. *Acta neurochirurgica.* 2006, 148(3):269-275.

[182] Attenello FJ, Mukherjee D, Datoo G, McGirt MJ, Bohan E, Weingart JD, Olivi A, Quinones-Hinojosa A, Brem H: Use of Gliadel (BCNU) wafer in the surgical treatment of malignant glioma: a 10-year institutional experience. *Annals of surgical oncology.* 2008, 15(10):2887-2893.

[183] McGirt MJ, Than KD, Weingart JD, Chaichana KL, Attenello FJ, Olivi A, Laterra J, Kleinberg LR, Grossman SA, Brem H et al.: Gliadel (BCNU) wafer plus concomitant temozolomide therapy after primary resection of glioblastoma multiforme. *Journal of neurosurgery.* 2009, 110(3):583-588.

[184] Bock HC, Puchner MJ, Lohmann F, Schutze M, Koll S, Ketter R, Buchalla R, Rainov N, Kantelhardt SR, Rohde V et al.: First-line treatment of malignant glioma with carmustine implants followed by concomitant radiochemotherapy: a multicenter experience. *Neurosurgical review.* 2010, 33(4):441-449.

[185] Noel G, Schott R, Froelich S, Gaub MP, Boyer P, Fischer-Lokou D, Dufour P, Kehrli P, Maitrot D: Retrospective Comparison of Chemoradiotherapy Followed by Adjuvant Chemotherapy, With or Without Prior Gliadel Implantation (Carmustine) After Initial Surgery in Patients With Newly Diagnosed High-Grade Gliomas. *International journal of radiation oncology, biology, physics.* 2011, Feb 5.

[186] Tysnes BB, Mahesparan R: Biological mechanisms of glioma invasion and potential therapeutic targets. *Journal of neuro-oncology.* 2001, 53(2):129-147.

[187] Louis DN: Molecular pathology of malignant gliomas. *Annual review of pathology.* 2006, 1:97-117.

[188] Comprehensive genomic characterization defines human glioblastoma genes and core pathways. *Nature.* 2008, 455(7216):1061-1068.

[189] Stupp R, Hegi ME, Gilbert MR, Chakravarti A: Chemoradiotherapy in malignant glioma: standard of care and future directions. *J. Clin. Oncol.* 2007, 25(26):4127-4136.

[190] Rich JN, Reardon DA, Peery T, Dowell JM, Quinn JA, Penne KL, Wikstrand CJ, Van Duyn LB, Dancey JE, McLendon RE et al.: Phase II trial of gefitinib in recurrent glioblastoma. *J. Clin. Oncol.* 2004, 22(1):133-142.

[191] Galanis E, Buckner JC, Maurer MJ, Kreisberg JI, Ballman K, Boni J, Peralba JM, Jenkins RB, Dakhil SR, Morton RF et al.: Phase II trial of temsirolimus (CCI-779) in recurrent glioblastoma multiforme: a North Central Cancer Treatment Group Study. *J. Clin. Oncol.* 2005, 23(23):5294-5304.

[192] Chang SM, Wen P, Cloughesy T, Greenberg H, Schiff D, Conrad C, Fink K, Robins HI, De Angelis L, Raizer J et al.: Phase II study of CCI-779 in patients with recurrent glioblastoma multiforme. *Investigational new drugs.* 2005, 23(4):357-361.

[193] Cloughesy TF, Wen PY, Robins HI, Chang SM, Groves MD, Fink KL, Junck L, Schiff D, Abrey L, Gilbert MR et al.: Phase II trial of tipifarnib in patients with recurrent malignant glioma either receiving or not receiving enzyme-inducing antiepileptic drugs: a North American Brain Tumor Consortium Study. *J. Clin. Oncol.* 2006, 24(22):3651-3656.

[194] Chi AS, Wen PY: Inhibiting kinases in malignant gliomas. *Expert opinion on therapeutic targets.* 2007, 11(4):473-496.

[195] Sathornsumetee S, Reardon DA, Desjardins A, Quinn JA, Vredenburgh JJ, Rich JN: Molecularly targeted therapy for malignant glioma. *Cancer.* 2007, 110(1):13-24.

[196] Stommel JM, Kimmelman AC, Ying H, Nabioullin R, Ponugoti AH, Wiedemeyer R, Stegh AH, Bradner JE, Ligon KL, Brennan C et al.: Coactivation of receptor tyrosine kinases affects the response of tumor cells to targeted therapies. *Science.* 2007, 318(5848):287-290.

[197] Furnari FB, Fenton T, Bachoo RM, Mukasa A, Stommel JM, Stegh A, Hahn WC, Ligon KL, Louis DN, Brennan C et al.: Malignant astrocytic glioma: genetics, biology, and paths to treatment. *Genes and development.* 2007, 21(21):2683-2710.

[198] Schmidt NO, Westphal M, Hagel C, Ergun S, Stavrou D, Rosen EM, Lamszus K: Levels of vascular endothelial growth factor, hepatocyte growth factor/scatter factor and basic fibroblast growth factor in human gliomas and their relation to angiogenesis. *International journal of cancer.* 1999, 84(1):10-18.

[199] Norden AD, Young GS, Setayesh K, Muzikansky A, Klufas R, Ross GL, Ciampa AS, Ebbeling LG, Levy B, Drappatz J et al.: Bevacizumab for recurrent malignant gliomas: efficacy, toxicity, and patterns of recurrence. *Neurology.* 2008, 70(10):779-787.

[200] Narayana A, Kelly P, Golfinos J, Parker E, Johnson G, Knopp E, Zagzag D, Fischer I, Raza S, Medabalmi P et al.: Antiangiogenic therapy using bevacizumab in recurrent high-grade glioma: impact on local control and patient survival. *Journal of neurosurgery.* 2009, 110(1):173-180.

[201] Nghiemphu PL, Liu W, Lee Y, Than T, Graham C, Lai A, Green RM, Pope WB, Liau LM, Mischel PS et al.: Bevacizumab and chemotherapy for recurrent glioblastoma: a single-institution experience. *Neurology.* 2009, 72(14):1217-1222.

[202] Poulsen HS, Grunnet K, Sorensen M, Olsen P, Hasselbalch B, Nelausen K, Kosteljanetz M, Lassen U: Bevacizumab plus irinotecan in the treatment patients with progressive recurrent malignant brain tumours. *Acta oncologica.* 2009, 48(1):52-58.

[203] Zuniga RM, Torcuator R, Jain R, Anderson J, Doyle T, Ellika S, Schultz L, Mikkelsen T: Efficacy, safety and patterns of response and recurrence in patients with recurrent

high-grade gliomas treated with bevacizumab plus irinotecan. *Journal of neuro-oncology.* 2009, 91(3):329-336.
[204] Pope WB, Lai A, Nghiemphu P, Mischel P, Cloughesy TF: MRI in patients with high-grade gliomas treated with bevacizumab and chemotherapy. *Neurology.* 2006, 66(8):1258-1260.
[205] Vredenburgh JJ, Desjardins A, Herndon JE, 2nd, Marcello J, Reardon DA, Quinn JA, Rich JN, Sathornsumetee S, Gururangan S, Sampson J et al.: Bevacizumab plus irinotecan in recurrent glioblastoma multiforme. *J. Clin. Oncol.* 2007, 25(30):4722-4729.
[206] Yung WK, Albright RE, Olson J, Fredericks R, Fink K, Prados MD, Brada M, Spence A, Hohl RJ, Shapiro W et al.: A phase II study of temozolomide vs. procarbazine in patients with glioblastoma multiforme at first relapse. *British journal of cancer.* 2000, 83(5):588-593.
[207] Friedman HS, Prados MD, Wen PY, Mikkelsen T, Schiff D, Abrey LE, Yung WK, Paleologos N, Nicholas MK, Jensen R et al.: Bevacizumab alone and in combination with irinotecan in recurrent glioblastoma. *J. Clin. Oncol.* 2009, 27(28):4733-4740.
[208] Kreisl TN, Kim L, Moore K, Duic P, Royce C, Stroud I, Garren N, Mackey M, Butman JA, Camphausen K et al.: Phase II trial of single-agent bevacizumab followed by bevacizumab plus irinotecan at tumor progression in recurrent glioblastoma. *J. Clin. Oncol.* 2009, 27(5):740-745.
[209] Vredenburgh JJ, Desjardins A, Kirkpatrick JP, Reardon DA, Peters KB, Herndon JE, 2nd, Marcello J, Bailey L, Threatt S, Sampson J et al.: Addition of Bevacizumab to Standard Radiation Therapy and Daily Temozolomide Is Associated with Minimal Toxicity in Newly Diagnosed Glioblastoma Multiforme. *International journal of radiation oncology, biology, physics.* 2010, Oct 30.
[210] Vredenburgh JJ, Desjardins A, Reardon DA, Peters KB, Herndon JE, 2nd, Marcello J, Kirkpatrick JP, Sampson JH, Bailey L, Threatt S et al.: The addition of bevacizumab to standard radiation therapy and temozolomide followed by bevacizumab, temozolomide, and irinotecan for newly diagnosed glioblastoma. *Clin. Cancer. Res*, 17(12):4119-4124.
[211] Macdonald DR, Cascino TL, Schold SC, Jr., Cairncross JG: Response criteria for phase II studies of supratentorial malignant glioma. *J. Clin. Oncol.* 1990, 8(7):1277-1280.
[212] Henson JW, Ulmer S, Harris GJ: Brain tumor imaging in clinical trials. *Ajnr.* 2008, 29(3):419-424.
[213] van den Bent MJ, Vogelbaum MA, Wen PY, Macdonald DR, Chang SM: End point assessment in gliomas: novel treatments limit usefulness of classical Macdonald's Criteria. *J. Clin. Oncol.* 2009, 27(18):2905-2908.
[214] Wen PY, Macdonald DR, Reardon DA, Cloughesy TF, Sorensen AG, Galanis E, Degroot J, Wick W, Gilbert MR, Lassman AB et al.: Updated response assessment criteria for high-grade gliomas: response assessment in neuro-oncology working group. *J. Clin. Oncol.* 2010, 28(11):1963-1972.
[215] Easaw JC, Mason WP, Perry J, Laperriere N, Eisenstat DD, Del Maestro R, Belanger K, Fulton D, Macdonald D: Canadian recommendations for the treatment of recurrent or progressive glioblastoma multiforme. *Current oncology.* 2011, 18(3):e126-e136.
[216] Roldan GB, Scott JN, McIntyre JB, Dharmawardene M, de Robles PA, Magliocco AM, Yan ES, Parney IF, Forsyth PA, Cairncross JG et al.: Population-based study of

pseudoprogression after chemoradiotherapy in GBM. *The Canadian journal of neurological sciences.* 2009, 36(5):617-622.

[217] Taal W, Brandsma D, de Bruin HG, Bromberg JE, Swaak-Kragten AT, Smitt PA, van Es CA, van den Bent MJ: Incidence of early pseudo-progression in a cohort of malignant glioma patients treated with chemoirradiation with temozolomide. *Cancer.* 2008, 113(2):405-410.

[218] Chamberlain MC, Glantz MJ, Chalmers L, Van Horn A, Sloan AE: Early necrosis following concurrent Temodar and radiotherapy in patients with glioblastoma. *Journal of neuro-oncology.* 2007, 82(1):81-83.

[219] Sanghera P, Perry J, Sahgal A, Symons S, Aviv R, Morrison M, Lam K, Davey P, Tsao MN: Pseudoprogression following chemoradiotherapy for glioblastoma multiforme. *The Canadian journal of neurological sciences.* 2010, 37(1):36-42.

[220] Brandes AA, Franceschi E, Tosoni A, Blatt V, Pession A, Tallini G, Bertorelle R, Bartolini S, Calbucci F, Andreoli A et al.: MGMT promoter methylation status can predict the incidence and outcome of pseudoprogression after concomitant radiochemotherapy in newly diagnosed glioblastoma patients. *J. Clin. Oncol.* 2008, 26(13):2192-2197.

In: Horizons in Cancer Research. Volume 54
Editor: Hiroto S. Watanabe

ISBN: 978-1-63321-389-0

Chapter 2

The Biology of the Interleukin-2 (IL-2)-Based Immunotherapies in Cancer and Autoimmune Disease

***André Ballesteros-Tato*[1] *and Troy D. Randall*[1*]**
From the Department of Medicine, Division of Clinical Immunology and Rheumatology, University of Alabama at Birmingham, Birmingham, AL, US

Abstract

Interleukin-2 (IL-2) is an important T cell growth factor with the capacity to promote T cell expansion. Consistent with this idea, IL-2 is used clinically to enhance T cell responses to viral and tumor antigens in both preclinical models and patients. However, the role of IL-2 in immune responses is far more complex than initially expected. In addition to its ability to promote immune responses, IL-2 signaling is essential for the differentiation of regulatory T cells (Tregs), which suppress immune responses. Thus, IL-2 signaling can both promote and inhibit immune responses depending on the context, the dose, and the nature of the IL-2/IL-2 receptor interactions. As a result, IL-2 therapies that selectively target Tregs may be useful for treating autoimmune diseases, whereas IL-2 therapies that selectively target effector T cells may improve cancer immunotherapy. In this chapter we summarize our current understanding of the biology of IL-2-based immunotherapies for cancer and autoimmune disease

Introduction

IL-2 was originally characterized as a soluble growth factor with ability to sustain long-term growth of T cells in culture [1-3]. Initial studies also demonstrated that IL-2 promoted NK cell activation [4-7], helped the expansion of T cells *in vivo* [8, 9], augmented the

* Correspondence: Troy Randall, PhD, Department of Medicine, Division of Clinical Immunology and Rheumatology, University of Alabama at Birmingham, Birmingham, AL, 35294. Email: randallt@uab.edu; Phone: 205-975-3323; Fax: 205-975-3322

cytotoxic activity of T cells [7, 8, 10] and mediated anti-tumor effects when administered in conjunction with immune lymphocytes [9, 11, 12]. Together, these early data suggested that IL-2 was a potent immune activating agent and, following the molecular cloning of IL-2 in 1983, a broad variety of IL-2-based immunotherapies were developed with the goal of enhancing immune responses to both tumors and viruses in pre-clinical and clinical studies [13, 14]. Unfortunately, although the administration of high-dose of rIL-2 increases long-term survival in certain cancer patients [15-17], the overall efficacy of IL-2-based immunotherapies in cancer is lower than expected and there is essentially no clinical benefit of rIL-2 in the treatment of chronic human virus infections. In part, the lack of clinical success in IL-2–based therapeutics may be attributed to the paradoxical ability of IL-2 to suppress, as well as activate, immune responses. In fact, IL-2 has potent immune suppressive effects on both T cell and B cell responses [18, 19]. In this review, we focus on our current understanding of the biology IL-2-based immunotherapies, the advantages and limitations of the present IL-2-based treatments and the future perspectives for IL-2 immunotherapy in cancer and autoimmune disease.

1. Pleiotropic and Dose-Dependent Effects of IL-2 in Regulating Immune Responses

1.1. Pleiotropic Effects of IL-2 Signaling

IL-2 is a member of the γ-chain family of cytokines, which includes IL-4, IL-7, IL-9, IL-15 and IL-21. IL-2 can deliver signals into the cells after binding to the intermediate-affinity IL-2 receptor (IL-2R), ($K_d \approx 1$ nM) or the high-affinity IL-2R ($K_d \approx 10$ pM) [20]. The intermediate-affinity IL-2R is a heterodimeric complex consisting of the β chain of the IL-2R (IL-2Rβ or CD122) and the common γ chain (CD132) [19-21], which is shared with the other members of the common cytokine receptor γ-chain family. In contrast, the high-affinity IL-2R is a heterotrimeric complex consisting of the non-covalent association of the IL-2Rα (CD25) with the aforementioned β and γ chains [19-21]. Although CD25 is not directly involved in signal transduction, binding of IL-2 to CD25 stabilizes a secondary binding site for IL-2, which facilitates the interaction of IL-2 with the IL-2Rβ and the subsequent recruitment of the γ chain to form the stable quaternary IL-2-IL-2R complex [20].

A broad range of cells expresses the intermediate-affinity IL-2R, including natural killer (NK) cells, NK T cells and memory $CD8^+$ T cells. In contrast, the high-affinity IL-2R is only constitutively expressed on FoxP3-expressing $CD4^+$ regulatory T-cells (Tregs) [22, 23]. Although IL-2 binding to the intermediate-affinity receptor is sufficient for IL-2-mediated signal transduction, T cells rapidly up-regulate CD25 expression following TCR activation [19, 20]. As a consequence, the majority of the biological effects of IL-2 on activated T cells are mediated by the high-affinity IL-2R. Similarly, other immune cells, such as dendritic cells (DCs) [24, 25] or NK T cells [26], also up-regulate CD25 after activation and receive signals through the high-affinity IL-2R.

IL-2 binding to the high-affinity IL-2R induces the phosphorylation of tyrosine residues in Janus-Activated Kinases (JAKs) that are associated with the cytoplasmic domains of the α and γ chains of the IL-2R (reviewed in [19, 27]). Ultimately, IL-2R signaling results in the activation of the transcription factor Signal Transducer and Activator of Transcription 5 (STAT5) [28-30]. In turn, STAT5 directly and indirectly regulates the expression and activity of a broad range of key transcription factors, such as the Signal Transducer and Activator of Transcription 3 (STAT3) [31, 32], forkhead box P3 (FOXP3) [33-35], eomesodermin (Eomes) [36], B Lymphocyte Induced Maturation Protein 1 (BLIMP1) [36], T-box Transcription Factor TBX21 (T-bet) [37, 38], Retinoic Acid-related Orphan Receptor γ (RORγ) [31, 32, 39] or the B Cell Lymphoma 6 protein (BCL6) [38, 40-43], all of which play critical, and often contradictory, roles in controlling immune responses. The broad range of effects triggered by IL-2 signaling is the basis of the multiple and paradoxical roles played by this cytokine in controlling immune homeostasis.

1.2. IL-2 and the Mainteinance of Peripheral Tolerance

The critical role of IL-2 in maintaining immune tolerance was first revealed by the phenotypic characterization of mice with a targeted disruption of the genes encoding IL-2 [44], or the α and β chain of the IL-2R [45-47]. Rather than being immunodeficient due to poor T cell proliferation as originally predicted, these animals developed severe autoimmunity characterized by aberrant lymphocyte expansion and extensive lymphocytic infiltration of tissues [44-47]. In a similar way, genetic deficiency in the α chain of the IL-2R gene is associated with autoimmune disease development in humans [48-50].

The principal mechanism by which IL-2 signaling prevents autoreactive immune responses is by supporting the development and maintenance of Foxp3-expressing Tregs [51-54], which suppress self-reactive T and B cell responses and contribute to the maintenance of peripheral tolerance in both mice [55, 56] and humans [57, 58]. Tregs constitutively express high levels of CD25 [22] and require IL-2/IL2R interactions for their generation, maintenance and function (reviewed in [23]). As a result, Tregs do not develop in IL-2-deficient and IL-2R-deficient mice leading to the uncontrolled expansion of autoreactive effector T and B cell responses observed in these animals [59, 60] . Supporting this conclusion, adoptive transfer of Tregs into IL-2Rβ-deficient mice, restores immune tolerance and prevents autoimmune pathology [60]. Since Tregs suppress self-reactive immune responses, IL-2 immunotherapy to promote Treg-mediated immunosuppression has been suggested to prevent graft rejection after transplantation [61, 62] and to treat autoimmune disorders [63].

1.3. Opposite Effects of IL-2 in Regulating T Cell Responses

Early studies indicated that IL-2 promoted $CD8^+$ T cell expansion *in vitro*, suggesting an important role for this cytokine in promoting T cell responses. However, this early paradigm has been challenged by more recent studies showing that primary $CD8^+$ T cell responses to pathogens do not require IL-2/IL-2R interactions [64-66], perhaps because the inflammatory milieu generated by innate immune cells during the infection overcomes the requirement for IL-2 as a growth factor. In contrast, late IL-2 signaling during the primary response is required for the sustained expansion of antigen-specific $CD8^+$ T cell, particularly within non-lymphoid tissues [65, 67, 68]. IL-2 also acts at later times during the primary response to promote the differentiation of functional memory $CD8^+$ and $CD4^+$ T cells [64, 68-72], suggesting that the requirement for IL-2 changes over time. Supporting this view, recent studies demonstrate that rIL-2 administration during the initial expansion phase of the primary response to Lymphocytic Choriomeningitis Virus (LCMV) did not affect the expansion of virus-specific $CD8^+$ T cell [73, 74]. In contrast, rIL-2 treatment during the contraction phase resulted in increased survival and proliferation of $CD8^+$ T cells [73]. Importantly, rIL-2 therapy leads to increased numbers of virus specific-$CD8^+$ T cells and an enhanced anti-viral response in mice with established chronic LCMV infection [73, 74], demonstrating that exogenous IL-2 administration can restore exhausted antiviral T-cell responses *in vivo.*

Although IL-2 can restore exhausted T cells under some conditions, under other conditions it may induce the opposite effect depending on the dose. For example, although some degree of IL-2 signaling is required for memory development, prolonged IL-2 signaling through the IL-2R leads to the terminal differentiation of effector T cells and prevents memory formation [36, 75]. Similarly, at the same time that IL-2 promotes effector T cell differentiation, sustained IL-2 signaling also enhances the susceptibility of T cells to activation-induced cell death [76]. Thus, IL-2 can have positive and negative effects on the same cell types.

IL-2 can also alter the differentiation program of effector T cells. For example, recent studies demonstrate that, whereas IL-2 signaling through the IL-2R favors Th1 and Th2 differentiation [36, 37, 77]; excessive IL-2 inhibits the formation of T follicular helper $CD4^+$ T cells (Tfh) [38, 40, 42, 43], which are required for long-term antibody responses [78, 43]. Furthermore, whereas infusion of relative high levels of IL-2 may support effector T cell responses [79], low doses of IL-2 may preferentially support Treg expansion and prevent T cell activation [62, 63, 80]. Collectively these results indicate that the role played by IL-2 in the control of immune homeostasis is far more complex than initially expected. IL-2 signaling has the ability to both, suppress, and support immune cell responses depending on the target cell, the timing and dose of administration, the nature of the antigen and the duration of the IL-2 signaling. Thus, the pleiotropic and dose effects of IL-2 signaling in controlling immune cell responses are important factors to consider when designing and evaluating IL-2 therapies.

2. IL-2 Immunotherapy to Treat Autoimmune Diseases

2.1. Genetic Defects in the IL-2 and IL-2R Genes and Development of Autoimmune Diseases

Single nucleotide polymorphisms (SNPs) in the IL-2 and IL-2 receptor genes are linked to various autoimmune diseases [81-83], including rheumatoid arthritis (RA) [84], type I diabetes (T1D) [81, 85, 86] and multiple sclerosis (MS) [83, 87, 88]. Polymorphisms in the IL-2 and IL-2R genes correlate with decreased IL-2 production and autoimmune susceptibility in mice and humans. In this regard, impaired IL-2 production by T cells is observed in murine models of Systemic lupus erythematosus (SLE) [89, 90] and in human SLE patients [81, 91-93]. Similarly, T cells obtained from RA patients show diminished IL-2 production when compared with T cells obtained from healthy donors [90, 94, 95]. Furthermore, acquired defects in IL-2 synthesis have been reported in patients with T1D [96-98], and studies using non-obese diabetic (NOD) mice indicate that the immune-mediated destruction of pancreatic beta-cells in these animals is associated with lower expression of IL-2 [81, 98, 99]. Interestingly, increased concentrations of a soluble form of CD25 have been also detected in the serum of some SLE [100-103], MS and T1D patients [88, 104]. Soluble CD25 prevents IL-2/IL-2R interactions and might act as a decoy receptor for circulating IL-2 [88, 105]. Thus, reductions in IL-2 signaling due to lowered IL-2 production or antagonism by soluble CD25 may both contribute to poor Treg activity and loss of immune tolerance.

2.2. IL-2 Therapy to Boost Treg Responses and Prevent Autoimmune Disorders

Treatment of autoimmune mice with rIL-2 improves disease in several experimental models. For example, treatment of lupus-prone mice with rIL-2 prevents disease progression and prolongs the survival of mice with established disease [89]. Similarly, treatment of NOD mice with low doses of IL-2 prevents diabetes in these animals [99, 106, 107]. Importantly, rIL-2 treatment promotes the expansion of Tregs in SLE mice [89] and increases the numbers of Tregs in the pancreas of IL-2-treated NOD mice [99, 106, 108]. Based on these data, it is generally believed that an unbalanced Treg response due to IL-2 shortage contributes to autoimmune susceptibility in mice and humans, and that IL-2 immunotherapy may improve disease by restoring Treg numbers and/or activity [89]. Importantly, although low doses of rIL-2 prevent the development of diabetes, administration of high doses of IL-2 increases the presence of myeloid cell infiltrates in the pancreas and rapidly accelerates the onset of diabetes in prediabetic NOD mice [80]. Thus, whereas infusion of a relative low dose of rIL-2 may preferentially support Tregs expansion and prevent disease, administration of high amounts of rIL-2 may boost effector responses and exacerbate autoimmune pathology.

The potential clinical effects of low-dose rIL-2 immunotherapy in human patients have been recently examined in clinical trials [62, 63]. Similar to what is observed in mice, low-dose rIL-2 administration leads to a significant expansion of Tregs in humans without significant adverse events [62, 63]. Correlating with the expansion of Tregs, low-dose rIL-2 treatment is also associated with a significant clinical improvement in hepatitis C virus (HCV)-induced vasculitis patients [63]. However, despite the potential benefit of low-dose rIL-2 immunotherapies, the optimal dose of IL-2 may be difficult to predict for heterogeneous populations of patients, which may limit the clinical applicability of this therapy. Interestingly, administration of IL-2 complexed with the anti-IL2 JES6-1 mAb induced preferential activation of cells expressing high levels of CD25 and, as a consequence, causes selective expansion of Tregs with little effect on other effector cells [109]. Thus, IL-2-JES6-1 complexes may represent a valuable alternative to low-dose IL-2 therapy to more selectively target Treg-mediated imunnosuppression and prevent autoimmune pathology. In fact, IL-2-JES6-1 complex injection expands Tregs and suppresses autoimmune pathology in several animal experimental models [110-112], suggesting the potential use of this therapy for the treatment autoimmune disorders.

2.3. Potential Use of IL-2-Immunotheraphy to Prevent Self-Reactive B Cell Responses

Tfh cells are a specialized subset of $CD4^+$ T cells that provide help to B cells and promote the formation and maintenance of the germinal centers (GCs) [78, 113-115]. With the help of Tfh cells, activated B cell in the GCs undergo a series of cellular and molecular changes that ultimately lead to the differentiation of memory B cells and long-lived plasma cells (PCs), which secrete high affinity antibodies (Abs) for extended periods of time [116-118]. Although the underlying mechanisms that drive autoimmune disease progression remain unclear, accumulating evidence indicate that aberrant GC activity and self-reactive Tfh cell expansion can contribute to autoantibody production, which play a major role in autoimmune immunopathology in some diseases [119-124]. Consistent with this idea, the expansion of self-reactive GC B cells [121, 125] and Tfh-like $CD4^+$ T cells [126-131] is observed in autoimmune patients. Furthermore, high frequencies of Tfh cells correlate with disease scores in some of these studies (reviewed in [132, 133]). Importantly blockade of factors, such as CD40 [119, 121, 134-136] or IL-21 [137-139], that promote Tfh differentiation and GC formation, also prevents disease progression in autoimmune mice, suggesting that targeting GC and Tfh cells may be a good strategy for treating autoimmune disorders.

In this regard, recent data indicate that prolonged signaling through the IL-2R prevents the expression of the transcription factor, Bcl6 [83-85], which is required for Tfh cell development [140-142]. As a result of IL-2 signaling, Tfh cells do not develop and GCs and long-lived antibody responses are reduced [43]. Although rIL-2 administration promotes the accumulation of Tregs in this experimental model, Tregs are not required for the ability of rIL-2 to repress influenza-specific Tfh cell responses. Based on these results, it is tempting to speculate that, in addition to promoting Treg expansion, IL-2 immunotherapy may also prevent autoimmune pathology by preventing self-reactive Tfh responses.

B cell depletion therapies are used to treat autoimmune disorders based on the rationale that the depletion of autoreactive B cells would reduce auto-antibody production and thereby reduce immunopathology [143-146]. However, current B-cell depleting agents do not substantially deplete GC B cells or long-lived Plasma cells (PCs), and their clinical efficacy is lower than expected, particularly in treating SLE [145, 147, 148]. It would be interesting to test whether rIL-2 administration synergizes with the current B-cell depleting drugs by preventing Tfh differentiation and impairing the generation and maintenance of autoreactive GCs and thereby reducing autoimmune pathology.

2.4. IL-2 Deficiency and Th17 Driven Autoimmune Disorders

Th17 cells play an important role in in the pathogenesis of inflammatory autoimmune disorders such as psoriasis, inflammatory bowel disease and experimental autoimmune encephalitis (EAE) and MS [149]. Similar to Tfh cells, IL-2 signaling also represses Th17 differentiation, in this case by preventing the expression of the transcription factor RORγ [31, 32, 39, 150]. In agreement with the role of IL-2 in preventing Th17 differentiation, IL-2-deficient mice exhibit elevated concentrations of IL-17 [31, 32]. Some studies suggest a positive correlation between IL-2 deficiency, excessive IL-17 responses and autoimmune disease development. For example, STAT3-deficiency prevents IL-17 responses in IL-2-deficient mice. Correlating with diminished IL-17 production, mice lacking both STAT3 and IL-2 show reduced inflammatory colitis and prolonged survival compared to mice lacking only IL-2 [31]. In addition, a recent study indicates that elevated levels of soluble CD25 enhance IL-17 responses and aggravate EAE in mice through sequestering extracellular IL-2 [105]. Thus, IL-2 deprivation might contribute to autoimmune disease susceptibility by favoring aberrant Th17 responses. Conversely, IL-2 immunotherapy may help to prevent autoimmune pathology by curtailing IL-17 production.

3. IL-2-Based Anti-Tumor Immunotherapies

3.1. IL-2 and Immunotherapy against Metastatic Cancer

Over the last three decades, researchers have devoted a considerable amount of effort and resources to study the potential clinical benefits of human rIL-2 (Aldesleukin or Proleukin) in the treatment of a wide variety of cancers. In 1985, a study developed in the Surgery Branch of the US National Cancer Institute demonstrated the clinical benefits of administrating high-doses of rIL-2 to patients with metastatic cancer [151]. Additional studies confirmed that treatment of metastatic renal cell carcinoma [15, 152-154] and metastatic melanoma [15, 155-157] with high doses of intravenous rIL-2 induced tumor regression in 6 to 10% of the patients. Two-thirds of metastatic kidney cancer patients that initially responded to rIL-2 therapy remained free of disease up to 20 years from the onset of the treatment [158]. Similarly, 60% of patients with metastatic melanoma who initially achieved complete remission remain progression-free after 8 years [155]. Based on its ability to mediate sustained tumor regression, the U.S. Food and Drug Administration (FDA) approved the use of high-dose bolus IL-2 for patients with metastatic renal cancer in 1992, and granted its use for treatment of patients with metastatic melanoma in 1998. Although, IL-2-based immunotherapy is only effective in a minority of good prognosis patients, it is still considered the only curative treatment available to patients with these forms of cancer [17, 159].

Despite the dramatic and sustained anti-tumor effects attributed to IL-2 in some patients, the clinical applicability of IL-2-based immunotherapy is strongly compromised due to its life-threatening toxicity, including vascular leak syndrome [159-161]. Currently, administration of high doses of rIL-2 requires clinical expertise and is restricted to selected patients with a good prognosis. In order to minimize the adverse effects of rIL-2 immunotherapy and allow more tolerable treatments, several groups have attempted low-dose intravenous rIL-2 administration regimens and subcutaneous rIL-2 injection, both alone [152, 162-164] or in combination with other therapeutic agents, such as IFN-α2b [153, 163, 165-169]. Although some studies indicate that low-dose rIL-2 treatments can be administrated with significantly less adverse effects, this protocol does not completely mimic the antitumor activity associated with high-dose rIL-2 administration. Thus, despite the reduced toxicity of low-dose rIL-2 regimens, high-dose bolus IL-2 still remains the preferred therapy for selected patients with metastatic renal cell carcinoma and metastatic melanoma.

3.2. Combined IL-2 and Rituximab Therapy

B cell depletion therapy with Rituximab, a chimeric monoclonal antibody that targets CD20, is currently approved to treat patients with non-Hodgkin's lymphoma, chronic lymphocytic leukemia and some autoimmune diseases, including RA [146]. Several preclinical models and phase I clinical trials indicate that rIL-2 administration enhances Rituximab efficacy against leukemias [170, 171] and lymphomas [172-176], perhaps by enhancing expansion and activation of natural killer (NK) cells [177, 178]. These data suggest a potential therapeutic benefit of rIL-2 administration in the treatment of these forms of cancer. However, a phase-2 study indicates that, despite the synergistic effects of IL-2 and Rituximab on antibody-dependent cellular cytotoxicity *in vitro*, the clinical benefits of the combination therapy against refractory indolent non-Hodgkin's lymphoma are low [174].

Interestingly, using a murine xenograft tumor model, a more recent study demonstrates that, when combined with Rituximab, targeted delivery of IL-2 into the lymphoma-associated subendothelial matrix induces complete remission of established localized lymphomas. In contrast, Rituximab alone, or in combination with conventional rIL-2 administration, fails to prevent tumor relapse [179]. In this case, targeted delivery of IL-2 into the lymphoma neovasculature is achieved using a fusion protein consisting of rIL-2 fused to a human single-chain Fv (scFv) antibody fragment directed against the extra-domain B (ED-B) of fibronectin [180] (L19-IL2). Additional studies suggest that L19-IL2 can be can be safely and repeatedly administered and indicate a promising therapeutic activity against several forms of tumors [180-184]. Thus, antibody-based delivery of IL-2 to the particular tumor microenvironment might represent an alternative to conventional rIL-2 administration to increase the efficacy of the current IL-2-based immunotherapies, particularly when combined with other therapeutic agents.

3.3. IL-2 to Help Anti-Tumor T-Cell Therapies

Adoptive cell therapy (ACT) is a promising approach to treat cancer. In such therapies, *in vitro*-expanded autologous tumor-infiltrating lymphocytes (TILs) or genetically engineered T cells are transferred into cancer patients [185]. rIL-2 is often used in ACT immunotherapies as a growth factor to expand TILs *in vitro*, but also to favor expansion of transferred T cells after infusing them back into the patient [186-190]. ACT therapy with autologous TILs in combination with rIL-2 administration has been recently shown to mediate durable complete responses in lympho-depleted patients with metastatic melanoma [190]. In this study, 22% of patients receiving TILs in combination with rIL-2 experienced complete tumor regression and 95% of these responding patients remain tumor-free after 3years.

The adjuvant-like activity of IL-2 has also been used to boost anti-tumor responses following vaccination with tumor antigens [79, 156, 191-194]. In this regard, a phase 2 clinical trial of 684 consecutive patients with metastatic melanoma indicated that administration of high-dose bolus i.v. rIL-2 in combination with the highly immunogenic gp209-217(210M) correlates with significant increase in response rates when compared to rIL-2 administration alone [156]. The conclusions in this study were recently confirmed in a randomized phase 3 clinical trial [79].

Exhaustion of tumor-specific effector $CD8^+$ T cells within the particular tumor microenvironment limits the clinical efficacy of current ACT immunotherapies and cancer vaccines [195, 196]. Over the last few years, multiple groups have studied the role molecular and cellular basis of T cell exhaustion and found that activation of certain inhibitory receptors, particularly Programmed Death-1 (PD-1) and Cytotoxic T Lymphocyte Antigen-4 (CTLA-4), is generally associated with exhaustion of T cells [195-198]. Importantly, anti-PD-1 and anti-CTLA4 Ab therapies, alone or combined with adoptive cell transfer and tumor vaccines, have shown promising results in preventing T cell exhaustion and promoting anti-tumor immunity in mice and cancer patients [197-200]. Using a murine model of chronic LCMV infection a recent study demonstrates that combined IL-2 and anti-PD-L1 therapy more efficiently reinvigorate exhausted T cells than IL-2 or anti-PD-L1 administration alone [74]. The results in this study suggest that combined administration of IL-2 and anti-PD-L1 Ab may represent a valid strategy to more efficiently prevent TIL exhaustion an increase the efficacy of current ACT-therapies and tumor-vaccines therapies.

Collectively, the aforementioned data support the notion that the ability of IL-2 to expand IL-2R expressing lymphocytes facilitates anti-tumor immune responses, thereby inhibiting tumor growth. However, IL-2 administration also promotes Treg expansion, which may limit the effectiveness of the IL-2 treatment. To circumvent this problem, recent studies using an engineered form of IL-2, named IL-2 "superkine" or "super-2", show increased affinity for CD122 [201]. As a result, when administrated *in vivo,* the mutant IL-2 form induces superior expansion of effector T cells, and proportionally less expansion of T regulatory cells than native rIL-2. Consistent with this idea, IL-2 "superkine" elicits better anti-tumor responses than rIL-2 [201]. In an alternative approach, other studies show that IL-2 complexed to the anti-IL2 S4B6 mAb forms CD122-specific IL-2/mAb complexes [202], and that these complexes more efficiently expand cytotoxic T cells and promote anti-tumor responses than IL-2 immunotherapy [109]. Together, these results indicate that therapeutic agents that selective activate the intermediate-affinity IL-2R could promote anti-tumor T cell responses without inducing undesirable Treg-mediated immunosuppression.

References

[1] Morgan DA, Ruscetti FW, Gallo R. Selective in vitro growth of T lymphocytes from normal human bone marrows. *Science* 1976; 193:1007-1008.

[2] Ruscetti FW, Morgan DA, Gallo RC. Functional and morphologic characterization of human T cells continuously grown in vitro. *J Immunol* 1977; 119:131-138.

[3] Mier JW, Gallo RC. Purification and some characteristics of human T-cell growth factor from phytohemagglutinin-stimulated lymphocyte-conditioned media. *Proceedings of the National Academy of Sciences of the United States of America* 1980; 77:6134-6138.

[4] Henney CS, Kuribayashi K, Kern DE, Gillis S. Interleukin-2 augments natural killer cell activity. *Nature* 1981; 291:335-338.

[5] Hefeneider SH, Conlon PJ, Henney CS, Gillis S. In vivo interleukin 2 administration augments the generation of alloreactive cytolytic T lymphocytes and resident natural killer cells. *J Immunol* 1983; 130:222-227.

[6] Kawase I, Brooks CG, Kuribayashi K et al. Interleukin 2 induces gamma-interferon production: participation of macrophages and NK-like cells. *J Immunol* 1983; 131:288-292.

[7] Kuribayashi K, Gillis S, Kern DE, Henney CS. Murine NK cell cultures: effects of interleukin-2 and interferon on cell growth and cytotoxic reactivity. *J Immunol* 1981; 126:2321-2327.

[8] Wagner H, Hardt C, Heeg K, Rollinghoff M, Pfizenmaier K. T-cell-derived helper factor allows in vivo induction of cytotoxic T cells in nu/nu mice. *Nature* 1980; 284:278-278.

[9] Cheever MA, Greenberg PD, Fefer A, Gillis S. Augmentation of the anti-tumor therapeutic efficacy of long-term cultured T lymphocytes by in vivo administration of purified interleukin 2. *The Journal of experimental medicine* 1982; 155:968-980.

[10] Kern DE, Gillis S, Okada M, Henney CS. The role of interleukin-2 (IL-2) in the differentiatin of cytotoxic T cells: the effect of monoclonal anti-IL-2 antibody and absorption with IL-2 dependent T cell lines. *J Immunol* 1981; 127:1323-1328.

[11] Mazumder A, Rosenberg SA. Successful immunotherapy of natural killer-resistant established pulmonary melanoma metastases by the intravenous adoptive transfer of syngeneic lymphocytes activated in vitro by interleukin 2. *The Journal of experimental medicine* 1984; 159:495-507.

[12] Mule JJ, Shu S, Schwarz SL, Rosenberg SA. Adoptive immunotherapy of established pulmonary metastases with LAK cells and recombinant interleukin-2. *Science* 1984; 225:1487-1489.

[13] Taniguchi T, Matsui H, Fujita T et al. Structure and expression of a cloned cDNA for human interleukin-2. *Nature* 1983; 302:305-310.

[14] Rosenberg SA, Grimm EA, McGrogan M et al. Biological activity of recombinant human interleukin-2 produced in Escherichia coli. *Science* 1984; 223:1412-1414.

[15] Rosenberg SA, Yang JC, Topalian SL et al. Treatment of 283 consecutive patients with metastatic melanoma or renal cell cancer using high-dose bolus interleukin 2. *JAMA : the journal of the American Medical Association* 1994; 271:907-913.

[16] Rosenberg SA, Mule JJ, Spiess PJ, Reichert CM, Schwarz SL. Regression of established pulmonary metastases and subcutaneous tumor mediated by the systemic administration of high-dose recombinant interleukin 2. *The Journal of experimental medicine* 1985; 161:1169-1188.

[17] Rosenberg SA. Raising the bar: the curative potential of human cancer immunotherapy. *Science translational medicine* 2012; 4:127ps128.

[18] Malek TR, Castro I. Interleukin-2 receptor signaling: at the interface between tolerance and immunity. *Immunity* 2010; 33:153-165.

[19] Malek TR. The biology of interleukin-2. *Annual review of immunology* 2008; 26:453-479.

[20] Wang X, Rickert M, Garcia KC. Structure of the quaternary complex of interleukin-2 with its alpha, beta, and gammac receptors. *Science* 2005; 310:1159-1163.

[21] Rickert M, Wang X, Boulanger MJ, Goriatcheva N, Garcia KC. The structure of interleukin-2 complexed with its alpha receptor. *Science* 2005; 308:1477-1480.

[22] Sakaguchi S, Sakaguchi N, Asano M, Itoh M, Toda M. Immunologic self-tolerance maintained by activated T cells expressing IL-2 receptor alpha-chains (CD25).

Breakdown of a single mechanism of self-tolerance causes various autoimmune diseases. *J Immunol* 1995; 155:1151-1164.

[23] Cheng G, Yu A, Malek TR. T-cell tolerance and the multi-functional role of IL-2R signaling in T-regulatory cells. *Immunological reviews* 2011; 241:63-76.

[24] Fukao T, Koyasu S. Expression of functional IL-2 receptors on mature splenic dendritic cells. *European journal of immunology* 2000; 30:1453-1457.

[25] Wuest SC, Edwan JH, Martin JF et al. A role for interleukin-2 trans-presentation in dendritic cell-mediated T cell activation in humans, as revealed by daclizumab therapy. *Nature medicine* 2011; 17:604-609.

[26] Godfrey DI, Kronenberg M. Going both ways: immune regulation via CD1d-dependent NKT cells. *The Journal of clinical investigation* 2004; 114:1379-1388.

[27] Gaffen SL. Signaling domains of the interleukin 2 receptor. *Cytokine* 2001; 14:63-77.

[28] Fujii H, Nakagawa Y, Schindler U et al. Activation of Stat5 by interleukin 2 requires a carboxyl-terminal region of the interleukin 2 receptor beta chain but is not essential for the proliferative signal transmission. *Proceedings of the National Academy of Sciences of the United States of America* 1995; 92:5482-5486.

[29] Johnston JA, Bacon CM, Finbloom DS et al. Tyrosine phosphorylation and activation of STAT5, STAT3, and Janus kinases by interleukins 2 and 15. *Proceedings of the National Academy of Sciences of the United States of America* 1995; 92:8705-8709.

[30] Gilmour KC, Pine R, Reich NC. Interleukin 2 activates STAT5 transcription factor (mammary gland factor) and specific gene expression in T lymphocytes. *Proceedings of the National Academy of Sciences of the United States of America* 1995; 92:10772-10776.

[31] Yang XP, Ghoreschi K, Steward-Tharp SM et al. Opposing regulation of the locus encoding IL-17 through direct, reciprocal actions of STAT3 and STAT5. *Nature immunology* 2011; 12:247-254.

[32] Laurence A, Tato CM, Davidson TS et al. Interleukin-2 signaling via STAT5 constrains T helper 17 cell generation. *Immunity* 2007; 26:371-381.

[33] Zorn E, Nelson EA, Mohseni M et al. IL-2 regulates FOXP3 expression in human CD4+CD25+ regulatory T cells through a STAT-dependent mechanism and induces the expansion of these cells in vivo. *Blood* 2006; 108:1571-1579.

[34] Murawski MR, Litherland SA, Clare-Salzler MJ, Davoodi-Semiromi A. Upregulation of Foxp3 expression in mouse and human Treg is IL-2/STAT5 dependent: implications for the NOD STAT5B mutation in diabetes pathogenesis. *Annals of the New York Academy of Sciences* 2006; 1079:198-204.

[35] Passerini L, Allan SE, Battaglia M et al. STAT5-signaling cytokines regulate the expression of FOXP3 in CD4+CD25+ regulatory T cells and CD4+CD25- effector T cells. *International immunology* 2008; 20:421-431.

[36] Pipkin ME, Sacks JA, Cruz-Guilloty F, Lichtenheld MG, Bevan MJ, Rao A. Interleukin-2 and inflammation induce distinct transcriptional programs that promote the differentiation of effector cytolytic T cells. *Immunity* 2010; 32:79-90.

[37] Liao W, Lin JX, Wang L, Li P, Leonard WJ. Modulation of cytokine receptors by IL-2 broadly regulates differentiation into helper T cell lineages. *Nature immunology* 2011; 12:551-559.

[38] Oestreich KJ, Mohn SE, Weinmann AS. Molecular mechanisms that control the expression and activity of Bcl-6 in TH1 cells to regulate flexibility with a TFH-like gene profile. *Nature immunology* 2012; 13:405-411.

[39] Chen Y, Haines CJ, Gutcher I et al. Foxp3(+) regulatory T cells promote T helper 17 cell development in vivo through regulation of interleukin-2. *Immunity* 2011; 34:409-421.

[40] Johnston RJ, Choi YS, Diamond JA, Yang JA, Crotty S. STAT5 is a potent negative regulator of TFH cell differentiation. *The Journal of experimental medicine* 2012; 209:243-250.

[41] Walker SR, Nelson EA, Frank DA. STAT5 represses BCL6 expression by binding to a regulatory region frequently mutated in lymphomas. *Oncogene* 2007; 26:224-233.

[42] Nurieva RI, Podd A, Chen Y et al. STAT5 protein negatively regulates T follicular helper (Tfh) cell generation and function. *The Journal of biological chemistry* 2012; 287:11234-11239.

[43] Ballesteros-Tato A, Leon B, Graf BA et al. Interleukin-2 inhibits germinal center formation by limiting T follicular helper cell differentiation. *Immunity* 2012; 36:847-856.

[44] Sadlack B, Merz H, Schorle H, Schimpl A, Feller AC, Horak I. Ulcerative colitis-like disease in mice with a disrupted interleukin-2 gene. *Cell* 1993; 75:253-261.

[45] Suzuki H, Duncan GS, Takimoto H, Mak TW. Abnormal development of intestinal intraepithelial lymphocytes and peripheral natural killer cells in mice lacking the IL-2 receptor beta chain. *The Journal of experimental medicine* 1997; 185:499-505.

[46] Sadlack B, Lohler J, Schorle H et al. Generalized autoimmune disease in interleukin-2-deficient mice is triggered by an uncontrolled activation and proliferation of CD4+ T cells. *European journal of immunology* 1995; 25:3053-3059.

[47] Suzuki H, Kundig TM, Furlonger C et al. Deregulated T cell activation and autoimmunity in mice lacking interleukin-2 receptor beta. *Science* 1995; 268:1472-1476.

[48] Sharfe N, Dadi HK, Shahar M, Roifman CM. Human immune disorder arising from mutation of the alpha chain of the interleukin-2 receptor. *Proceedings of the National Academy of Sciences of the United States of America* 1997; 94:3168-3171.

[49] Caudy AA, Reddy ST, Chatila T, Atkinson JP, Verbsky JW. CD25 deficiency causes an immune dysregulation, polyendocrinopathy, enteropathy, X-linked-like syndrome, and defective IL-10 expression from CD4 lymphocytes. *The Journal of allergy and clinical immunology* 2007; 119:482-487.

[50] Roifman CM. Human IL-2 receptor alpha chain deficiency. *Pediatric research* 2000; 48:6-11.

[51] Fontenot JD, Rasmussen JP, Gavin MA, Rudensky AY. A function for interleukin 2 in Foxp3-expressing regulatory T cells. *Nature immunology* 2005; 6:1142-1151.

[52] Setoguchi R, Hori S, Takahashi T, Sakaguchi S. Homeostatic maintenance of natural Foxp3(+) CD25(+) CD4(+) regulatory T cells by interleukin (IL)-2 and induction of autoimmune disease by IL-2 neutralization. *The Journal of experimental medicine* 2005; 201:723-735.

[53] Brandenburg S, Takahashi T, de la Rosa M et al. IL-2 induces in vivo suppression by CD4(+)CD25(+)Foxp3(+) regulatory T cells. *European journal of immunology* 2008; 38:1643-1653.

[54] Furtado GC, Curotto de Lafaille MA, Kutchukhidze N, Lafaille JJ. Interleukin 2 signaling is required for CD4(+) regulatory T cell function. *The Journal of experimental medicine* 2002; 196:851-857.

[55] Kim JM, Rasmussen JP, Rudensky AY. Regulatory T cells prevent catastrophic autoimmunity throughout the lifespan of mice. *Nature immunology* 2007; 8:191-197.

[56] Brunkow ME, Jeffery EW, Hjerrild KA et al. Disruption of a new forkhead/winged-helix protein, scurfin, results in the fatal lymphoproliferative disorder of the scurfy mouse. *Nature genetics* 2001; 27:68-73.

[57] Bennett CL, Christie J, Ramsdell F et al. The immune dysregulation, polyendocrinopathy, enteropathy, X-linked syndrome (IPEX) is caused by mutations of FOXP3. *Nature genetics* 2001; 27:20-21.

[58] Wildin RS, Ramsdell F, Peake J et al. X-linked neonatal diabetes mellitus, enteropathy and endocrinopathy syndrome is the human equivalent of mouse scurfy. *Nature genetics* 2001; 27:18-20.

[59] Almeida AR, Legrand N, Papiernik M, Freitas AA. Homeostasis of peripheral CD4+ T cells: IL-2R alpha and IL-2 shape a population of regulatory cells that controls CD4+ T cell numbers. *J Immunol* 2002; 169:4850-4860.

[60] Malek TR, Yu A, Vincek V, Scibelli P, Kong L. CD4 regulatory T cells prevent lethal autoimmunity in IL-2Rbeta-deficient mice. Implications for the nonredundant function of IL-2. *Immunity* 2002; 17:167-178.

[61] Koreth J, Matsuoka K, Kim HT et al. Interleukin-2 and regulatory T cells in graft-versus-host disease. *The New England journal of medicine* 2011; 365:2055-2066.

[62] Matsuoka K, Koreth J, Kim HT et al. Low-dose interleukin-2 therapy restores regulatory T cell homeostasis in patients with chronic graft-versus-host disease. *Science translational medicine* 2013; 5:179ra143.

[63] Saadoun D, Rosenzwajg M, Joly F et al. Regulatory T-cell responses to low-dose interleukin-2 in HCV-induced vasculitis. *The New England journal of medicine* 2011; 365:2067-2077.

[64] Williams MA, Tyznik AJ, Bevan MJ. Interleukin-2 signals during priming are required for secondary expansion of CD8+ memory T cells. *Nature* 2006; 441:890-893.

[65] D'Souza WN, Lefrancois L. IL-2 is not required for the initiation of CD8 T cell cycling but sustains expansion. *J Immunol* 2003; 171:5727-5735.

[66] Yu A, Zhou J, Marten N et al. Efficient induction of primary and secondary T cell-dependent immune responses in vivo in the absence of functional IL-2 and IL-15 receptors. *J Immunol* 2003; 170:236-242.

[67] D'Souza WN, Schluns KS, Masopust D, Lefrancois L. Essential role for IL-2 in the regulation of antiviral extralymphoid CD8 T cell responses. *J Immunol* 2002; 168:5566-5572.

[68] Peperzak V, Xiao Y, Veraar EA, Borst J. CD27 sustains survival of CTLs in virus-infected nonlymphoid tissue in mice by inducing autocrine IL-2 production. *The Journal of clinical investigation* 2010; 120:168-178.

[69] Feau S, Arens R, Togher S, Schoenberger SP. Autocrine IL-2 is required for secondary population expansion of CD8(+) memory T cells. *Nature immunology* 2011; 12:908-913.

[70] Bachmann MF, Wolint P, Walton S, Schwarz K, Oxenius A. Differential role of IL-2R signaling for CD8+ T cell responses in acute and chronic viral infections. *European journal of immunology* 2007; 37:1502-1512.
[71] Dooms H, Wolslegel K, Lin P, Abbas AK. Interleukin-2 enhances CD4+ T cell memory by promoting the generation of IL-7R alpha-expressing cells. *The Journal of experimental medicine* 2007; 204:547-557.
[72] Dooms H, Kahn E, Knoechel B, Abbas AK. IL-2 induces a competitive survival advantage in T lymphocytes. *J Immunol* 2004; 172:5973-5979.
[73] Blattman JN, Grayson JM, Wherry EJ, Kaech SM, Smith KA, Ahmed R. Therapeutic use of IL-2 to enhance antiviral T-cell responses in vivo. *Nature medicine* 2003; 9:540-547.
[74] West EE, Jin HT, Rasheed AU et al. PD-L1 blockade synergizes with IL-2 therapy in reinvigorating exhausted T cells. *The Journal of clinical investigation* 2013; 123:2604-2615.
[75] Kalia V, Sarkar S, Subramaniam S, Haining WN, Smith KA, Ahmed R. Prolonged interleukin-2Ralpha expression on virus-specific CD8+ T cells favors terminal-effector differentiation in vivo. *Immunity* 2010; 32:91-103.
[76] Lenardo MJ. Interleukin-2 programs mouse alpha beta T lymphocytes for apoptosis. *Nature* 1991; 353:858-861.
[77] Liao W, Schones DE, Oh J et al. Priming for T helper type 2 differentiation by interleukin 2-mediated induction of interleukin 4 receptor alpha-chain expression. *Nature immunology* 2008; 9:1288-1296.
[78] Crotty S. Follicular helper CD4 T cells (TFH). *Annual review of immunology* 2011; 29:621-663.
[79] Schwartzentruber DJ, Lawson DH, Richards JM et al. gp100 peptide vaccine and interleukin-2 in patients with advanced melanoma. *The New England journal of medicine* 2011; 364:2119-2127.
[80] Baeyens A, Perol L, Fourcade G et al. Limitations of IL-2 and rapamycin in immunotherapy of type 1 diabetes. *Diabetes* 2013; 62:3120-3131.
[81] Yamanouchi J, Rainbow D, Serra P et al. Interleukin-2 gene variation impairs regulatory T cell function and causes autoimmunity. *Nature genetics* 2007; 39:329-337.
[82] Brand OJ, Lowe CE, Heward JM et al. Association of the interleukin-2 receptor alpha (IL-2Ralpha)/CD25 gene region with Graves' disease using a multilocus test and tag SNPs. *Clinical endocrinology* 2007; 66:508-512.
[83] Matesanz F, Fedetz M, Collado-Romero M et al. Allelic expression and interleukin-2 polymorphisms in multiple sclerosis. *Journal of neuroimmunology* 2001; 119:101-105.
[84] Genome-wide association study of 14,000 cases of seven common diseases and 3,000 shared controls. *Nature* 2007; 447:661-678.
[85] Vella A, Cooper JD, Lowe CE et al. Localization of a type 1 diabetes locus in the IL2RA/CD25 region by use of tag single-nucleotide polymorphisms. *American journal of human genetics* 2005; 76:773-779.
[86] Lowe CE, Cooper JD, Brusko T et al. Large-scale genetic fine mapping and genotype-phenotype associations implicate polymorphism in the IL2RA region in type 1 diabetes. *Nature genetics* 2007; 39:1074-1082.
[87] Hafler DA, Compston A, Sawcer S et al. Risk alleles for multiple sclerosis identified by a genomewide study. *The New England journal of medicine* 2007; 357:851-862.

[88] Maier LM, Anderson DE, Severson CA et al. Soluble IL-2RA levels in multiple sclerosis subjects and the effect of soluble IL-2RA on immune responses. *J Immunol* 2009; 182:1541-1547.

[89] Humrich JY, Morbach H, Undeutsch R et al. Homeostatic imbalance of regulatory and effector T cells due to IL-2 deprivation amplifies murine lupus. *Proceedings of the National Academy of Sciences of the United States of America* 2010; 107:204-209.

[90] Wofsy D, Dauphinee MJ, Kipper SB, Talal N. Interleukin-2 deficiency in murine systemic lupus erythematosus. *Transactions of the Association of American Physicians* 1981; 94:341-348.

[91] Lieberman LA, Tsokos GC. The IL-2 defect in systemic lupus erythematosus disease has an expansive effect on host immunity. *Journal of biomedicine & biotechnology* 2010; 2010:740619.

[92] Solomou EE, Juang YT, Gourley MF, Kammer GM, Tsokos GC. Molecular basis of deficient IL-2 production in T cells from patients with systemic lupus erythematosus. *J Immunol* 2001; 166:4216-4222.

[93] Linker-Israeli M, Bakke AC, Kitridou RC, Gendler S, Gillis S, Horwitz DA. Defective production of interleukin 1 and interleukin 2 in patients with systemic lupus erythematosus (SLE). *J Immunol* 1983; 130:2651-2655.

[94] Kitas GD, Salmon M, Farr M, Gaston JS, Bacon PA. Deficient interleukin 2 production in rheumatoid arthritis: association with active disease and systemic complications. *Clinical and experimental immunology* 1988; 73:242-249.

[95] Kashiwado T, Miossec P, Oppenheimer-Marks N, Ziff M. Inhibitor of interleukin-2 synthesis and response in rheumatoid synovial fluid. *Arthritis and rheumatism* 1987; 30:1339-1347.

[96] Zier KS, Leo MM, Spielman RS, Baker L. Decreased synthesis of interleukin-2 (IL-2) in insulin-dependent diabetes mellitus. *Diabetes* 1984; 33:552-555.

[97] Kaye WA, Adri MN, Soeldner JS et al. Acquired defect in interleukin-2 production in patients with type I diabetes mellitus. *The New England journal of medicine* 1986; 315:920-924.

[98] Hulme MA, Wasserfall CH, Atkinson MA, Brusko TM. Central role for interleukin-2 in type 1 diabetes. *Diabetes* 2012; 61:14-22.

[99] Tang Q, Adams JY, Penaranda C et al. Central role of defective interleukin-2 production in the triggering of islet autoimmune destruction. *Immunity* 2008; 28:687-697.

[100] Tokano Y, Murashima A, Takasaki Y, Hashimoto H, Okumura K, Hirose S. Relation between soluble interleukin 2 receptor and clinical findings in patients with systemic lupus erythematosus. *Annals of the rheumatic diseases* 1989; 48:803-809.

[101] Sawada S, Hashimoto H, Iijma S et al. Increased soluble IL-2 receptor in serum of patients with systemic lupus erythematosus. *Clinical rheumatology* 1993; 12:204-209.

[102] Ward MM, Dooley MA, Christenson VD, Pisetsky DS. The relationship between soluble interleukin 2 receptor levels and anti double stranded DNA antibody levels in patients with systemic lupus erythematosus. *The Journal of rheumatology* 1991; 18:235-240.

[103] ter Borg EJ, Horst G, Limburg PC, Kallenberg CG. Changes in plasma levels of interleukin-2 receptor in relation to disease exacerbations and levels of anti-dsDNA and

complement in systemic lupus erythematosus. *Clinical and experimental immunology* 1990; 82:21-26.
[104] Maier LM, Lowe CE, Cooper J et al. IL2RA genetic heterogeneity in multiple sclerosis and type 1 diabetes susceptibility and soluble interleukin-2 receptor production. *PLoS genetics* 2009; 5:e1000322.
[105] Russell SE, Moore AC, Fallon PG, Walsh PT. Soluble IL-2Ralpha (sCD25) exacerbates autoimmunity and enhances the development of Th17] responses in mice. *PloS one* 2012; 7:e47748.
[106] Grinberg-Bleyer Y, Baeyens A, You S et al. IL-2 reverses established type 1 diabetes in NOD mice by a local effect on pancreatic regulatory T cells. *The Journal of experimental medicine* 2010; 207:1871-1878.
[107] Shapiro AM, Suarez-Pinzon WL, Power R, Rabinovitch A. Combination therapy with low dose sirolimus and tacrolimus is synergistic in preventing spontaneous and recurrent autoimmune diabetes in non-obese diabetic mice. *Diabetologia* 2002; 45:224-230.
[108] Liston A, Siggs OM, Goodnow CC. Tracing the action of IL-2 in tolerance to islet-specific antigen. *Immunology and cell biology* 2007; 85:338-342.
[109] Krieg C, Letourneau S, Pantaleo G, Boyman O. Improved IL-2 immunotherapy by selective stimulation of IL-2 receptors on lymphocytes and endothelial cells. *Proceedings of the National Academy of Sciences of the United States of America* 2010; 107:11906-11911.
[110] Webster KE, Walters S, Kohler RE et al. In vivo expansion of T reg cells with IL-2-mAb complexes: induction of resistance to EAE and long-term acceptance of islet allografts without immunosuppression. *The Journal of experimental medicine* 2009; 206:751-760.
[111] Liu R, Zhou Q, La Cava A, Campagnolo DI, Van Kaer L, Shi FD. Expansion of regulatory T cells via IL-2/anti-IL-2 mAb complexes suppresses experimental myasthenia. *European journal of immunology* 2010; 40:1577-1589.
[112] Lee SY, Cho ML, Oh HJ et al. Interleukin-2/anti-interleukin-2 monoclonal antibody immune complex suppresses collagen-induced arthritis in mice by fortifying interleukin-2/STAT5 signalling pathways. *Immunology* 2012; 137:305-316.
[113] Goodnow CC, Vinuesa CG, Randall KL, Mackay F, Brink R. Control systems and decision making for antibody production. *Nature immunology* 2010; 11:681-688.
[114] Vinuesa CG, Linterman MA, Goodnow CC, Randall KL. T cells and follicular dendritic cells in germinal center B-cell formation and selection. *Immunological reviews* 2010; 237:72-89.
[115] Yu D, Vinuesa CG. The elusive identity of T follicular helper cells. *Trends in immunology* 2010; 31:377-383.
[116] Cyster JG. B cell follicles and antigen encounters of the third kind. *Nature immunology* 2010; 11:989-996.
[117] Allen CD, Okada T, Cyster JG. Germinal-center organization and cellular dynamics. *Immunity* 2007; 27:190-202.
[118] Vinuesa CG, Linterman MA, Goodnow CC, Randall KL. T cells and follicular dendritic cells in germinal center B-cell formation and selection. *Immunological reviews* 2010; 237:72-89.

[119] Grammer AC, Slota R, Fischer R et al. Abnormal germinal center reactions in systemic lupus erythematosus demonstrated by blockade of CD154-CD40 interactions. *The Journal of clinical investigation* 2003; 112:1506-1520.
[120] Craft JE. Follicular helper T cells in immunity and systemic autoimmunity. *Nature reviews Rheumatology* 2012; 8:337-347.
[121] Chang A, Henderson SG, Brandt D et al. In situ B cell-mediated immune responses and tubulointerstitial inflammation in human lupus nephritis. *J Immunol* 2011; 186:1849-1860.
[122] Linterman MA, Rigby RJ, Wong RK et al. Follicular helper T cells are required for systemic autoimmunity. *The Journal of experimental medicine* 2009; 206:561-576.
[123] Odegard JM, Marks BR, DiPlacido LD et al. ICOS-dependent extrafollicular helper T cells elicit IgG production via IL-21 in systemic autoimmunity. *The Journal of experimental medicine* 2008; 205:2873-2886.
[124] Vinuesa CG, Cook MC, Angelucci C et al. A RING-type ubiquitin ligase family member required to repress follicular helper T cells and autoimmunity. *Nature* 2005; 435:452-458.
[125] Pugh-Bernard AE, Silverman GJ, Cappione AJ et al. Regulation of inherently autoreactive VH4-34 B cells in the maintenance of human B cell tolerance. *J Clin Invest* 2001; 108:1061-1070.
[126] Simpson N, Gatenby PA, Wilson A et al. Expansion of circulating T cells resembling follicular helper T cells is a fixed phenotype that identifies a subset of severe systemic lupus erythematosus. *Arthritis Rheum* 2010; 62:234-244.
[127] Luo C, Li Y, Liu W et al. Expansion of circulating counterparts of follicular helper T cells in patients with myasthenia gravis. *Journal of neuroimmunology* 2013; 256:55-61.
[128] Zhu C, Ma J, Liu Y et al. Increased frequency of follicular helper T cells in patients with autoimmune thyroid disease. *The Journal of clinical endocrinology and metabolism* 2012; 97:943-950.
[129] Liu R, Wu Q, Su D et al. A regulatory effect of IL-21 on T follicular helper-like cell and B cell in rheumatoid arthritis. *Arthritis research & therapy* 2012; 14:R255.
[130] Ma J, Zhu C, Ma B et al. Increased frequency of circulating follicular helper T cells in patients with rheumatoid arthritis. *Clinical & developmental immunology* 2012; 2012:827480.
[131] Wang J, Shan Y, Jiang Z et al. High frequencies of activated B cells and T follicular helper cells are correlated with disease activity in patients with new-onset rheumatoid arthritis. *Clinical and experimental immunology* 2013; 174:212-220.
[132] Ma CS, Deenick EK. Human T follicular helper (Tfh) cells and disease. *Immunology and cell biology* 2013.
[133] King C, Tangye SG, Mackay CR. T follicular helper (TFH) cells in normal and dysregulated immune responses. *Annual review of immunology* 2008; 26:741-766.
[134] Mohan C, Shi Y, Laman JD, Datta SK. Interaction between CD40 and its ligand gp39 in the development of murine lupus nephritis. *J Immunol* 1995; 154:1470-1480.
[135] Ma J, Xu J, Madaio MP et al. Autoimmune lpr/lpr mice deficient in CD40 ligand: spontaneous Ig class switching with dichotomy of autoantibody responses. *J Immunol* 1996; 157:417-426.

[136] Daikh DI, Finck BK, Linsley PS, Hollenbaugh D, Wofsy D. Long-term inhibition of murine lupus by brief simultaneous blockade of the B7/CD28 and CD40/gp39 costimulation pathways. *J Immunol* 1997; 159:3104-3108.

[137] Rankin AL, Guay H, Herber D et al. IL-21 receptor is required for the systemic accumulation of activated B and T lymphocytes in MRL/MpJ-Fas(lpr/lpr)/J mice. *J Immunol* 2012; 188:1656-1667.

[138] Bubier JA, Sproule TJ, Foreman O et al. A critical role for IL-21 receptor signaling in the pathogenesis of systemic lupus erythematosus in BXSB-Yaa mice. *Proc Natl Acad Sci U S A* 2009; 106:1518-1523.

[139] Herber D, Brown TP, Liang S, Young DA, Collins M, Dunussi-Joannopoulos K. IL-21] has a pathogenic role in a lupus-prone mouse model and its blockade with IL-21R.Fc reduces disease progression. *Journal of immunology* 2007; 178:3822-3830.

[140] Yu D, Rao S, Tsai LM et al. The transcriptional repressor Bcl-6] directs T follicular helper cell lineage commitment. *Immunity* 2009; 31:457-468.

[141] Nurieva RI, Chung Y, Martinez GJ et al. Bcl6 mediates the development of T follicular helper cells. *Science* 2009; 325:1001-1005.

[142] Johnston RJ, Poholek AC, DiToro D et al. Bcl6 and Blimp-1] are reciprocal and antagonistic regulators of T follicular helper cell differentiation. *Science* 2009; 325:1006-1010.

[143] Ramos-Casals M, Sanz I, Bosch X, Stone JH, Khamashta MA. B-cell-depleting therapy in systemic lupus erythematosus. *Am J Med* 2012; 125:327-336.

[144] Lund FE, Randall TD. Effector and regulatory B cells: modulators of CD4(+) T cell immunity. *Nat Rev Immunol* 2010; 10:236-247.

[145] Sanz I, Lee FE. B cells as therapeutic targets in SLE. *Nature reviews Rheumatology* 2010; 6:326-337.

[146] Edwards JC, Szczepanski L, Szechinski J et al. Efficacy of B-cell-targeted therapy with rituximab in patients with rheumatoid arthritis. *The New England journal of medicine* 2004; 350:2572-2581.

[147] Calero I, Sanz I. Targeting B cells for the treatment of SLE: the beginning of the end or the end of the beginning? *Discov Med* 2010; 10:416-424.

[148] Cambridge G, Leandro MJ, Teodorescu M et al. B cell depletion therapy in systemic lupus erythematosus: effect on autoantibody and antimicrobial antibody profiles. *Arthritis Rheum* 2006; 54:3612-3622.

[149] Weaver CT, Hatton RD, Mangan PR, Harrington LE. IL-17 family cytokines and the expanding diversity of effector T cell lineages. *Annual review of immunology* 2007; 25:821-852.

[150] Pandiyan P, Conti HR, Zheng L et al. CD4(+)CD25(+)Foxp3(+) regulatory T cells promote Th17 cells in vitro and enhance host resistance in mouse Candida albicans Th17 cell infection model. *Immunity* 2011; 34:422-434.

[151] Rosenberg SA, Lotze MT, Muul LM et al. Observations on the systemic administration of autologous lymphokine-activated killer cells and recombinant interleukin-2 to patients with metastatic cancer. *The New England journal of medicine* 1985; 313:1485-1492.

[152] Yang JC, Topalian SL, Parkinson D et al. Randomized comparison of high-dose and low-dose intravenous interleukin-2 for the therapy of metastatic renal cell carcinoma:

an interim report. *Journal of clinical oncology : official journal of the American Society of Clinical Oncology* 1994; 12:1572-1576.
[153] Atzpodien J, Lopez Hanninen E, Kirchner H et al. Multiinstitutional home-therapy trial of recombinant human interleukin-2 and interferon alfa-2 in progressive metastatic renal cell carcinoma. *Journal of clinical oncology : official journal of the American Society of Clinical Oncology* 1995; 13:497-501.
[154] Fyfe G, Fisher RI, Rosenberg SA, Sznol M, Parkinson DR, Louie AC. Results of treatment of 255 patients with metastatic renal cell carcinoma who received high-dose recombinant interleukin-2 therapy. *Journal of clinical oncology : official journal of the American Society of Clinical Oncology* 1995; 13:688-696.
[155] Atkins MB, Lotze MT, Dutcher JP et al. High-dose recombinant interleukin 2 therapy for patients with metastatic melanoma: analysis of 270 patients treated between 1985 and 1993. *Journal of clinical oncology : official journal of the American Society of Clinical Oncology* 1999; 17:2105-2116.
[156] Smith FO, Downey SG, Klapper JA et al. Treatment of metastatic melanoma using interleukin-2 alone or in conjunction with vaccines. *Clinical cancer research : an official journal of the American Association for Cancer Research* 2008; 14:5610-5618.
[157] Rosenberg SA, Yang JC, White DE, Steinberg SM. Durability of complete responses in patients with metastatic cancer treated with high-dose interleukin-2: identification of the antigens mediating response. *Annals of surgery* 1998; 228:307-319.
[158] Klapper JA, Downey SG, Smith FO et al. High-dose interleukin-2 for the treatment of metastatic renal cell carcinoma : a retrospective analysis of response and survival in patients treated in the surgery branch at the National Cancer Institute between 1986 and 2006. *Cancer* 2008; 113:293-301.
[159] McDermott DF, Atkins MB. Interleukin-2 therapy of metastatic renal cell carcinoma predictors of response. *Seminars in oncology* 2006; 33:583-587.
[160] Schwartz RN, Stover L, Dutcher J. Managing toxicities of high-dose interleukin-2. *Oncology (Williston Park)* 2002; 16:11-20.
[161] Schwartzentruber DJ. Guidelines for the safe administration of high-dose interleukin-2. *J Immunother* 2001; 24:287-293.
[162] Sleijfer DT, Janssen RA, Buter J, de Vries EG, Willemse PH, Mulder NH. Phase II study of subcutaneous interleukin-2 in unselected patients with advanced renal cell cancer on an outpatient basis. *Journal of clinical oncology : official journal of the American Society of Clinical Oncology* 1992; 10:1119-1123.
[163] Lopez Hanninen E, Kirchner H, Atzpodien J. Interleukin-2 based home therapy of metastatic renal cell carcinoma: risks and benefits in 215 consecutive single institution patients. *The Journal of urology* 1996; 155:19-25.
[164] Yang JC, Sherry RM, Steinberg SM et al. Randomized study of high-dose and low-dose interleukin-2 in patients with metastatic renal cancer. *Journal of clinical oncology : official journal of the American Society of Clinical Oncology* 2003; 21:3127-3132.
[165] Trehu EG, Mier JW, Dubois JS et al. Phase I trial of interleukin 2 in combination with the soluble tumor necrosis factor receptor p75] IgG chimera. *Clinical cancer research : an official journal of the American Association for Cancer Research* 1996; 2:1341-1351.
[166] Du Bois JS, Trehu EG, Mier JW et al. Randomized placebo-controlled clinical trial of high-dose interleukin-2 in combination with a soluble p75 tumor necrosis factor

receptor immunoglobulin G chimera in patients with advanced melanoma and renal cell carcinoma. *Journal of clinical oncology : official journal of the American Society of Clinical Oncology* 1997; 15:1052-1062.

[167] McDermott DF, Trehu EG, Mier JW et al. A two-part phase I trial of high-dose interleukin 2 in combination with soluble (Chinese hamster ovary) interleukin 1 receptor. *Clinical cancer research : an official journal of the American Association for Cancer Research* 1998; 4:1203-1213.

[168] Negrier S, Escudier B, Lasset C et al. Recombinant human interleukin-2, recombinant human interferon alfa-2a, or both in metastatic renal-cell carcinoma. Groupe Francais d'Immunotherapie. *The New England journal of medicine* 1998; 338:1272-1278.

[169] McDermott DF, Regan MM, Clark JI et al. Randomized phase III trial of high-dose interleukin-2 versus subcutaneous interleukin-2 and interferon in patients with metastatic renal cell carcinoma. *Journal of clinical oncology : official journal of the American Society of Clinical Oncology* 2005; 23:133-141.

[170] Pautas C, Merabet F, Thomas X et al. Randomized study of intensified anthracycline doses for induction and recombinant interleukin-2 for maintenance in patients with acute myeloid leukemia age 50 to 70 years: results of the ALFA-9801 study. *Journal of clinical oncology : official journal of the American Society of Clinical Oncology* 2010; 28:808-814.

[171] Goodman M, Spector N, Rodrigues G, Cassileth PA. Interleukin-2 therapy for advanced chronic myeloid leukemia. *Leukemia* 1998; 12:1682-1684.

[172] Friedberg JW, Neuberg D, Gribben JG et al. Combination immunotherapy with rituximab and interleukin 2 in patients with relapsed or refractory follicular non-Hodgkin's lymphoma. *British journal of haematology* 2002; 117:828-834.

[173] Gluck WL, Hurst D, Yuen A et al. Phase I studies of interleukin (IL)-2 and rituximab in B-cell non-hodgkin's lymphoma: IL-2 mediated natural killer cell expansion correlations with clinical response. *Clinical cancer research : an official journal of the American Association for Cancer Research* 2004; 10:2253-2264.

[174] Khan KD, Emmanouilides C, Benson DM, Jr. et al. A phase 2 study of rituximab in combination with recombinant interleukin-2 for rituximab-refractory indolent non-Hodgkin's lymphoma. *Clinical cancer research : an official journal of the American Association for Cancer Research* 2006; 12:7046-7053.

[175] Lopes de Menezes DE, Denis-Mize K, Tang Y et al. Recombinant interleukin-2 significantly augments activity of rituximab in human tumor xenograft models of B-cell non-Hodgkin lymphoma. *J Immunother* 2007; 30:64-74.

[176] Eisenbeis CF, Grainger A, Fischer B et al. Combination immunotherapy of B-cell non-Hodgkin's lymphoma with rituximab and interleukin-2: a preclinical and phase I study. *Clinical cancer research : an official journal of the American Association for Cancer Research* 2004; 10:6101-6110.

[177] Gluck WL, Hurst D, Yuen A et al. Phase I studies of interleukin (IL)-2 and rituximab in B-cell non-hodgkin's lymphoma: IL-2 mediated natural killer cell expansion correlations with clinical response. *Clinical cancer research : an official journal of the American Association for Cancer Research* 2004; 10:2253-2264.

[178] Carson WE, Parihar R, Lindemann MJ et al. Interleukin-2 enhances the natural killer cell response to Herceptin-coated Her2/neu-positive breast cancer cells. *European journal of immunology* 2001; 31:3016-3025.

[179] Schliemann C, Palumbo A, Zuberbuhler K et al. Complete eradication of human B-cell lymphoma xenografts using rituximab in combination with the immunocytokine L19-IL2. *Blood* 2009; 113:2275-2283.
[180] Halin C, Rondini S, Nilsson F et al. Enhancement of the antitumor activity of interleukin-12 by targeted delivery to neovasculature. *Nature biotechnology* 2002; 20:264-269.
[181] Johannsen M, Spitaleri G, Curigliano G et al. The tumour-targeting human L19-IL2 immunocytokine: preclinical safety studies, phase I clinical trial in patients with solid tumours and expansion into patients with advanced renal cell carcinoma. *Eur J Cancer* 2010; 46:2926-2935.
[182] Eigentler TK, Weide B, de Braud F et al. A dose-escalation and signal-generating study of the immunocytokine L19-IL2 in combination with dacarbazine for the therapy of patients with metastatic melanoma. *Clinical cancer research : an official journal of the American Association for Cancer Research* 2011; 17:7732-7742.
[183] Gutbrodt KL, Schliemann C, Giovannoni L et al. Antibody-based delivery of interleukin-2 to neovasculature has potent activity against acute myeloid leukemia. *Science translational medicine* 2013; 5:201ra118.
[184] Moschetta M, Pretto F, Berndt A et al. Paclitaxel enhances therapeutic efficacy of the F8-IL2 immunocytokine to EDA-fibronectin-positive metastatic human melanoma xenografts. *Cancer research* 2012; 72:1814-1824.
[185] Restifo NP, Dudley ME, Rosenberg SA. Adoptive immunotherapy for cancer: harnessing the T cell response. *Nature reviews Immunology* 2012; 12:269-281.
[186] Rosenberg SA, Yannelli JR, Yang JC et al. Treatment of patients with metastatic melanoma with autologous tumor-infiltrating lymphocytes and interleukin 2. *Journal of the National Cancer Institute* 1994; 86:1159-1166.
[187] Rosenberg SA, Dudley ME. Cancer regression in patients with metastatic melanoma after the transfer of autologous antitumor lymphocytes. *Proceedings of the National Academy of Sciences of the United States of America* 2004; 101 Suppl 2:14639-14645.
[188] Overwijk WW, Theoret MR, Finkelstein SE et al. Tumor regression and autoimmunity after reversal of a functionally tolerant state of self-reactive CD8+ T cells. *The Journal of experimental medicine* 2003; 198:569-580.
[189] Dudley ME, Wunderlich JR, Robbins PF et al. Cancer regression and autoimmunity in patients after clonal repopulation with antitumor lymphocytes. *Science* 2002; 298:850-854.
[190] Rosenberg SA, Yang JC, Sherry RM et al. Durable complete responses in heavily pretreated patients with metastatic melanoma using T-cell transfer immunotherapy. *Clinical cancer research : an official journal of the American Association for Cancer Research* 2011; 17:4550-4557.
[191] Rosenberg SA, Yang JC, Schwartzentruber DJ et al. Immunologic and therapeutic evaluation of a synthetic peptide vaccine for the treatment of patients with metastatic melanoma. *Nature medicine* 1998; 4:321-327.
[192] Schwaab T, Schwarzer A, Wolf B et al. Clinical and immunologic effects of intranodal autologous tumor lysate-dendritic cell vaccine with Aldesleukin (Interleukin 2) and IFN-{alpha}2a therapy in metastatic renal cell carcinoma patients. *Clinical cancer research : an official journal of the American Association for Cancer Research* 2009; 15:4986-4992.

[193] Nacsa J, Edghill-Smith Y, Tsai WP et al. Contrasting effects of low-dose IL-2 on vaccine-boosted simian immunodeficiency virus (SIV)-specific CD4+ and CD8+ T cells in macaques chronically infected with SIVmac251. *J Immunol* 2005; 174:1913-1921.

[194] Chapman PB. Combining a peptide vaccine with high-dose interleukin-2. *Journal of clinical oncology : official journal of the American Society of Clinical Oncology* 2008; 26:2250-2251.

[195] Virgin HW, Wherry EJ, Ahmed R. Redefining chronic viral infection. *Cell* 2009; 138:30-50.

[196] Wherry EJ. T cell exhaustion. *Nature immunology* 2011; 12:492-499.

[197] Weber J. Immune checkpoint proteins: a new therapeutic paradigm for cancer--preclinical background: CTLA-4 and PD-1 blockade. *Seminars in oncology* 2010; 37:430-439.

[198] Pardoll DM. The blockade of immune checkpoints in cancer immunotherapy. *Nature reviews Cancer* 2012; 12:252-264.

[199] Topalian SL, Hodi FS, Brahmer JR et al. Safety, activity, and immune correlates of anti-PD-1 antibody in cancer. *The New England journal of medicine* 2012; 366:2443-2454.

[200] John LB, Devaud C, Duong CP et al. Anti-PD-1 Antibody Therapy Potently Enhances the Eradication of Established Tumors By Gene-Modified T Cells. *Clinical cancer research : an official journal of the American Association for Cancer Research* 2013; 19:5636-5646.

[201] Levin AM, Bates DL, Ring AM et al. Exploiting a natural conformational switch to engineer an interleukin-2 'superkine'. *Nature* 2012; 484:529-533.

[202] Boyman O, Kovar M, Rubinstein MP, Surh CD, Sprent J. Selective stimulation of T cell subsets with antibody-cytokine immune complexes. *Science* 2006; 311:1924-1927.

In: Horizons in Cancer Research. Volume 54
Editor: Hiroto S. Watanabe
ISBN: 978-1-63321-389-0

Chapter 3

OFF or ON: RNA Interference (RNAi) / RNA Activation (RNAa) for Cancer Therapeutics

Sorah Yoon and John J. Rossi
Department of Molecular and Cellular Biology, Beckman Research Institute of City of Hope, Duarte, California, US

Abstract

Small double-stranded RNAs (dsRNAs) have emerged as main key regulators of gene expression. The small RNA molecules which suppress their target gene expression have been termed RNA interference (RNAi). The ability of transcriptional upregulation has been referred to RNA activation (RNAa). New evidences have shown that silencing hyperactive genes or activating genes targeted against the specific promoter region induce significant tumor responses. The recent preclinical animal model studies show strong evidence that dsRNA can be effective in treating liver cancer. The advanced technologies of nucleic acid therapeutics make small dsRNAs promising cancer therapeutics. We describe here strategies to turn genes off or on with small RNAs along with their tumor-specific delivery for the treatment of cancer. Given the potential of RNAs as druggable therapeutics, dsRNAs-based drugs can be exploited in fast growing therapeutic market.

1. Background

Small duplex RNAs (dsRNA) are powerful tools to regulate gene expression which is silencing or activating. The first experimentally shown silencing effect was in *C.elegans* and it was identified that 21 to 25-nucleotide short interfering RNAs (siRNA) are the key factors of RNAi [1]. The Scientists who discovered the RNAi phenomenon were awarded the Nobel Prize in Physiology and Medicine 2006 [2]. This phenomenon was also observed in other species like vertebrates [3, 4]. Since the first discovery of RNAi phenomenon, the silence effects of dsRNA have been evaluated for the therapeutic efficacy in clinical trials [5-7]. For the potential therapeutic use, RNAi is ideal to treat disorders that are caused by the expression of mutant genes encoding dominant-negative proteins, aberrant splicing isoforms, or overexpressed genes leading to gain-of-function effects [8]. siRNAs theoretically can be ideal drugs for the specific inhibition of overexpressed genes in cancer.

Two research papers were reported in 2006 and 2007 that short RNAs to specific promoter regions of certain genes up-regulate expression at the transcriptional level without altering the genome in human cells [9, 10]. This phenomenon has been termed RNA activation (RNAa/saRNA). RNAa/saRNA is conserved in non-human primate cells [11]. Contrary to the antagonism of a specific target genes offered by siRNA, the activation of molecular targets is also crucial to control cancer effectively by providing gain of function.

2. siRNA for Cancer Therapeutics

RNAi which is RNA-dependent regulation functions generally to silent homologous sequences of target genes by sequence-specific manner. Since the first discovery of gene silencing effects, the great efforts are depicted to develop siRNA based cancer therapeutics in numerous cancers. There are many novel druggable targets in cancer therapy. Additionally, the specificity of RNAi would be greater therpaeutics other than many current approaches. In here, we describe the representative studies of *in vivo* or clinical trials along with delivery and applications. Currently, few publications have emerged dealing with clinical experiments, the clinical trials information have been collected from the US National Institutes of Health trials http://www.clinicaltrials.gov. The summary is in Table 1.

KRAS has long been underlined as a beneficial target for cancer therapeutics, because its activation drives many of the tumor-cell-related traits, especially growth and proliferation [12]. Genetic alterations in the KRAS signaling pathway are involved in over 90% of pancreatic cancer cases [13]. Khvalevsky et al. proved that silencing KRAS is effective in controlling pancreatic cancer proliferation [14]. In the study, they exploited the advantage of siRNA as a cancer therapeutic and the slow-release of siRNA in biodegradable polymer matrix (siG12D LODER) *in vitro* and *in vivo*. The results demonstrated that siRNA-KRAS significantly inhibit the tumor growth. siG12D LODER, Silenseed Ltd, is in a phase I to test single dose study and a phase II clinical trial combination with chemotherapies.

Alnylam Pharmaceutics et al. have published Phase I trial results of lipid nanoparticle (LNP)-formulated RNAi therapeutics named ALN-VSP in the treatment of solid tumors with liver involvement [15]. The target genes are VEGF-A (vascular endothelial growth factor A) and KSP (kinesin spindle protein). To reduce immunostimulatory effects, both siRNA is chemically modified. Their objective was to evaluate the safety, tolerability and pharmacokinetics of I.V. injection in VEGF overexpression tumors such as renal cell cancer, endometrial cancer, pancreatic neuroendocrine tumor, and angiosarcoma. In this study, they showed that target downregulation and anti-tumor activity including complete regression of liver metastases in endometrial cancer. It is very promising results demonstrating the therapeutic effects of the systemically delivered siRNA in human cancers. This is the first trial showing that two siRNAs can be safely delivered to cancer patients.

PKN3 (Protein Kinase N3) expressed in the vascular endothelium has been identified as a promising cancer therapeutic target for inhibiting tumor progression and lymph node metastasis [16].

Table 1. The summary of siRNA

Gene Symbol	Full Name	Species	Cancer	Reference
KRAS	V-Ki-ras2 Kirsten rat sarcoma viral oncogene homolog	Human	Pancreatic cancer ****	14
MK	midkine	Human	Pancreatic cancer *	69
HOXB7	Homeobox-containing genes encode DNA-binding proteins	Human	Pancreatic cancer	70
survivin	baculoviral inhibitor of apoptosis repeat-containing 5	Human	Breast cancer ** Pancreatic cancer **	71
VEGF-A, KSP	(vascular endothelial growth factor A, kinesin spindle protein	Human	Clinical trials/ Liver cancer ***	15
PKN3	protein kinase N3	Human	Clinical trials/Solid tumor ***	17-19
EphA2	tyrosine kinase receptor	Human	Clinical trials recruiting/ Ovarian cancer *	25,26
RRM2	ribonucleotide reductase M2	Human	Clinical trials/Solid tumor ***	29

* *in vivo* experiments done.
** *in vivo* experiments done and combination therapy with doxorubicin.
*** Clinical trials

Recently, PKN3 has been considered as a suitable therapeutics target for modulating tumor-associated angiogenesis [17]. Atu027 is cationic lipoplexes containing chemically stabilized siRNA targeting PKN3 and Silence Ltd. holds the license. Preclinical data of Atu027 reported in 2008 [18]. It showed that Atu027 mediated inhibition of PKN3 impairs tube formation on extracellular matrix and cell migration *in vitro*. It also revealed that systemic administration of Atu027 silences PKN3 expression in mice, rat and nonhuman primates *in vivo*. The orthotropic mouse models for prostate and pancreatic cancers significantly inhibit the tumor growth and lymph node metastasis. Santel et al. reported that Atu027 inhibites hematogenous metastasis to the target organ lung in four different preclinical mouse models in 2010 [19]. Recently, the phase I clinical trial data in advanced solid tumors released that a total of 24 patients received Atu027 as a single 4h-infusion with 3 weeks, thereafter, they were treated twice weekly for a period of 4 weeks [17]. Although some adverse events are reported, Atu027 is well-tolerated in this study. In case of two patients with neuroendocrine cancer, one patient showed disease stabilization for 9 months and the other one showed partial regression of pulmonary metastasis. The combinational therapy with Atu027 and Gemcitabine in advanced or metastatic pancreatic cancer is under recruiting for clinical trials.

EphA2 is a tyrosine kinase receptor in the ephrin family that plays a key role in neural development [20]. The high rate of overexpression in ovarian cancer is associated with poor clinical outcomes [21]. The down regulation of EphA2 reduces tumorigenicity in preclinical studies of breast and pancreatic cancer [22-24]. Landen et al. reported that the therapeutic effects of neutral Liposomal siRNA EphA2 in ovarian cancer *in vivo* [25]. In the study, they showed the tumor growth reduction in orthotopic mouse model of ovarian cancer. Another paper came out that is the therapeutic synergy between microRNA and siRNA in ovarian cancer treatment [26]. In this paper, they identified that miR-520d-3p is considerably less expressed and directly targets EphA2 in human ovarian cancer patients. miR-520d-3p acts as a tumor suppressor upstream of EphA2. Restoring miRNA-520d-3p prominently decreased EphA2 level and suppressed tumor growth, migration, and invasion both *in vitro* and *in vivo*. The combination therapy miR-520d-3p with siRNA EphA2 showed synergistic inhibition and boosts antitumor effects *in vitro* and *in vivo*. The phase I clinical trial of siRNA-EphA2 in advanced cancers is recruiting.

RRM2, ribonucleotide reductase subunit M2, is only expressed during DNA replication [27]. RRM2 is increased in tumors and tumor cell lines [28]. CALAA-01, employing the CDP-based anti-RRM2 siRNA, is under the license at Calando Ltd. Anti-RRM2 siRNA exhibited significant anti-proliferation effects in a broad spectrum of cancer types [29].

3. saRNA in Developing Cancer Therapeutics

Since the first report of the saRNA, the potentials for the cancer therapeutic have been tested in different type of cancers. The first saRNA targeting noncoding regulatory regions in gene promoters are E-cadherin, p21 and VEGF promoter [9]. It showed the induction of target genes in various human cell lines. This paper also described that RNAa is sensitive to target location [9]. Importantly, IFN response is not involved in transcriptional activation by RNAa. Another interesting paper was reported that the chromosome-targeted RNAs activate gene expression [10]. Target gene was progesterone receptor (PR) and the length of RNA is 19-21 mer. Based on above two interesting results, the application of RNAa as cancer therapeutics has been developed in different type of cancers. The summary is in Table 2.

Table 2. The summary of saRNA

Gene Symbol	Full Name	Species	Cell line/Cancer	Reference
CDH1	E-cadherin	Human	Cervical cancer	9
CDKN1A(p21)	Cyclin-dependent kinase inhibitor 1A	Human	Prostate cancer, Breast cancer, Cervical cancer, Bladder cancer Pancreatic cancer * Non-small-cell lung carcinoma Liver cancer	9 32 42 31
VEGF	Vascular endothelial growth factor	Human	Cervical cancer	9
PGR(PR)	Progestrone receptor	Human	Breast cancer	10
MVP	Major valut protein	Human	Breast cancer	10
KLF4	Kruppel-like factor 4	Human	Prostate cancer	33
C/EBPa	CCAAT/enhancer-binding protein a	Human	Liver cancer *	30
PAWR	PRKC apoptosis WT1 regulator	Human	Bladder cancer Prostate cancer	43
NKX3-1	NK3 homeobox 1	Human	Prostate cancer *	39

* *in vivo* experiments done.

3.1. Liver Cancer

C/EBPa (CCAAT/enhancer-binding protein-a) is a transcriptional factor and a leucine zipper protein. This factor is enriched in hepatocytes and known to upregulate p21 which is a inhibitor of cell proliferation [30]. Reebye et al. described that saRNA targeting C/EBPa increase albumin secretion and decrease cell proliferation in HepG2 cells. *In vivo* cirrhotic model, intravenous injection of C/EBPa-saRNA improved liver function and decreased tumor burden [30]. Furthermore, they identified the pathway of C/EBPa-saRNA involving which is up-regulation of tumor suppressor genes and down-regulation of liver cancer related genes. These findings have important implications that C/EBPa-saRNA might be druggable. Another paper showed that p21-saRNA has anti-growth effects on HCC cells *in vitro* [31].

3.2. Pancreatic Cancer

p21 is cyclin-dependent kinase inhibitor and well known tumor suppressor genes which is mediator of cell proliferation, differentiation, and senescence. p21-saRNA induces the inhibitory effect of cell proliferation and apoptosis in PANC-1 cell *in vitro*. It also has tumor growth inhibitory effects *in vivo* [32].

3.3. Prostate Cancer

KLF4 (Krupple-like factor) is a member of the Krupple-like factor subfamily of zinc finger proteins and is significantly down-regulated in prostate cancer cell lines compared with non-tumor prostate cells. RNAa-mediated overexpression of KLF4 inhibits prostate cancer cell proliferation and survival. Even better, it inhibits migration and invasion of proststе cancer cells. saRNA against KLFs alters the expression of several downstream cell-cycle-related genes such as CCNB1, members of the cyclin-dependent kinase inhibitor family which are p21,p27, and p57 [33].

NKX3-1, NK3 homeobox 1, is transcription factor known to bind to the consensus sequence "TAAGTA" [34] and is regarded as a prostate specific tumor suppressor [35, 36]. Deletion of NKx3.1 in mouse model causes hyperplasia and dysplasia [37, 38]. Ren et al. reported that NKX3.1-saRNA induces the activation of target gene from 1.5 to 2 fold and inhibits the cancer cell growth and survival *in vitro* and anti-tumor effects *in vivo* [39]. The cellular mechanism responsible for anti-proliferative effects is by induction apoptosis and cell cycle arresting which are up-regulation of p21 and p27 and reduction of VEGFC (vascular endothelial growth factor C).

3.4. Lung Cancer

The functional loss of p21 can mediate a drug-resistance phenotype in tumor therapy [40, 41]. Wei et al. approached a very interesting way of application of saRNA in chemosensitivity [42]. In the study, they showed that p21-saRNA not only inhibits cell growth and enhances chemosensitivity to cisplatin in non-small-cell lung carcinoma *in vitro* and *in vivo*. These results suggest another therapeutic strategy for chemoresistance lung carcinoma.

3.5. Cervical and Bladder Cancer

The first report describing transcriptional activation by saRNA is about E-cadherin, VEGF, and p21 in cervical cancer cells and p21 in bladder cancer cells. PAWR (PRKC apoptosis WT1 regulator) gene encodes a leucine zipper domain protein undergoing apoptosis [43]. Yang et al. described that saRNA-PAWR induces activation of target gene and inhibits cell growth in bladder cancer *in vitro* [43]. In down-stream pathways to identify mechanism, they showed that Bcl-2, apoptosis regulator, is down-regulated.

Although the exact mechanism of activation remains unclear, few studies have provided several important aspects of RNAa. To have functions as RNAa, Li et al. performed quite interesting experiments [9]. They shortened or extended 5 bp from the 3' end of the antisense strand. They both failed the induction of transcription, suggesting that 21nt in size is a key element for RNAa. This group also found that 5' portion of the antisense strand is critical to initiate the transcriptional activation and Ago2 is indispensable for RNAa mechanism. Based on the criteria of siRNA, the efficiency of saRNA is predictable. However, less-than-optimal scores should not discourage targeting of promoter sequences [10]. Because it could simply mean that promoter becomes more GC rich. It is not known which strand guides recognition, both strands must be considered to design. Distinct kinetics of RNAa is that the gene activation by transfecting promoter-targeting saRNA is delayed by 24-48 h in comparision to RNAi, because RNAa is nuclear process acting on gene transcription [44]. Another peculiar feature of RNAa is its prolonged effect. The gene activation can last for nearly 2 weeks in certain cell lines and mismatches in regions out of seed sequence are tolerable [44]. To maximize the RNAa effects, two most important aspects should be considered: concentration and duration. A higher concentration of saRNA is needed compared to siRNA and peak gene activation does not appear till 4-5 days pos-transfection [44]. It is advised that observing gene activation is between 3 and 5 days [45].

4. Delivery into Tumors

Arguably, the biggest challenges have been safe and effective deliveries. Herein, we describe the representative delivery vehicles. For successful application to use as cancer drugs, the application routes should be considered. Also, to maximize the anti-tumor effects and minimize side effects, cancer specific delivery system is needed to develop.

4.1. Aptamer Mediated Delivery

For targeted delivery in cancers, Aptamer is the best vehicle of delivery of siRNA and saRNA into tumors. Aptamer-targeted siRNA/saRNA, unlike antibodies, can be synthesized in a chemical process providing a more straightforward and cost-effective manufacturing and regulatory approval process to generate clinical-grade reagents [46]. The chemically synthesized aptamer-siRNAs reduce the risk of immunogenicity and enhance the feasibility of generating reagents suitable for clinical use [46]. For Aptamer targeting of siRNA/saRNA to cancer cells, binding of the aptamer-siRNA/saRNA conjugate against cancer cells internalizes and translocates to the cytoplasm. The first report regarding aptamer-siRNA conjugate is in 2006 by McNamara et al. In the study, they developed cell-type specific delivery siRNA with PMSA aptamer in prostate cancer [47].

4.2. Nanoparticle-Based Delivery

The termed, LODER (local drug eluter), was employed for the slow-release and the tumor growth is assessed in s.c. to test siRNA in pancreatic cancer [14]. The lipofectamine based intratumor injection in pancreatic cancer [32], lipid nanoparticle based intratumor injection in prostate cancer [39] and dendrimer based tail vein injection in hepatocarcinoma are performed [30] *in vivo* test of saRNA. The good advantage which is relevant for RNAi/RNAa based therapeutics for cancer is that several siRNA/saRNA can be combined simultaneously targeting multiple organs.

4.3. Cell Penetrating Peptides (CPPs) Mediated Delivery

It has been twenty years since the first discovery of CPP in 1988 by Frankel and Green. They found that the transactivator of transcription (TAT) protein in HIV can cross cell membranes and be internalized in cells [48]. Even though CPPs have a great sequence variety, it is possible to divided into three subgroups defined by their physical-chemical properties: cationic, amphipathic and hydrophoibic [49]. Crombez et al. developed a secondary amphipathic peptide (CADY) for siRNA delivery into human osteosarcoma, U_2OS cells. The CADY mediated delivery of siRNA significantly knockdown the target gene with nanomolar range at both the mRNA and protein levels. Importantly, it is not toxic and enters cells through a mechanism which is independent of endosomal pathway [50]. Recently, Christopher et al. enhanced siRNA delivery by exploiting a cell surface binding synergism between ligands and CPPs [51]. They showed the synergies between the activity of cell surface binding ligands, folate and penetratin, and cell internalizing ligands and improve their target gene silencing efficacy in tumor models by intratumor injection.

In vivo delivery can be achieved either through intratumor injection or systemic administration through i.v. Importantly, unmodified naked RNAs are not stable in biofluids due to nuclease degradation. Local intratumor administration increase bioavailablity at target sites. However, this approach is limited to a short list of cancers. Theoretically, systemic delivery is the best option to provide a simple route for siRNA administration to all tissues by blood vessels. When systemically administrated through i.v., the naked nucleic acids generally accumulate in the organs such as the liver, lung, spleen and kidneys [52, 53]. The naked siRNAs accumulate in the kidneys of mice and are detectable in the urine as early as 5 minutes after i.v. injection [52, 54]. This means that siRNAs are susceptible to glomerular filtration in the kidney and excretion in the urine. Besides of the safe and effective delivery, the rapid clearance when systemically applied through i.v. is the biggest challenge to overcome for cancer therapeutic development.

5. Strategies to Improve Small RNA Based Cancer Therapeutics

To address the strategies, we need to know problems, such as stability, uptake, pharmacokinetics and immunostimulations. The design of sequence is important to improve efficacy to reduce off-target effects and avoid immune response. The rules for predicting the efficiency of siRNA have been developed [55]. The criteria to design siRNA include the followings: 30-52% C+G content, at least three A or U at positions 15-19 of the sense strand, an A at the position 19 of the sense strand, a U at position 10 of the sense strand, a base other than C or U at position 19 of the sense strand and a base other than G at position 13.

Off-Target effects by small interfering RNAs were described by Jackson et al. in 2003, which could result in sequence specific and extensive silencing of nontargeted transcripts [56]. They noted that complementarity to the first 8 nucleotides of the 5'-end of siRNAs is most important for off-targeting. In principle, any region of mRNA can be targeted. However, it should be pointed out that complementarity often found in the 3'-UTR induces the off-target sequences. Furthermore, sequence complementarity between the 5' end of guide strand and the mRNA is known to be the key to off-target silencing. Additionally, intronic sequences must be avoided since RNAi is a cytoplasmic process [57]. Interestingly, Fedorov et al. found that there is differences in sensitivity to siRNA off-targeting between the cervical, prostate, and breast cancer cell lines; normal diploid cells with all native responses intact may show even more pronounced off-target effect and innate immune responses [58].

The GU rich sequence seems to be a common feature among the immunostimulatory motifs: UGUGU and GUCCUUCAA. However, it is important to note that several immunostimulatory siRNAs do not contain either of these motifs, wherase others are not stimulatory despite being U and G rich [59]. A number of Wab-based softwares have been developed to identify the efficient siRNA sequences. Since the rules that cover efficient siRNA-directed silencing are still unknown, researchers looking for silence gene expression should be synthesize several siRNA candidates to a target gene and validate the efficiency. To make sure that the chosen siRNA sequence targets a single gene, the selected sequence should be searched against sequence database.

Synthetic RNA duplex of 27-nt, which are Dicer substrate dsRNA (DsiRNA), have been shown to be up to 100-fold more potent than traditional 21-nt siRNA [60]. DsiRNA induce enhanced and prolonged gene silencing at lower concentrations than those of conventional 21-nt siRNA.

6. Chemical Modification

To improve the medical properties for both of small duplex RNA, identifying chemical modification is necessary. Backbone modifications and 2'-ribose modification not only increase nuclease stability but also confer increased binding affinity or duplex stabilization

[61]. Modifications at the 2'position have been most extensively studied such as 2'O-methyl RNA (2'OMe), 2'-O-methoxyethly (2'MOE), locked nucleic acids (LNA), 2'-fluro (2'F), 2'-fluro-b-D-arabinonucleotide (FANA). 2'-OMe is a naturally occurring nucleotide and no toxicity has been reported from its use [62]. Unlocked nucleic acids (UNA), lacking a C2-C3 bond in the ribose ring, were described [63] and combining with LNAs improved the relative stability of siRNA termini [63]. Exploiting chemical modifications in combination is a good way to improve the properties of RNA based drug for clinical application. Overcoming nuclease degradation is a challenge when administrating siRNA through i.v. *in vivo*.

Chemical modifications can rescue off-target effects of RNAi [64]. Blocking the 5'-OH of the passenger strand in synthetic saRNA has been shown to reduce off-target effects [45]. Modification to the 2'backbone such as 2'-OMe, 2'-Fluoro, and LNA, are tolerated by saRNA/duplexes [44]. Methyl-groups added to the 2' position of the ribosyl ring of the second base of the siRNA significantly reduced off-targeting [65]. Interestingly, this RNA oligonucleotides modification does not affect the silencing effect [66]. 2'-OMe modification is much more effective at reducing the off-target effect when it is added to the position 1 of the siRNA [67].

Conclusion Remarks and Future Perspectives

Suppressing the overexpressed genes by RNAi or restoring the expression of silenced genes by RNAa, it is one of good strategies to develop cancer therpeutics. To develop the effective RNAi/RNAa based cancer therapeutics, finding druggable target genes is the first step to be considered very important. The target genes can be mRNA, long non-coding RNA, miRNA and promotor regions. So far, only two oligonucleotide-based therapeutics, Vitravene and Macugen, have reached the market. None of RNAi/RNAa based cancer therapeutics have approved by FDA. Regardless ON or OFF of gene expression, RNAi and RNAa have a lot of potentials and are faster in drug development than those of conventional drug or protein therapeutics for cancer therapeutics. Although there is a belief that RNAi is dead due to the reduction by pharmaceutical industry [68], we have no doubt that RNAi/RNAa based cancer therapeutics will be shown in the market.

References

[1] Pushparaj, P.N., Aarthi, J.J., Kumar, S.D. & Manikandan, J. RNAi and RNAa--the yin and yang of RNAome. *Bioinformation* 2, 235-237 (2008).

[2] Couzin, J. Nobel Prize in Physiology or Medicine. Method to silence genes earns loud praise. *Science* 314, 34 (2006).

[3] Hannon, G.J. RNA interference. *Nature* 418, 244-251 (2002).

[4] Hannon, G.J. & Conklin, D.S. RNA interference by short hairpin RNAs expressed in vertebrate cells. *Methods in molecular biology* 257, 255-266 (2004).

[5] Braasch, D.A. & Corey, D.R. Novel antisense and peptide nucleic acid strategies for controlling gene expression. *Biochemistry* 41, 4503-4510 (2002).

[6] Eckstein, F. Small non-coding RNAs as magic bullets. *Trends in biochemical sciences* 30, 445-452 (2005).

[7] Dykxhoorn, D.M., Palliser, D. & Lieberman, J. The silent treatment: siRNAs as small molecule drugs. *Gene therapy* 13, 541-552 (2006).

[8] Aigner, A. Gene silencing through RNA interference (RNAi) in vivo: strategies based on the direct application of siRNAs. *Journal of biotechnology* 124, 12-25 (2006).

[9] Li, L.C., et al. Small dsRNAs induce transcriptional activation in human cells. *Proceedings of the National Academy of Sciences of the United States of America* 103, 17337-17342 (2006).

[10] Janowski, B.A., et al. Activating gene expression in mammalian cells with promoter-targeted duplex RNAs. *Nature chemical biology* 3, 166-173 (2007).

[11] Huang, V., et al. RNAa is conserved in mammalian cells. *PloS one* 5, e8848 (2010).

[12] Friday, B.B. & Adjei, A.A. K-ras as a target for cancer therapy. *Biochimica et biophysica acta* 1756, 127-144 (2005).

[13] Maitra, A. & Hruban, R.H. Pancreatic cancer. *Annual review of pathology* 3, 157-188 (2008).

[14] Zorde Khvalevsky, E., et al. Mutant KRAS is a druggable target for pancreatic cancer. *Proceedings of the National Academy of Sciences of the United States of America* 110, 20723-20728 (2013).

[15] Tabernero, J., et al. First-in-humans trial of an RNA interference therapeutic targeting VEGF and KSP in cancer patients with liver involvement. *Cancer discovery* 3, 406-417 (2013).

[16] Leenders, F., et al. PKN3 is required for malignant prostate cell growth downstream of activated PI 3-kinase. *The EMBO journal* 23, 3303-3313 (2004).

[17] Strumberg, D., et al. Phase I clinical development of Atu027, a siRNA formulation targeting PKN3 in patients with advanced solid tumors. *International journal of clinical pharmacology and therapeutics* 50, 76-78 (2012).

[18] Aleku, M., et al. Atu027, a liposomal small interfering RNA formulation targeting protein kinase N3, inhibits cancer progression. *Cancer research* 68, 9788-9798 (2008).

[19] Santel, A., et al. Atu027 prevents pulmonary metastasis in experimental and spontaneous mouse metastasis models. *Clinical cancer research : an official journal of the American Association for Cancer Research* 16, 5469-5480 (2010).

[20] Sulman, E.P., et al. ECK, a human EPH-related gene, maps to 1p36.1, a common region of alteration in human cancers. *Genomics* 40, 371-374 (1997).

[21] Thaker, P.H., et al. EphA2 expression is associated with aggressive features in ovarian carcinoma. *Clinical cancer research : an official journal of the American Association for Cancer Research* 10, 5145-5150 (2004).

[22] Noblitt, L.W., et al. Decreased tumorigenic potential of EphA2-overexpressing breast cancer cells following treatment with adenoviral vectors that express EphrinA1. *Cancer gene therapy* 11, 757-766 (2004).

[23] Dobrzanski, P., et al. Antiangiogenic and antitumor efficacy of EphA2 receptor antagonist. *Cancer research* 64, 910-919 (2004).

[24] Duxbury, M.S., Ito, H., Zinner, M.J., Ashley, S.W. & Whang, E.E. EphA2: a determinant of malignant cellular behavior and a potential therapeutic target in pancreatic adenocarcinoma. *Oncogene* 23, 1448-1456 (2004).

[25] Landen, C.N., Jr., et al. Therapeutic EphA2 gene targeting in vivo using neutral liposomal small interfering RNA delivery. *Cancer research* 65, 6910-6918 (2005).

[26] Nishimura, M., et al. Therapeutic synergy between microRNA and siRNA in ovarian cancer treatment. *Cancer discovery* 3, 1302-1315 (2013).

[27] Engstrom, Y., et al. Cell cycle-dependent expression of mammalian ribonucleotide reductase. Differential regulation of the two subunits. *The Journal of biological chemistry* 260, 9114-9116 (1985).

[28] Jensen, R.A., Page, D.L. & Holt, J.T. Identification of genes expressed in premalignant breast disease by microscopy-directed cloning. *Proceedings of the National Academy of Sciences of the United States of America* 91, 9257-9261 (1994).

[29] Heidel, J.D., et al. Potent siRNA inhibitors of ribonucleotide reductase subunit RRM2 reduce cell proliferation in vitro and in vivo. *Clinical cancer research : an official journal of the American Association for Cancer Research* 13, 2207-2215 (2007).

[30] Reebye, V., et al. Novel RNA oligonucleotide improves liver function and inhibits liver carcinogenesis in vivo. *Hepatology* (2013).

[31] Kosaka, M., Kang, M.R., Yang, G. & Li, L.C. Targeted p21WAF1/CIP1 activation by RNAa inhibits hepatocellular carcinoma cells. *Nucleic acid therapeutics* 22, 335-343 (2012).

[32] Zhang, Z., et al. Up-regulation of p21WAF1/CIP1 by small activating RNA inhibits the in vitro and in vivo growth of pancreatic cancer cells. *Tumori* 98, 804-811 (2012).

[33] Wang, J., et al. Prognostic value and function of KLF4 in prostate cancer: RNAa and vector-mediated overexpression identify KLF4 as an inhibitor of tumor cell growth and migration. *Cancer research* 70, 10182-10191 (2010).

[34] Steadman, D.J., Giuffrida, D. & Gelmann, E.P. DNA-binding sequence of the human prostate-specific homeodomain protein NKX3.1. *Nucleic acids research* 28, 2389-2395 (2000).

[35] Bieberich, C.J., Fujita, K., He, W.W. & Jay, G. Prostate-specific and androgen-dependent expression of a novel homeobox gene. *The Journal of biological chemistry* 271, 31779-31782 (1996).

[36] Kim, M.J., et al. Nkx3.1 mutant mice recapitulate early stages of prostate carcinogenesis. *Cancer research* 62, 2999-3004 (2002).

[37] Bhatia-Gaur, R., et al. Roles for Nkx3.1 in prostate development and cancer. *Genes & development* 13, 966-977 (1999).

[38] Schneider, A., Brand, T., Zweigerdt, R. & Arnold, H. Targeted disruption of the Nkx3.1 gene in mice results in morphogenetic defects of minor salivary glands: parallels to glandular duct morphogenesis in prostate. *Mechanisms of development* 95, 163-174 (2000).

[39] Ren, S., et al. Targeted induction of endogenous NKX3-1 by small activating RNA inhibits prostate tumor growth. *The Prostate* 73, 1591-1601 (2013).

[40] Cariou, S., et al. Down-regulation of p21WAF1/CIP1 or p27Kip1 abrogates antiestrogen-mediated cell cycle arrest in human breast cancer cells. *Proceedings of the National Academy of Sciences of the United States of America* 97, 9042-9046 (2000).

[41] Giannakakou, P., Robey, R., Fojo, T. & Blagosklonny, M.V. Low concentrations of paclitaxel induce cell type-dependent p53, p21 and G1/G2 arrest instead of mitotic arrest: molecular determinants of paclitaxel-induced cytotoxicity. *Oncogene* 20, 3806-3813 (2001).

[42] Wei, J., et al. p21WAF1/CIP1 gene transcriptional activation exerts cell growth inhibition and enhances chemosensitivity to cisplatin in lung carcinoma cell. *BMC cancer* 10, 632 (2010).
[43] Yang, K., et al. Promoter-targeted double-stranded small RNAs activate PAWR gene expression in human cancer cells. *The international journal of biochemistry & cell biology* 45, 1338-1346 (2013).
[44] Portnoy, V., Huang, V., Place, R.F. & Li, L.C. Small RNA and transcriptional upregulation. *Wiley interdisciplinary reviews. RNA* 2, 748-760 (2011).
[45] Place, R.F., Noonan, E.J., Foldes-Papp, Z. & Li, L.C. Defining features and exploring chemical modifications to manipulate RNAa activity. *Current pharmaceutical biotechnology* 11, 518-526 (2010).
[46] Gilboa, E. Expression of new antigens on tumor cells by inhibiting nonsense-mediated mRNA decay. *Immunologic research* 57, 44-51 (2013).
[47] McNamara, J.O., 2nd, et al. Cell type-specific delivery of siRNAs with aptamer-siRNA chimeras. *Nature biotechnology* 24, 1005-1015 (2006).
[48] Koren, E. & Torchilin, V.P. Cell-penetrating peptides: breaking through to the other side. *Trends in molecular medicine* 18, 385-393 (2012).
[49] Wang, F., et al. Recent progress of cell-penetrating peptides as new carriers for intracellular cargo delivery. *Journal of controlled release : official journal of the Controlled Release Society* 174, 126-136 (2014).
[50] Crombez, L., et al. A new potent secondary amphipathic cell-penetrating peptide for siRNA delivery into mammalian cells. *Molecular therapy : the journal of the American Society of Gene Therapy* 17, 95-103 (2009).
[51] Cheng, C.J. & Saltzman, W.M. Enhanced siRNA delivery into cells by exploiting the synergy between targeting ligands and cell-penetrating peptides. *Biomaterials* 32, 6194-6203 (2011).
[52] van de Water, F.M., et al. Intravenously administered short interfering RNA accumulates in the kidney and selectively suppresses gene function in renal proximal tubules. *Drug metabolism and disposition: the biological fate of chemicals* 34, 1393-1397 (2006).
[53] Braasch, D.A., et al. Biodistribution of phosphodiester and phosphorothioate siRNA. *Bioorganic & medicinal chemistry letters* 14, 1139-1143 (2004).
[54] Santel, A., et al. A novel siRNA-lipoplex technology for RNA interference in the mouse vascular endothelium. *Gene therapy* 13, 1222-1234 (2006).
[55] Reynolds, A., et al. Rational siRNA design for RNA interference. *Nature biotechnology* 22, 326-330 (2004).
[56] Jackson, A.L., et al. Expression profiling reveals off-target gene regulation by RNAi. *Nature biotechnology* 21, 635-637 (2003).
[57] Dykxhoorn, D.M., Novina, C.D. & Sharp, P.A. Killing the messenger: short RNAs that silence gene expression. *Nature reviews. Molecular cell biology* 4, 457-467 (2003).
[58] Fedorov, Y., et al. Off-target effects by siRNA can induce toxic phenotype. *Rna* 12, 1188-1196 (2006).
[59] De Paula, D., Bentley, M.V. & Mahato, R.I. Hydrophobization and bioconjugation for enhanced siRNA delivery and targeting. *Rna* 13, 431-456 (2007).
[60] Kim, D.H., et al. Synthetic dsRNA Dicer substrates enhance RNAi potency and efficacy. *Nature biotechnology* 23, 222-226 (2005).

[61] Watts, J.K., Deleavey, G.F. & Damha, M.J. Chemically modified siRNA: tools and applications. *Drug discovery today* 13, 842-855 (2008).
[62] Rettig, G.R. & Behlke, M.A. Progress toward in vivo use of siRNAs-II. *Molecular therapy : the journal of the American Society of Gene Therapy* 20, 483-512 (2012).
[63] Langkjaer, N., Pasternak, A. & Wengel, J. UNA (unlocked nucleic acid): a flexible RNA mimic that allows engineering of nucleic acid duplex stability. *Bioorganic & medicinal chemistry* 17, 5420-5425 (2009).
[64] Snove, O., Jr. & Rossi, J.J. Chemical modifications rescue off-target effects of RNAi. *ACS chemical biology* 1, 274-276 (2006).
[65] Jackson, A.L., et al. Position-specific chemical modification of siRNAs reduces "off-target" transcript silencing. *Rna* 12, 1197-1205 (2006).
[66] Amarzguioui, M., Holen, T., Babaie, E. & Prydz, H. Tolerance for mutations and chemical modifications in a siRNA. *Nucleic acids research* 31, 589-595 (2003).
[67] Brennecke, J., Stark, A., Russell, R.B. & Cohen, S.M. Principles of microRNA-target recognition. *PLoS biology* 3, e85 (2005).
[68] Krieg, A.M. Is RNAi dead? *Molecular therapy : the journal of the American Society of Gene Therapy* 19, 1001-1002 (2011).
[69] Yu, L., et al. Suppression of metastasis of human pancreatic cancer cells to the liver by small interfering RNA-mediated targeting of the midkine gene. *Oncology letters* 6, 1338-1342 (2013).
[70] Chile, T., et al. HOXB7 mRNA is overexpressed in pancreatic ductal adenocarcinomas and its knockdown induces cell cycle arrest and apoptosis. *BMC cancer* 13, 451 (2013).
[71] Ghosh, S.K., et al. Sequence-dependent combination therapy with doxorubicin and a survivin-specific small interfering RNA nanodrug demonstrates efficacy in models of adenocarcinoma. *International journal of cancer. Journal international du cancer* (2013).

In: Horizons in Cancer Research. Volume 54
Editor: Hiroto S. Watanabe
ISBN: 978-1-63321-389-0

Chapter 4

Melanoma Progression to Metastatic Disease: The Role of the PI3K/AKT and Wnt/β-Catenin Pathways

Jaskiran Sidhu, Geetha Venkateswaran and Sujata Persad*
Department of Pediatrics Faculty of Medicine and Dentistry University of Alberta, Edmonton, Alberta, Canada

Abstract

Worldwide, melanoma has the most rapidly rising incidence rate of any human cancer. It arises from the malignant transformation of the melanocyte cells of the skin. Due to the inefficacy of present chemotherapeutic regimens and the resistance of melanocyte cells to radiotherapy, 95% of stage IV metastatic melanoma patients die within five years of diagnosis. Metastasis, the spread of a cancer from the site of the primary tumour to distant sites of the body, makes melanoma very hard to treat. Risk factors associated with malignant melanoma include excessive sun exposure and associated mutations in specific genes and deregulation of signal transduction pathways.

Malignant melanoma is characterized by frequent metastasis; however, specific changes that cause this malignancy are yet to be characterized. Several oncogenes, tumour suppressor genes, and pathways are implicated in melanoma; for example, NRAS, which activates RAF kinases in response to growth factors is overactive in 15–20% of melanomas. P16 (INK4A) tumour suppressor expression is lost by mutation, deletion, or transcriptional silencing of the CDKN2A locus in many melanomas. BRAF mutations are often found alongside P16 mutations. Phosphatase and tensin homolog (PTEN) mutations and deletions are also present in a significant number of melanomas, coinciding with BRAF mutations. Since these two mutations often occur together PTEN loss reflects the importance of two RAS-effector pathways in melanoma. Another genomic aberration associated with melanoma is the amplification of microphthalmia-associated transcription factor (MITF).

* Correspondence to: Dr. Sujata Persad Associate Professor, Department of Pediatrics Faculty of Medicine and Dentistry University of Alberta 3020 Katz Group Centre for Pharmacy and Health Research Edmonton, Alberta, Canada T6G 2E1 TEL: 780 492 5201 E-mail: sujata.persad@ualberta.ca.

The occurrence of several different mutations implies that several signal transduction pathways are perturbed in melanoma. Of particular interest to this review are mutations in the Wnt/β-catenin pathway as well as the PI3K pathway. Elevated levels of nuclear β-catenin are observed in ~30% of human melanomas. In fact, melanoma is one of the first cancer types associated with β-catenin/Wnt signaling mutations. Mutations in the Wnt signaling pathway that result in over-activation of β-catenin signaling are readily observed in melanomas, but the functional implications of these mutations in melanoma progression remain unclear.

The PI3K pathway is likely the most frequently deregulated pathway in melanoma, although the mechanism underlying the over-activation in most cases remains largely elusive. Growth factor stimulation of receptor tyrosine kinases (RTK) and/or non-RTKs results in the activation of PI3K and the conversion of phosphatidylinositol-bis-phosphate (PIP2) to phosphatidylinositol-tri- phosphate (PIP3). The presence of PIP3 mediates the phosphorylation and activation of Akt/PKB by PDK1/PDK2 at Threonine 308 (T308) and Serine 473 (S473). Activated Akt (phosphorylated Akt [P-Akt]) is the central effector of many downstream signaling pathways regulating protein synthesis, cell cycle, cell death, cell growth, and cell survival. In Melanoma, the loss of the tumour suppressor protein and negative regulator of the PI3K/Akt pathway, PTEN, is a common event leading to the constitutive activation of PI3K/Akt signaling. The consitutive activation of this pathway with PTEN loss and the resulting elevation of the P-AKT signaling axis may be a method for promoting/sustaining melanoma progression. This includes modes of regulation between PI3K/Akt and other pathways such as 1) cross-talk with the Wnt/GSK3β/β- catenin pathway, 2) cross-talk with FOXO family of transcription factors and 3) mammalian target of rapamycin (mTOR).

This review will discuss the current evidence available for PI3K/PTEN/Akt and Wnt-β-catenin mediated signaling in melanoma progression.

Section 1. PI3K/AKT Signaling Pathway and Its Components

1.1. Overview

The Phosphatidylinositol-3-kinase/AKT (Protein Kinase B) pathway (PI3K) serves a role in altering cellular functions in response to extracellular signals, and it is a central integrator of metabolism, survival and growth signals [1]. With respect to metabolism, various studies have shown PI3K pathway's role in insulin sensitivity [2]. Several membrane receptors, in particular receptor tyrosine kinases (RTKs), G-protein coupled receptors (GPCR) and cytokine receptors activate PI3Ks. A number of the components of the pathway have been found mutated or deregulated in a wide variety of human cancers highlighting the key role of this pathway in cellular transformation and further in tumourigenesis [3]. The PI3K pathway has been shown to be prominently involved in tumour development and also in the tumour's potential response to cancer treatment. Many of the new "targeted agents" have been specifically designed to act on PI3Krelated targets [4].

1.2. Components of the PI3K Pathway

1.2.1. PI3K Isoforms

PI3K is a member of a large family of lipid kinases that are characterized by their ability to phosphorylate the inositol ring 3'-OH group in inositol phospholipids [4]. They are sub-classified based on their structure and preferred substrates [5]. The PI3Ks are comprised of three classes, Class I, II and III. The three classes differ in structure, substrate preference, tissue distribution, mechanism of activation and, ultimately, in function [6]. Class I serves an important role in cancer development through its role in cell growth regulation. Class II and III PI3Ks, on the other hand, are less studied and are recognized for their involvement in membrane trafficking and receptor internalization, and vesicle trafficking, respectively [7, 8, 1]. In this review, we will focus mainly on Class IA PI3K as they have been shown to be most relevant in cell growth regulation and cancer development. Although frequent genetic alterations in the PI3K group of enzymes and the pathway effectors makes this pathway the most frequently deregulated pathway in cancer, only the Class IA PI3Ks have been implicated in human cancer [9]. Throughout this review we will be refer to Class IA PI3K as PI3K unless otherwise stated.

Class I PI3Ks (PI3Ks) are divided into four members based on their mechanism of activation. They present as a heterodimeric complex comprising of a regulatory subunit p85α and any of three catalytic subunits; p110α, p110β and p110δ. The p110 isoforms (α, β, δ) have the same basic structure, a p85 binding domain, a kinase domain and a C2 domain for membrane anchoring [10]. The p110α subunit additionally has a Ras-binding domain (Ras-BD) and a helical domain [11]. The regulatory subunit contains SH2 and SH3 domains, which are involved in associating with target proteins that have the appropriate binding sites [12]. In particular, the p85α subunit of PI3Ks encodes an adaptor-like protein that has two SH2 domains and an inter-SH2 domain that binds constitutively to the p110 catalytic subunit [10]. The regulatory subunits are subject to further splicing. The two splice variants (p55α and p50α) retain such regions but lacks an amino terminal SH3 domain (mediates the binding of proline rich sequences) and a breakpoint cluster region (BCR) homology domain (a protein-protein interaction motif) [10]. PI3K p110α domain isoform is the most mutated amongst cancers, causing the kinase to be more active [13, 14, 15] and perpetuating a constitutively active PI3K pathway.

1.2.2. Phosphatase and Tensin Homologue Deleted on Chromosome 10 (PTEN)

The tumour suppressor, PTEN, is a negative regulator of the PI3K pathway. PTEN is a dual phosphatase that acts on Tyr, Ser and Thr residues on lipid and protein substrates [16]. The lipid phosphatase-hydrolysing activity of PTEN occurs at position 3' from phosphoinositides [17]. PTEN can dephosphorylate the D3 position of PIP_3 thus antagonizing signaling through the PI3K pathway [18]. The lipid phosphatase role of PTEN effectively reduces the activation of Protein Kinase B (PKB/AKT) and prevents the downstream signaling events that are controlled by AKT [12]. This therefore controls the activity of the PI3K pathway in regulating cell survival and growth via signaling from growth factor receptors and components of the extracellular matrix [17].

Loss of PTEN is observed in many cancers [19] and further germline alterations are associated with a group of syndromes known as PTEN hamartoma tumour syndromes, which are characterized by the presence of developmental and neurological defects and cancer susceptibility. Along with PTEN loss, mutations in AKT and RTK amplifications, presents a class of frequent genomic aberrations that promotes tumourigenesis through upregulation of the PI3K signaling axis [9]. Loss of PTEN results in suppression of apoptosis and accelerated cell cycle progression [20].

PTEN is tightly regulated at the transcriptional level as well as by post translational modification, primarily ubiquitylation. Incidentally, the activity of PTEN is also controlled by the PI3K pathway. Transcriptionally, the levels of PTEN are controlled by PI3K through the regulation of the transcription factor NF-κB, while PPARβ/δ agonists and TNFα repress PTEN expression [1, 21]. In p85 conditional knockout mice, the loss of p85 resulted in PTEN activity, while loss of p110δ isoform regulated PTEN activity through a RhoA-ROCK-dependent signaling [1, 22]. Currently, NEDD4-1 is the first and only identified E3 ligase for PTEN [1, 23]. Similar to PTEN, NEDD4-1 is also regulated by the PI3K pathway, thus representing a positive feedback for PTEN degradation and PI3K activation [1, 24]. More often than not, heterozygous alterations of PTEN are most common in the initial steps of tumourigenesis. Surprisingly, complete PTEN deletion does not have pro-tumourigenic effect.

1.2.3. AKT

The formation of PIP_3 is the central initiating event which functions to recruit plekstrin homology (PH) domain containing proteins to the plasma membrane. Of relevance here, is AKT/PKB, as it is the critical mediator of signal transduction events downstream of the PI3K cascade. There are three members of the AKT family (AKT1, AKT2, and AKT3) with AKT1 being the major isoform implicated in cancers. AKT2 is known for its involvement in insulin signaling and glucose transport whereas AKT3 is thought to play specific roles in brain tissue [13, 25].

The AKT gene encodes a serine/threonine kinase with an amino-terminal PH domain, a central catalytic domain, and a carboxyl-terminal regulatory domain. The regulation of AKT function is two- fold, requiring its translocation to the plasma membrane and its sequential phosphorylation at Threonine 308 (T308) and Serine 473 (S473). In unstimulated cells, AKT is constitutively phosphorylated at S124 and T450. When PIP_3 is generated it interacts directly with AKT via the PH domain which recruits AKT to the plasma membrane. Here, PDK1 phosphorylates AKT on T308 which is the priming event to mediate the phosphorylation of S473 by PDK2, which is thought to be mammalian target of rapamycin complex 2 (mTORC2). This secondary phosphorylation event is necessary for maximal activation of AKT increasing the kinase activity 10-fold [13, 26, 27]. AKT has multiple substrates within the cytoplasm and nucleus and the activation of AKT regulates many cellular processes including cell proliferation and survival, cell size and glucose homeostasis, metabolism, angiogenesis, and tissue invasion [13].

Phosphorylation of AKT in response to various stimuli can lead to an anti-apoptotic response. This is affected through a series of phosphorylation/inhibition of key pro-apoptotic proteins including, BAD, MDM2 and members of the Forkhead family of proteins. AKT also phosphorylates the pro-death enzyme, caspase 9, and inhibits its catalytic activity. An indirect mechanism by which AKT regulates apoptosis is mediated by the NF-κB and p53 pathways. Specifically, phosphorylation and activation of IκB kinase (IκK) results in the degradation of the NF-κB inhibitor, IκB. This causes the nuclear translocation of NF-κB and the expression of anti-apoptotic genes. The pro-apoptotic effects of p53 tumour suppressor protein are also mediated by phosphorylation of the p53 binding protein, MDM2 by AKT. MDM2 is a negative regulator of p53 function as it targets p53 for ubiquitin mediated proteosomal degradation through its E3 ubiquitin ligase activity. The phosphorylation of MDM2 increases the efficiency by which MDM2 translocates to the nucleus and thereby enhancing p53 degradation [13].

The proliferative effects of AKT activation can also be attributed to the inhibition of the enzyme, glycogen synthase kinase (GSK) 3β at its Serine 9 phosphorylation site as well as its role in inactivating the cell cycle inhibitor p27 and p21. AKT has an important role in preventing cyclin D1 degradation by inhibiting GSK3β, which phosphorylates cyclin D1, thereby increasing cyclin D1 levels resulting in cell cycle progression. The regulation of cell cycle progression is regulated throughcyclin-dependent kinase (CDK) complexes and CDK inhibitors (CKI). p27 and p21 are CKIs that become phosphorylated by AKT and through indirect mechanisms, can modulate the expression of CKIs as well as their activities. Cyclin D1 expression is also tightly controlled by the transcription factor FOXO3A, in that FOXO3A is a transcriptional repressor of the Cyclin D1 gene. When AKT phosphorylates FOXO3A, it is removed from the nucleus resulting in decreased transcriptional repression and thus increased cyclin D1 expression [28].

1.3. PI3K Pathway Activation and Downstream Targets

The activity of PI3K is regulated within the cell by growth factor-receptor interactions [9]. In a quiescent cell, PI3K is inactive and localized in the cytoplasm, far removed from its plasma membrane substrates. Under such unstimulated conditions p85 binds to p110 resulting in the inhibition of its kinase activity. Moreover, only a small fraction of these PI3Ks become activated upon growth factor stimulation [9]. PI3K is activated upon receptor occupation by several growth factors, including fibroblast growth factor (FGF), vascular endothelial cell growth factor (VEGF), human growth factor (HGF), angiopoietin I (Ang1), insulin like growth factor 1 (IGF-1), and insulin. The growth factor activated receptors are receptor tyrosine kinase (RTK) that undergo transphosphorylation and activation upon binding their respective growth factor ligands. Upon growth factor stimulation, the SH2 domain (Roussarcoma-oncogene homology-2 domains) of p85 binds to phosphorylated tyrosine in YxxM motifs in RTKs or their substrate adaptor proteins. This binding relieves the inhibition of p110 and mediates recruitment of the catalytic subunit of PI3K in close proximity to its lipid substrates at the plasma membrane [29].

In the simplest scenario, phosphorylated residue on receptor becomes a docking site for the p85 subunit of heterodimeric PI3K. In some cases, however, receptor phosphorylation mediates the recruitment of an adaptor protein. For example, when insulin activates the insulin receptor, the insulin receptor substrate protein (IRS) must be recruited to facilitate PI3K binding. Similarly, focal adhesion kinase (FAK) serves as an adaptor protein, docking PI3K via its p85 regulatory domain when integrins (instead of RTK) are activated. In each case, an SH2 or SH3 domain of the p85 subunit of PI3K binds to the adaptor protein at an autophosphorylated site [12].

The preferred substrates of PI3K are the non-phosphorylated phosphatidylinositol (PI), inositol monophosphate (PI(4)P), and phosphatidyl-bis-phosphate (PI(4,5)P_2). PI3Ks mediate the addition of a phosphate group in the D-3 position of the inositol ring to generate PI(3)P, PIP_2, and PIP_3, respectively [30, 31]. PI-3,4-bisphosphate promotes cell proliferation (growth) and resistance to apoptosis (survival), unlike its precursor PI-4-phosphate. Finally, PIP_2 is converted to PI-3,4,5-trisphosphate (PIP_3), which modulates cell adhesion, growth, and survival [12]. PIP_3 serves to recruit proteins containing the pleckstrin homology (PH) domain. The PH domains are diverse in their structure, providing varying degrees of selectivity. This interaction controls the timing and localization of protein-membrane association and in this way regulates protein activity. The interaction of the protein with the lipid may also change protein conformation to alter protein function. The generation of PIP_3 promotes the movement of the PH domain-containing enzyme phosphoinositide-dependent kinase 1 (PDK1) to the plasma membrane [12]. AKT/Protein Kinase B (PKB), a PH domain containing protein, is a central protein involved in normal and pathological signaling. Upon recruitment to the plasma membrane, AKT is phosphorylated at two sites, specifically at Thr 308 by PDK1 and Ser 473 by PDK2. However, the exact mechanism of these phosphorylations is yet unclear [4]. Phosphorylated-AKT (pAKT) results in a cascade involving various downstream signaling proteins [32, 33, 34]. A high level of pAKT is correlated with poor prognosis of many cancers, whereas pAKT is mostly undetectable in normal tissue [35]. Along with several downstream effectors as mentioned in the previous section, activated AKT inhibits GSK3β, which normally prevents up-regulation of cell proliferation due to increased cyclin D1 degradation. Also, inhibition of GSK3β is shown to spare free β-catenin from degradation in cancer cells [35]. Further, increased β-catenin can bind and stabilize cyclin D1 mRNA, which leads to enhanced expression of the latter protein and promotion of G1-phase/S-phase progression [36]. Another key effector downstream of PI3K is mTOR [37, 38]. It has been shown that mTOR is a serine/threonine kinase that plays a central role in protein translation, cell proliferation and evasion of apoptosis [37]. Components of this pathway have been implicated in carcinogenesis and cancer progression at many levels such as excessive growth signals, insensitivity to growth inhibitory signals, evasion of apoptosis, limitless replicative potential, sustained angiogenesis, and tissue invasion and metastasis [39]. AKT, through the phosphorylation of these target proteins, fulfills a role as a key regulator of a variety of critical cell functions including glucose metabolism, cell proliferation and survival [40].

1.4. PI3K in Cancer

Activating mutations in PIK3CA, the gene encoding the p110α catalytic subunit of PI3K, were recently identified as novel mechanisms of inducing oncogenic PI3K signaling [41]. PI3K gene amplifications are frequently seen in ovarian and gastric tumours, and mutations of PI3K are common in breast and colorectal cancer [29]. The most frequent mutations of PI3K are in its kinase domain and helical domain causing different impacts on PI3K targets [42]. Deregulation of the pathway is usually caused by oncogenic activation of the RTKs upstream of PI3K. Alternatively, amplifications of genes encoding the catalytic unit of PI3K, and activating mutations in the regulatory subunit of PI3K, also cause excessive activation of the pathway [3].

Section 2. PI3K Pathway in Melanoma

2.1. Melanoma

2.1.1. Overview

Worldwide, melanoma has the most rapidly rising incidence rate of any human cancer. It arises from the malignant transformation of melanocyte cells of the skin. Due to the inefficacy of present chemotherapeutic regimens and the resistance of melanoma cells to radiotherapy, 95% of stage IV metastatic melanoma patients die within five years of diagnosis [43, 44, 45]. Metastasis, the spread of a cancer from the site of the primary tumour to distant sites of the body, makes melanoma very hard to treat. A risk factor associated with malignant melanoma is sun exposure which can cause mutations in specific genes and deregulation of signal transduction pathways.

2.1.2. Stages of Melanoma

Malignant melanoma is characterized by the uncontrollable proliferation of melanocytes, cells originating from neural crest cells. The liver, brain, and lungs are the most common targets of melanoma metastasis, and patients with metastasized melanoma have a median survival of six months [46].

Melanocytes are located in the basal layer of the epidermis surrounded by keratinocytes. Keratinocytes maintain controlled growth of melanocytes through (1) extracellular communication through paracrine growth factors, (2) intracellular communication through second messengers and signal transduction, and (3) intercellular communication through cell–cell adhesion molecules, cell–matrix adhesion, and gap junctional intercellular communication [47]. Perturbations in the cellular environment can lead to alterations in molecules involved in cell-cell adhesion and cell communication, leading to melanoma development [48]. Uncontrolled proliferation, homeostatic balance perturbation through deregulation of signal transduction, and loss in cell adhesion can all lead to melanoma progression to metastasis.

Normal melanocytes are transformed to malignant melanocytes through distinct phenotypic changes, as they progress through the process of Epithelial to Mesenchymal Transition (EMT). This is characterized by a disruption in adherens junctions of melanocytes as a result of the down regulation of the epithelial E-cadherin and up regulation of the mesenchymal N-cadherin (the "cadherin switch") [49]. The result is a loss of cell adhesion and an increase in cell mobility. Loss of E-cadherin allows melanocytes to escape from keratinocyte growth control and allows malignant melanocytes to escape from the primary tumour focus [50]. EMT must take place for cells to progress to a metastatic stage, as cells must shed their epithelial phenotype and gain a mesenchymal phenotype. To gain metastatic potential, cells must invade the basement membrane and make their way into the bloodstream.

The American Joint Committee on Cancer (AJCC) has devised a system to categorize melanoma. This system incorporates tumour thickness, nodal status, and metastatic disease [51]. Melanoma progresses through distinct phases, clustering of cells on the skin begins with a benign nevus stage, which can be defined as a mole. This then progresses to a dysplastic nevus, and with further proliferation to a radial growth phase. As cells progress through EMT, changes in cells cause invasion into the sub-epidermal tissue in a vertical fashion, known as the vertical growth phase. The final stage of melanoma is a metastatic stage, when cells invade through the basement membrane and travel through the vascular system to distant tissues/organs and survive as single cells or colonies at these sites. The most common sites of metastasis by melanoma are lung, liver, brain and bone [52].

2.1.3. Melanoma and Common Mutations of Signaling Pathways

Several oncogenes, tumour suppressor genes, and pathways are known to be deregulated in melanoma; for example, NRAS, which activates RAF kinases in response to growth factors, is overactive in 15–20% of melanomas [53, 54]. P16 (INK4A) tumour suppressor expression is also lost by mutation, deletion, or transcriptional silencing of the CDKN2A locus in many melanomas [55]. BRAF mutations are often found with P16 mutations. PTEN mutations and deletions are also present in some melanomas, coinciding with BRAF mutations [55, 56, 57]. The frequent occurrence of these two mutations together is likely a reflection of the importance of two RAS-effector pathways (PI3K and Mitogen Activation Protein Kinase Pathway (MAPK) in melanomagenesis and progression [58]. Another genomic aberration associated with melanoma is the amplification of microphthalmia-associated transcription factor (MITF) [58]. The high incidence and low survival rate of melanoma, makes it an important area of study. Elucidation of the changes and dysregulation occurring in signal transduction pathways that leads to metastasis will allow identification of molecular targets and thus the design of efficacious therapies to treat metastatic disease [59]. Melanoma was one of the first cancer types which was associated with mutations in the β-catenin/Wnt signaling pathway [60]. However, the exact role of these mutations in melanoma has remained elusive [61]. Mutations in the Wnt signaling pathway that result in over-activation of β-catenin signaling are readily observed in melanomas, but the functional implications are still unclear [62]. Several *in vivo* and *in vitro* models have been established to study the implications of a deregulated Wnt signaling pathway in melanoma. Overactive β-catenin signaling along with a constitutively active PI3K pathway was shown to facilitate melanoma development in a mouse model [62]. Elevated levels of nuclear β-catenin are observed in ~30% of human melanomas [63]. The occurrence of multiple mutations in melanoma implies that several signal transduction pathways are likely perturbed and involved in melanoma progression. Although the PI3K pathway is one of the most frequently deregulated pathways in melanoma, the mechanism underlying the over-activation in most cases remains largely elusive [64].

2.2. PI3K and Melanoma Progression

Malignant melanoma is characterized by frequent metastasis; however, specific changes that cause this malignancy are yet to be characterized [62]. Deregulation of the PI3K pathway is used by many tumours to attain growth advantage and survival [65]. The PI3K pathway is one of the most deregulated pathways in melanoma. PTEN mutations are found in 30-40% of melanoma cell lines and 5-20% of primary melanomas [66, 67]. Loss of expression or function of PTEN is not only due to mutation and allelic loss [66, 67], but functional inactivation by epigenetic silencing [68] or altered subcellular localization [69]. Ectopic expression of PTEN has been demonstrated to suppress melanoma cell growth and melanoma tumourigenicity and metastasis [70]. Absence or inactivity of PTEN deregulates the PI3K pathway and constitutively activates the downstream effector, AKT via its phosphorylation at two critical amino acids: Serine (Ser) 473 and Threonine (Thr) 308 [71]. This results in sustained proliferative and anti-apoptotic cellular response. The importance of the PI3K pathway in malignant melanoma is underscored by the fact that over 60% of melanomas exhibit activated AKT [72] and overexpression of AKT has been shown to convert radial growth melanoma to vertical growth melanoma [73]. Further the PI3K pathway has been shown to be overactive in preclinical models of melanoma.

Upregulation of cellular processes such as cellular growth, metabolism and proliferation due to a deregulated PI3K pathway in melanoma are controlled through downstream effectors which regulate cell cycle, angiogenesis, inflammation and invasiveness [64]. A positive correlation has been determined in melanoma progression and phosphorylated/activated AKT levels. Levels of phospho-AKT correlate inversely with disease-free survival and directly with poor prognosis [70]. PI3K triggers a network that positively regulates G1/S cell cycle progression and increases cyclin D1 expression. Loss of the G1/S phase checkpoint is often seen in melanoma and allows cells to pass into the stage of cell proliferation without control [74]. In this regard, mTOR has been the target of several phase I and II trials using its inhibitor rapamycin in various cancers, including melanoma [73, 75].

Section 3. PI3K Mediated Crosstalk in Melanoma Progression

In this section we will discuss the crosstalk between the PI3K pathway and other pathways that are altered in melanoma. There are several putative areas of crosstalk involving pathways such as the Mitogen Activated Protein Kinase (MAPK), Wnt-β catenin, Nuclear Factor kappaB (NF-κB), Transforming Growth Factor beta (TGF-β), JAK-STAT and Notch pathways. The crosstalk between the PI3K and Wnt-β catenin pathway will not be discussed in this section and will be discussed in detail in section 4.

3.1. PI3K – MAPK Crosstalk

MAPK pathway is one of the most commonly deregulated pathways in melanoma. MAPK pathway regulates important cellular processes and hence deregulation of this pathway plays a key role in cancer progression. In mammals there are 4 major isoforms of MAPK namely, the extracellular signal regulated kinase (ERK1/2), c-Jun amino (N)-terminal kinases (JNK 1/2/3), p38 isoforms (α, β, γ, δ) and ERK5. Although the signaling pathways originating from each MAPK isoform includes very specific components, the general route of the signaling occurs via a common three tier kinase cascade consisting of MAPK kinase kinase (MAP3K), MAPK kinase (MAP2K) and MAPK [76, 77, 78]. Among the four MAPK signaling pathways, the JNK and ERK modules are most frequently reported to be deregulated in melanoma and hence we will focus on these two modules in this section.

ERK 1/2 Module

ERK 1/2 is activated by several growth factors, cytokines as well as in response to stress. ERK 1/2 signaling begins with the activation of RTK or GPCR leading to transphosphorylation of Tyrosine residues in the intracellular domain. These phosphorylated residues serve as binding site for adaptor proteins like Grb2, which recruits Sos (a GEF, Guanine nucleotide exchange factor) to the plasma membrane. Sos mediates the exchange of Ras-GDP to the active Ras-GTP, resulting in the activation of MAP3K, Raf (A-Raf, B-Raf, Raf-1). Raf activation leads to the activation of the MAP2K (MEK 1/2) which in turn phosphorylates MAPK (ERK 1/2) at its Thr-Glu-Tyr motif leading to the activation ERK 1/2 [76, 77]. Once activated, ERK 1/2 translocates from cytoplasm to nucleus, where it induces transcription of its target genes [77, 78].

JNK Module

JNKs are MAPKs activated in response to stress and has three isforms JNK 1, 2, 3. The MAP2K components of JNK pathway are MKK4 and MKK7. MAP3K components are MEKK1-4, MLK-2 and 3, Tpl-2, DLK, TAO 1 and 2, TAK1 and ASK 1/2 with each MAP3K being induced specifically by different stimuli. Scaffold proteins like filamin, β-arrestin and JNK interacting protein (JIP) plays an important role in regulating the activation of JNK by optimizing the interaction of component kinases of JNK signaling module. Like ERK, JNK also requires phosphorylation of conserved Thr-Pro-Tyr motifs within its activation loop. Once activated JNK enters the nucleus where it acts on its substrates, mostly transcription factors. c-jun is the most important nuclear substrate of JNK, which when phosphorylated at Ser 63 and 73 dimerizes with c-fos to form the active AP-1 transcription factor complex. P53, ATF-2, STAT3, c-myc, Jun-B are other transcription factors that are activated by JNK [77, 78].

The PI3K and MAPK pathways are significant in cancer progression and studies have shown that treatment with PI3K inhibitor Wortmannin induced inhibiton of MAPK pathway, suggestive of potential crosstalk between these two pathways [79]. A review by Edita et al. shows experimental data and computer simulations to support several points of crosstalks between these two independent parallel pathways [80]. Ras is a prominent point for crosstalk as both MAPK and PI3K are effector pathways downstream of Ras [81]. Another point of crosstalk is at Raf. PIP_3 produced from an activated PI3K pathway leads to sequential activation of GEF, Rac (small GTPase) and finally PAK (P-21 activated kinase), an effector of Rac [82, 83]. Chaudhary et al. proposed that PAK activates Raf-1 by the phosphorylation at Ser 338 [84]. However, this is contradicted by Antonio et al. who show that S338 phosphorylation of Raf-1 is independent of PI3K and PAK [85]. Raf is also activated by AKT at Ser 259 [86] and this Raf-AKT crosstalk is regulated in a concentration and ligand dependent manner [87]. AKT is also shown to inhibit the Raf/ERK pathway by phosphorylating the Ser428 and Thr439 residues in the amino terminal regulatory domain of B-Raf [88]. Alternatively, constitutive activation of Raf/MAPK has been shown to inhibit AKT and cell cycle arrest specifically through MEK-1 [89]. Another point of crosstalk between the PI3K and MAPK pathway is via PDK1, which targets MEK1 and MEK2 by phosphorylation at Ser222 and Ser226, respectively [90].

Studies have also suggested crosstalk between PI3K and JNK signaling pathway. JNK2 has been reported to convey Src/PI3K signal for growth and metastasis by enhancing GAB2 (Grb2 associated binding protein 2) expression in 4TI mammary tumour cells [91]. A study by Logan et al. showed that dominant negative PI3K as well as Wortmannin blocked EGF induced JNK activation, suggesting crosstalk between PI3K/JNK pathways [92]. Studies done in nasopharyngeal cancer (NPC) has shown that activity of Matrix metalloprotease-9 (MMP9) is blocked only upon combined inhibition of PI3K and JNK, alluding to importance of JNK/PI3K crosstalk in NPC progression [93].

Hyperactivation of Ras signaling has been observed in melanoma and this attributes to alterations in both upstream and downstream components of the Ras pathway. Two important effectors of the Ras signaling are the MAPK and PI3K pathways. The significance of crosstalk between PI3K and MAPK in melanoma is supported by work of Merighi et al. in which the binding of an agonist to A3 adenosine receptor is shown to activate PLC-PI3K, which in turn reduces the pERK1/2 levels (MAPK) that is necessary for proliferation [94]. B-Raf is one of the most commonly mutated genes in melanoma. Potential mechanisms of B-Raf involvement in melanoma progression features crosstalk between AKT and ^{V600E}B-Raf. The frequently observed B-Raf mutation, ^{V600E}B-Raf results in the increased activation of MAPK that leads to senescence. On the other hand, phosphorylation at Ser^{364} and Ser^{428} of ^{V600E}B-Raf due to aberrant activity of AKT, as in case of melanoma promotes melanoma progression [95]. Brenden et al. proposes that ^{V600E}B-Raf negatively regulates AKT through its interaction with mTORC2. In cells with wild type AKT signaling, ^{V600E}B-Raf interacts with mTORC2 exerting a negative effect on AKT phosphorylation which prevent cell survival. However, in cells with aberrantly activated AKT signaling (due to PTEN loss leading to PI3K activation) as in case of melanoma, the effect of the negative impact from ^{V600E}B-Raf interaction with mTORC2 on AKT is countered by strong upstream signals that activate AKT signaling and lead to cell survival and melanoma progression [96]. Crosstalk between PI3K and MAPK is also mediated via PTEN. Studies with animal model have shown that ^{V600E}B-Raf expression alone was not sufficient to cause development of melanoma. However expression of ^{V600E}B-Raf in the background of PTEN silencing resulted in melanomagenesis and progression [97].

3.2. PI3K – NF-κB Cross Talk

NFκB signaling pathway is a key player in cancer. The NFκB family proteins comprises of two subfamilies: NFκB proteins (p105, p100) and Rel proteins (RelA, RelB, c-Rel) and its activity is tightly regulated by its interaction with inhibitory proteins I-κB. NFκB remains inactive in the cytoplasm by the inhibitory effect of I-κB. When I-κis phosphorylated by I-κB kinase (IKK), it is targeted for degradation resulting in the activation of NFκB. Once activated, NFκB enters the nucleus and activates the transcription of downstream targets that are involved in cell survival, apoptosis and cell migration and hence is implicated in tumour progression [98]. Several mechanisms of cross talk between PI3K and NFκB pathways have been reported in many cancers. NFκB was shown to be activated by AKT-induced activation of the IKK complex upon stimulation by Tumour Necrosis Factor (TNF-α) and Platelet Derived Growth Factor (PDGF) [99, 100]. Alternatively, Sizemore et al. show that AKT activates the p65/Rel A subunit of NFκB in a PI3K dependent manner in the absence ofdegradation of I-κB by IKK complex [101]. Another mechanism of crosstalk is proposed in a study by Madrid. V et al. which illustrates that the stimulation of transactivation of p65/Rel A by AKT requires IKK and p38 MAPK [102]. The PI3K-NFκB cross talk is reported to promote cell survival by suppressing apoptosis [103, 104, 105, 106, 107] and inducing EMT and metastasis [108, 109] in various cancers.

In melanoma, constitutive activation of IKK activity and enhanced degradation of I-κB was found to significantly activate NFκB compared to normal skin [110, 111, 112, 113, 114]. The nuclear levels of NFκB has been shown to increase with disease progression from dysplastic nevi to primary melanoma and metastatic melanoma, indicating that up-regulation of NFκB plays a role in enhancing melanoma progression [115]. NFκB was also shown to promote angiogenesis and metastasis in melanoma [110]. Punita et al. showed that crosstalk between the PI3K and NFκB pathways resulted in constitutive activation of AKT that resulted in up-regulation of NFκB and prevention of apoptosis in melanoma cells [72].

3.3. PI3K – TGFβ Pathway Crosstalk

TGFβ constitutes a superfamily of cytokines that regulate developmental processes and deregulation of this pathway has been shown to promote cancer genesis and progression. Binding of TGFβ to its trans-membrane Ser-Thr kinase receptor complex (TGFβR1, TGFβR2) activates intracellular mediators called Smads. There are three types of Smads; the regulatory or R-Smads (Smad – 1, 2, 3, 5, 8), co-smad (Smad-4) and inhibitory Smad (Smad 7). In the nucleus, R-Smads and co-Smad bind to various co-activators or co-repressors and regulate gene expression [116]. A comparison of the levels of different isoforms of TGFβ in normal melanocyte, nevi and melanoma showed that while TGFβ-1 is expressed in only some melanocytes, it is expressed uniformly in nevi as well as primary and metastatic melanoma. TGFβ-2 and TGFβ-3 isoforms were not expressed in melanocytes but were expressed in nevi, primary and metastatic melanoma [117]. Elevated levels of TGFβ-1 and TGFβ-2 have also been reported in patients with disseminated melanoma [118]. Inhibition of TGFβ pathway was shown to reduce bone metastasis in melanoma [119] and expression of TGFβ2 was shown to be critical for metastasis and invasiveness in melanoma [120]. Further, over-expression of Smad-7 was shown to decrease tumourigenicity and metastasis [121, 122,123]. Collectively, these reports highlight the significance of TGFβ signaling pathway in melanoma. Crosstalk between TGFβ and PI3K pathway was recently reported in a study by Fang et al., where stimulation of Nodal (member of TGFβ superfamily) was accompanied with increased levels of phospho-AKT leading to Snail-mediated EMT in melanoma [124].

3.4. PI3K – Notch Pathway Crosstalk

Notch signaling regulates the normal development of many tissues and hence perturbations in the pathway contribute to cancer development. Canonical Notch signaling involves the activation of the Notch receptor by ligands Delta and Jagged/Serate. The binding of ligands leads to the intra-membranal proteolysis of the intact receptor, releasing within the cytoplasm a soluble fragment containing intracellular domain called Notch intracellular domain (NICD). NICD has a nuclear localization sequence which allows the protein to enter the nucleus and regulates the transcription of target genes [125]. Gene expression studies support a role of Notch signaling in melanoma [126, 127]. The expression of Notch receptors and ligands are up-regulated in dysplastic nevi and melanoma compared to normal melanocytic nevi [128, 129]. Although Notch 1 signaling is elevated in melanoma, AKT and hypoxic conditions are required for melanomagenesis to occur [130]. Further, a role of Notch 1 signaling in promoting vertical growth phase of primary melanoma to aggressive phenotype was shown to be mediated by activation of AKT and MAPK pathways. This is underscored by the observation that effect of the Notch 1 signaling in melanoma progression is reversed with inhibition of either MAPK or the AKT pathways [131]. Collectively, these studies support the importance of crosstalk between PI3K and Notch signaling pathway in promoting melanomagenesis and progression.

3.5. PI3K – JAK-STAT Pathway Crosstalk

Janus kinase – signal transducer and activator of transcription (JAK-STAT) pathway conveys the information from polypeptide signals. Upon ligand binding, JAK activates the members of STAT family of proteins by phosphorylation of a single tyrosine moiety. When activated, STATs form dimers and enter the nucleus, where they bind to response elements on promoter regions of target genes and regulate their transcription [132, 133]. Reports indicate that the JAK-STAT pathway is associated with survival of melanoma cells. Different components of JAK-STAT pathway are observed to be defective in melanoma cell lines resistant to the anti-proliferative effect of interferon, highlighting a key role of this pathway in mediating the anti-proliferative signals from interferon [134]. However, this is contradicted with the study by David et al. which shows presence of the components of JAK-STAT pathway in MeWo melanoma cell line that is resistant to interferon response [135]. Melanoma cells are shown to have Interleukin-29 (IL-29) receptors on the surface, which when activated by IL-29 leads to apoptosis via JAK-STAT signaling [136]. Crosstalk between the PI3K and JAK-STAT pathways was reported in a study by M Krasilnikov et al., who showed that inhibition of MAPK and PI3K pathways led to down-regulation of JAK-STAT pathway and increased sensitivity to apoptosis [137].

3.6. PI3K- mTOR Crosstalk

The mTOR signaling pathway regulates cell growth, proliferation, survival and division in response to nutrients and growth factors via the regulation of protein synthesis. mTOR is a downstream effector of many pathways but is primarily activated by the PI3K pathway. mTOR comprises of two multiprotein complexes namely mTORC1 and mTORC2. mTORC1 is sensitive to rapamycin and mediates protein translation by activating S6K1 and 4EBP1 via signaling pathways like PI3K, MAPK and AMPK. mTORC2 is insensitive to rapamycin and regulates the actin cytoskeleton by activating PKC-α and AKT [138]. mTORC1 has five components; mTOR, the catalytic domain, regulatory-associated protein of mTOR (Raptor), mammalian lethal with Sec13 protein 8 (mLST8), proline rich AKT substrate 40 (PRAS40) and DEP domain containing mTOR interacting protein (Deptor). PRAS40 and Deptor are negative regulators, whereas mLST8 positively regulates mTOR kinase activity. mTORC2 has six components; rapamycin insensitive companion of mTOR (Rictor), mammalian stress activated protein kinase interacting protein (mSIN1), protein observed with Rictor-1 (Proctor-1), mLST8 and Deptor [139]. Activation of mTOR by PI3K pathway is the prototypic mechanism. However, there are several other AKT-independent mechanisms of activation. Since this section is focussed on crosstalk with the PI3K pathway, we will selectively discuss the AKT dependent mechanism/s of activation. As previously mentioned AKT is activated upon its phosphorylation by PDK 1 and PDK 2 (mTORC2 is now accepted as a PDK2) proteins. Phosphorylated AKT further activates mTORC1 in a tuberous sclerosis protein-2 (TSC-2)-dependent or independent manner. TSC-2 suppresses the activity of Ras-related GTPase Rheb, an activator of mTORC1. Hence, inhibition of TSC-2 by AKT leads to activation of mTORC1. AKT can also bind directly to PRAS40, thereby attenuating its inhibitory effect on mTORC1 leading to mTORC1 activation independent of TSC2 [140]. Activated mTORC1 promotes translation by inhibiting 4EBP1 (inhibitor of translation) or activating the S6K1.

mTOR signaling plays a role in various facets of cancer progression such as cell motility, and apoptosis and this has been supported with several studies. Increased mRNA levels of Rictor, mTOR and Raptor has been observed in advanced stages of colorectal cancer (CRC) and CRC metastasis was shown to be reduced with inhibition of mTORC1 and mTORC2, highlighting the significance of mTOR signaling in cancer progression and metastasis [141]. An *in vivo* mouse model study showed that CRC metastasis is inhibited upon treatment with rapamycin (mTOR inhibitor) and this is mainly due to reduction of VEGF levels. This prompts a role of mTOR in angiogenesis [142]. The importance of mTOR signaling in various cancers such as prostate cancer [143], ovarian cancer [144, 145], leukemia [146], breast cancer [147], colorectal cancer [148], hematologic malignancies [149], lung cancer [150], oral cancer [151] has been reported.

Many studies support the role of PI3K/ mTOR pathway in melanoma. mTOR is shown to be activated in malignant melanoma (73%) compared to benign nevi (4%) [152] and activated mTOR pathway in melanoma was associated with poor prognosis [153]. Study by Aziz et al. shows the co-expression of mTOR and PI3K, especially the p110 catalytic subunit in melanoma, signifying the role of PI3K/mTOR pathway [154]. Chemo-sensitivity of melanoma cells was shown to improve with inhibition of PI3K/ mTOR pathway [155], which highlights the importance of the PI3K/ mTOR pathway in supporting and promoting melanoma.

This section outlined the crosstalk of several signal transduction pathways with the PI3K pathway leading to melanoma progression. Section 4 will focus on the canonical Wnt signaling pathway and its crosstalk with the PI3K pathway in melanoma. The crosstalk between these two pathways is of significant interest to this review due to the role of these pathways independently and their putative crosstalk in melanoma progression.

Section 4. Wnt/β-Catenin and PI3K Pathway

4.1. β-Catenin

4.1.1. Structure and Function

β-catenin is a 781 amino acid protein encoded by the CTNNB1 gene that is highly conserved throughout species and shares 67% homology to the Drosophila Armadillo protein [156]. β-catenin's primary structure is composed of two terminal domains; the N-terminal

(NTD) and C-terminal (CTD) domains, and a central Armadillo (ARM) domain. β-catenin's structure allows binding of specific partners at distinct sites across the terminal domains and the central domain. The ARM domain is characteristic of the Armadillo/catenin family of proteins, and is distinguished by a positively charged groove of densely packed α-helices [157] comprising of 12 imperfect repeats of 42 amino acids (total 550 amino acids) [158, 157].

The crystal structure of the ARM repeat domain shows that each repeat consists of three helices, H1, H2, and H3 [157] and the repeats pack against one another to form a positively charged superhelix. This positively charged groove is ideal for β-catenin to bind its various negatively charged partners. When these interactors are post-translationally modified by phosphorylation, effectively increasing the magnitude of the negative charge, β-catenin's binding affinity with these interactors is augmented [159]. The ARM domain folds into a single structural unit where its surface serves to bind the majority of β-catenin's partners, such as cadherins, TCF/LEF transcription factors and APC [158].

The NTD and CTD of β-catenin are less evolutionarily conserved relative to the central ARM domain. The NTD is important for the stability of the cytoplasmic levels of β-catenin while both the NTD and CTD are significant in β-catenin's role as a co-activator/transactivator of TCF/LEF transcriptional activity. The established role of the CTD in recruiting factors required for regulation of gene expression is dependent on the interaction with cellular partners at the proximal structured elements of this region, such as helix C, which directly follows the 12th arm repeat [160]. The functions for the more distal unstructured region of the CTD remain poorly defined. Furthermore, the acidic charge distribution of the NTD and CTD creates a tertiary structure that brings the NTD and CTD in close proximity to the largely basic ARM domain. Since the NTD and CTD are highly negatively charged and the structural groove of the ARM domain is highly positively charged it is likely that both the NTD and CTD tails of β-catenin interact with the groove of the ARM domain through non-specific charge interactions [158]. The NTD and CTD serve as intramolecular chaperones of the ARM repeat domain which increases the binding specificity and prevents the self-aggregation of the armadillo repeat domain region [158]. Post-translational modifications, such as phosphorylation pattern which change the charge of β-catenin may further result in conformational change or stabilization of the N and/or C tails causing a regulation in binding specific interactors [158].

The CTD also plays a role in the interaction of β-catenin with a number of nuclear factors including, TATA Binding Protein (TBP) [161] Sox 17 and 13, histone deacetylase, SMAD4, the retinoic acid receptor, the CREB binding protein and related proteins [162] as well as transcriptional inhibitors such as ICAT, and Chibby [163, 164].

At Cellular Membrane

At the cell membrane, β-catenin is an important component of the adherens junctions, where it links E-cadherin and α-catenin to the actin cytoskeleton. The adherens junction is essential in maintaining the seamless cell-cell interaction of the epithelial phenotype and provides the cell with structural integrity. The binding of E-cadherin to β-catenin spans the entire ARM region [159] although the actual sites of interaction are concentrated within ARM repeats 4-12 [165]. Tyrosine (Tyr) modification of β-catenin regulates the disassembly of adherens junctions and is regulated by phosphorylation of Tyr-654 of the final armadillo repeat which leads to decreased binding of E-cadherin and β-catenin [166]. A possible mechanism by Piedra and colleagues suggests that this may be due to decreased interaction between ARM and CTD with the phosphorylation of Tyr-654 [162]. Interestingly, this phosphorylation neither affect the association of nuclear factors such as TBP (binding site 639-729), nor TCF-4 (T-cell factor 4) at the CTD. This supports the fact that the CTD is an integral regulatory component which facilitates the interactions of β-catenin with E-cadherin [162].

In the Cytoplasm and Nucleus

While β-catenin linked to E-cadherin is deemed to be highly stable, the cytosolic and nuclear pools are quite dynamic. The subcellular localization of β-catenin is largely regulated by direct competition of β-catenin's binding to E-cadherin and TCF. The N-terminal of TCF forms extensive contacts at ARM 3-9 of β-catenin which bears structural similarities to the E-cadherin-β-catenin interaction. To this end, overexpression of cadherins has been shown to inhibit the transcriptional activity of β-catenin [167]. Furthermore, binding to cadherins can effectively sequester β-catenin within the plasma membrane/cytoplasm and inhibit its signaling efficacy [168].

4.1.2. β-Catenin/Canonical Wnt Pathway

β-catenin is a dual function protein. It plays a role in intercellular adhesion and in regulating gene expression. The latter role is associated with its oncogenic properties. Its second role is as a transcriptional co-activator of the canonical Wnt signaling pathway. The Wnt signal transduction pathway is an essential regulatory pathway that directs cell proliferation, cell polarity and cell fate determination [168]. β-catenin's fate as an adhesion molecule or a transcriptional activator is determined by its intracellular stability. The Wnt pathway largely regulates the intracellular stability of β-catenin.

In the absence of Wnt occupancy of its receptor, free cytoplasmic β-catenin levels are regulated by a multi-protein destruction complex comprising the scaffold protein Axin, the tumour suppressor Adenomatous Polyposis Coli (APC), GSK3β and Casein Kinase-1 (CK-1). Axin is a central protein of the destruction complex that functions as a scaffold that brings all the components into close proximity. APC plays a key role in the regulation of β-catenin turnover since cells containing a mutant APC have elevated β-catenin levels. GSK3β binds a central region within Axin, with a single Axin helix fitting into a hydrophobic groove in the C-terminus of GSK3β, leaving the GSK3β active site free to phosphorylate β-catenin [169]. CK1 binds Axin and phosphorylates β-catenin at Ser45 in order to prime the N-terminal for phosphorylation at residues Ser33, Ser37 and Thr41 by GSK3β [170, 171, 172]. This phosphorylation creates a site for ubiquitination of β-catenin by E3 ubiquitin ligase β-transducin repeat-containing protein (β-Trcp), resulting in β-catenin's subsequent proteosomal degradation [168].

Wnts are secreted glycoproteins that bind to frizzled (Fz) seven-transmembrane spanned receptors. There are 19 known Wnt ligands, three of which are known to stimulate the canonical Wnt pathway in humans, namely Wnt 1, 3 and Wnt8 [168]. Particular Wnt ligands are responsible for embryonic development in several different species. A complete listing of the particular Wnts is described by Dr. Roel Nusse's laboratory [173]. Wnt ligands bind to Fz receptors which are coupled with heterotrimeric G proteins. In the canonical pathway, LRP

5/6, low-density lipoprotein receptors, are co-receptors of Wnt ligands. Upon binding of Wnt ligands, the activated Fz recruits the intracellular protein dishevelled (Dvl), which in recruits the GSK3β-Axin complex. Following recruitment of this complex to the plasma membrane LRP6 is phosphorylated [174]. Wnt-induced LRP6 phosphorylation is a key event in receptor activation [175]. These phosphorylated sites serve as docking sites for Axin complex [176, 175] thereby recruiting Axin to LRP6 upon Wnt stimulation [177]. Further phosphorylation of LRP6 by CK-1 (Davidson et al. 2005; Zeng et al. 2008) results in the clustering of various proteins—including LRP6, Dvl, and Axin—to form what has been referred to as the LRP6 signalosome [178]. Formation of this complex from the phosphorylation of LRP5/6 leads to inhibition of the "destruction complex". Deactivation of the destruction complex results in stabilization of β-catenin within the cytoplasm and its targeted entry into the nucleus, where it binds to the T-cell factor (TCF)/Lymphoid Enhancer Factor (LEF) family of transcription factors leading to transcriptional activation of Wnt target genes [179].

Within the nucleus, the CTD of β-catenin interacts with the TCF family of proteins, which anchor β-catenin to specific promoters for the transcription of Wnt target genes [180]. Many of these target genes, such as cMyc, Cyclin D1, vascular endothelial growth factor A (VEGFA) and matrix metalloproteases (MMPs) have implications in cell survival, cell proliferation, growth, cell cycle progression and invasion along with several others that can be found on the following page: http://www.stanford.edu/group/nusselab/cgi-bin/wnt/target_genes [173]. Since the canonical Wnt pathway regulates transcription of genes involved in cell cycle, growth and survival, uncontrolled activation of the pathway is highly significant in disease pathophysiology. Constitutive activation of the canonical Wnt pathway results in positive regulation of cell survival and negative regulation on cell death/apoptosis. These changes in cellular properties associated with elevated cellular β-catenin are associated with poor prognosis in many human cancers including adenocarcinoma of the prostate and breast as well as melanoma [168].

4.1.3. Active β-Catenin

Upon Canonical Wnt pathway activation, GSK3β associated with the axin scaffold is inhibited allowing β-catenin to evade degradation. The cytoplasmic accumulation of β-catenin is thought to ultimately result in its translocation to the nucleus. However, this translocation alone is not sufficient for β-catenin/TCF transcriptional activity [181, 182]. Staal and colleagues demonstrated that the increased half-life of β-catenin upon Wnt signaling was not a direct consequence of its stability [182]. The phosphorylation status of the NTD of β-catenin upon Wnt signaling independently affected the signaling properties and half-life of β-catenin. In fact, it is not so much the accumulation of β-catenin per se but the dephosphorylation of specific amino acids at the NTD of β-catenin that is important in generating a transcriptionally active form of β-catenin [182, 160]. Maher and colleagues demonstrated that the cadherin free form of β-catenin unphosphorylated at S37 and T41 (transcriptionally active- β-catenin (ABC)) is largely monomeric and located mainly within the nucleus. Active-β-catenin is found to be intrinsically more transcriptionally active than the non-phosphorylated β-catenin [160]. The predominant nuclear accumulation of the active-β-catenin is due to its low concentration within the cell, which renders it less likely to be bound by the cadherins and α-catenin [160]. Furthermore, β-catenin phosphorylated at three sites; S33, S37 and T41 is found to be more retained within the cytosol, as well as subject to increased nuclear export. Maher and colleagues also established that β-catenin phosphorylated at T41/S45 strongly co-localizes with active-β-catenin within the nucleus and is largely a cadherin-free form of β-catenin. This suggests that the nuclear form of β-catenin phosphorylated at Ser45 may also be a signaling/active form of β-catenin. Referring back to the Wnt pathway, β-catenin is phosphorylated at Ser45 by CK1 in a priming mechanism, allowing subsequent phosphorylation by GSK3β at Ser 33, 37 and T41 [171]. Therefore, it is possible that the priming of β-catenin at S45 by CK1 may be a temporal regulatory mechanism that couples β-catenin phosphorylation and degradation to β-catenin nuclear signaling. The fact that β-catenin phosphorylated at the three sites of phosphorylation by GSK3β does not completely overlap with β-catenin phosphorylated at serine 45 and threonine 41, suggests a possible spatial separation of the two kinase activities of GSK3β and CK1 [160]. In addition to serving as a priming site for phosphorylation, the phosphorylation at Serine 45 may facilitate the phosphorylation pattern of β-catenin making it transcriptionally active. However, this has to be investigated further as this idea is yet primitive [160]. High levels of nuclear phospho-β-catenin are associated with significantly worse overall survival [70]. Using a phosphorylation specific antibody Kielhorn and colleagues determined that nuclear β-catenin staining was more prevalent in advanced melanomas [183]. This may be due to the specific phosphorylation pattern of β-catenin having specificity for TCF thereby allowing transcription of cancer causing genes.

4.1.4. Localization

β-catenin is present in the cytoplasmic compartment as well as the nucleus. A well-defined feature of active-β-catenin is that it is located exclusively in the nucleus [182]. However, the mechanism of the nuclear localization of β-catenin is currently unknown. β-catenin does not contain a nuclear localization sequence (NLS) nor utilize the importin transport machinery [184]. However, nuclear export of β-catenin is established to be mediated by an intrinsic export signal and its interaction with APC. The retention of β-catenin within the nucleus is thought to be due to its interaction within the nucleus with TCF, BCL-9 and pygopous [184]. However, these interactions are not a prerequisite for β-catenin's localization into the nucleus as it has been demonstrated that the protein can successfully localize to the nucleus in the absence of these interactions. Overexpression of LEF/TCF has been shown to lead to β-catenin's accumulation in the nucleus [185, 186]. It has been suggested that the nuclear import of the β-catenin/LEFcomplex is mediated by the NLS provided by LEF/TCF proteins. However, elevations in nuclear levels of β-catenin are observed even when the levels of LEF/TCF are low [186, 187]. Therefore, mechanisms independent of LEF/TCF are likely to be important for regulating the nuclear import of β-catenin *in vivo* [188]. Two groups have independently demonstrated a direct importin-independent nuclear import of β-catenin in a semi-permeabilized cell model [189, 190]. However, to date no mandatory chaperone essential to the nuclear transport of β-catenin has been identified. In summary, within the nucleus, β-catenin specifically active-β-catenin, has an oncogenic role as it serves as a transcriptional co-activator of cancer promoting target genes.

4.1.5. β-Catenin in Cancer

In carcinomas, the loss of β-catenin-E-cadherin complexes is an important step in disease progression. Loss of organization by disruption of epithelial complexes at adherens junctions is a common feature of invasiveness. Furthermore, deregulation of the Wnt signaling pathway at various levels, often leads to metastasis and cancer progression as Wnt target genes are responsible for controlling the regulation of cell cycle, proliferation and inhibition of apoptosis. A common effect of deregulated/activated Wnt pathway components is an over-expression of β-catenin. Many common cancers including, colorectal cancer (CRC) [191], hepatocellular carcinoma [192], adrenal cancers [193, 194], breast cancer [195], Wilm's tumour [196], several hematological malignancies [197] and melanomas [63] have been found to have a deregulated Wnt pathway. Some of the causative factors of this deregulation are the loss of function mutations in APC or Axin [197], or mutations in the amino acids at the NTD of β-catenin which interfere with its phosphorylation and proteosomal degradation [191]. Truncating mutations in Axin cause nuclear accumulation of β-catenin in hepatocellular carcinomas [198]. Furthermore, APC is mutated in 85% of familial and sporadic CRCs [199]. Mutations have also been found to occur in exon 3 of the β-catenin gene, affecting sites of phosphorylation by GSK3β, making β-catenin refractory to degradation [200]. The result of mutations in the Wnt pathway is an elevation of total cellular levels of β-catenin and the activation of β-catenin dependent TCF/LEF transcription which mediates its oncogenic effect in various tissues. Over activation of the canonical Wnt signaling pathway results in up regulation of several cell growth regulatory proteins and processes, consequently resulting in cancer progression.

4.1.6. β-Catenin in Melanoma

Wnt-β-catenin signaling is up regulated in melanoma, and approximately 30% of melanoma exhibit increased nuclear β-catenin [63]. The high frequency of nuclear accumulation is not all attributable to mutations in the Wnt pathway. The discrepancy between these datasets prompts the investigation of putative mechanisms responsible for the excessive accumulation of nuclear β-catenin. The mechanism that regulates β-catenin's transcriptional activity of Wnt target genes needs further investigation. Determining how this nuclear pool of β-catenin is regulated by the Wnt pathway alongside other pathways to orchestrate the transcription of target genes is an area of study that needs much anticipated investigation. This would be a leap into the study of melanoma formation and tumour progression [63]. A thorough understanding of the pathway will provide a look into cell specific molecular mechanisms involved in initiation and progression of melanoma. β-catenin expression in melanoma has been shown to be different than many other cancers. Several studies using melanoma cell lines show a decrease in nuclear and cytoplasmic staining in malignant cell lines compared to a benign nevus stage [201]. This creates contradiction of β-catenin's expression pattern in other cancers where β-catenin levels are elevated as the cancer progresses, such as hepatoma, gastric and bladder cancers [201]. Little is known specifically about changes in active-β-catenin in melanoma progression, the pool of β-catenin relevant in the transcription of genes for the proteins that promote metastasis. Demunter and colleagues showed that post-translational modifications of β-catenin rather than mutations in the CTNNB1 gene itself are responsible for the altered distribution of β-catenin in the cell (Demunter et al., 2002). The fact that β-catenin serves many roles in the cell and has variability in its phosphorylation pattern may be an explanation as to why many studies measuring overall levels of β-catenin show an inverse relationship in melanoma progression and β-catenin levels. The fact that phospho-β-catenin is more prevalent in metastatic melanomas is consistent with the fact that β-catenin serves different roles and functions in a cell [202]. Kiehlhorn and colleagues suggests that phosphorylation specific antigen of β-catenin is correlated with a better marker of disease progression than overall levels, which are masked with different pools of β-catenin. However, high transcriptional activity of β-catenin in certain disease conditions cannot be attributed to mutations in β-catenin or components of the Wnt pathway. In support of this, β-catenin, recently identified as a candidate gene for melanoma progression, was found to be mutated in 5% of melanomas but constitutively active (nuclear expression and transcriptional activity) in 40-50% of melanomas [63]. This suggests that alternate regulatory mechanisms/pathways in controlling the oncogenic/transcriptional properties of β-catenin are involved. Although the canonical Wnt pathway is well characterized in the regulation of cellular β-catenin levels, several investigations suggest that β-catenin may also be regulated by other signal transduction pathways via potential cross talk. In particular, the phosphotidylinositol-3 kinase (PI3K) pathway has been significantly implicated in the regulation of β-catenin [203].

4.2. Crosstalk between the PI3K and Canonical Wnt Pathways in Melanoma Progression

There are divergent views on the role of the PI3K pathway in the regulation of β-catenin. There are several different hypotheses around how these two pathways may be linked. The regulation of β-catenin by the two pathways may be through direct crosstalk via a common component. Since GSK3β is a common component of both pathways, several studies suggest that the inactivation of GSK3β by AKT links the PI3K pathway to the Wnt pathway in a bipartite mechanism which subsequently regulates the cytoplasmic levels of β-catenin [204]. However, other studies propose that the Wnt and PI3K pathways remain distinct and variably regulate alternate pools of GSK3β [205]. Other components such as AKT, TGFβ1, mTOR and PI3K have also been suggested as linkers between the Wnt and PI3K pathways.

4.2.1. GSK3β As a Potential Candidate to Mediate Crosstalk between Wnt/β-Catenin and PI3K Pathways

There are two schools of thought regarding PI3K/Wnt crosstalk. One hypothesis states that both pathways signal through a common pool of GSK3β while an alternative hypothesis suggests two segregated pools of GSK3β. There is evidence supporting both hypotheses: Sharma et al. [206] saw that increased levels of PI3K signaling correspond to nuclear accumulation of β-catenin in what was assumed to be a GSK3β dependent mechanism since GSK3β is deactivated via AKT phosphorylation. They noted that inhibition of PI3K reduces AKT and GSK3β phosphorylation and subsequently decreases nuclear accumulation of β-catenin. However, many other studies suggest a more segregated pool of GSK3β linking the PI3K and Wnt systems.

The PI3K pathway, via AKT, elicits cellular responses through an array of downstream effectors, one of which is GSK3β. In this pathway GSK3β serves various roles such as protein synthesis, glycogen metabolism and cell cycle regulation [207, 208]. Insulin stimulation of the PI3K pathway results in downstream phosphorylation by AKT at Ser 9 of GSK3β and Ser 21 of GSK3α, resulting in the inactivation of GSK3β [209]. This inactivation further dephosphorylates and activates glycogen synthase (GS), which promotes the synthesis of glycogen (Nature 378, 785-789). By this mechanism, the phosphorylation of GSK3β turns off its catalytic activity thereby deregulating GSK3β and activating downstream targets that are normally repressed by GSK3β.

It has been suggested that interactions of GSK3β with a specific pathway may effectively shield GSK3β from the influences from other alternate pathways resulting in its specificity of effects to any one particular pathway at any one time. Ding et al. saw that the effect of each signaling pathway is highly specific, and changes to GSK3β activity in one pathway may not affect the downstream events of the components of the other pathway [210]. Another reason that may cause differential regulation may be a difference in post-translational modification of the GSK3β. The serine 9 phosphorylation of GSK3β is specific to PI3K signaling, and is not affected by the Wnt pathway activity. As Ding and colleagues showed Wnt stimulation does not cause phosphorylation of AKT at Thr-308 or Ser-473, nor phosphorylation of GSK3β on Ser-9 [210], therefore AKT is not the mediator of endogenous Wnt signals disrupting the destruction complex. Patel and colleagues also looked at the effect on β-catenin levels following activation of the PI3K pathway via insulin stimulation, which resulted in a decrease in overall GSK3β activity. Although there was a change in GSK3β activity they saw no change in β-catenin levels and therefore concluded that β-catenin regulation is "insulated from other signaling pathways" [211]. Further support comes from Ng and colleagues who reported that the Axin bound pool of GSK3β, which comprises 3-5% of total cellular GSK3β, compartmentalizes the pools involved in the wnt pathway [205]. This sequestration of the GSK3β prevents the Wnt pathway associated GSK3 and the subsequent Wnt-induced transcriptional activity from being affected by PI3K pathway [205]. It is possible that, although GSK3β downstream of PI3K and Wnt may be segregated, activation of AKT can affect both pools of GSK3β. The resulting reduction in activity of both pools of GSK3β may then contribute synergistically to the cellular accumulation β-catenin. However, this decrease must be in the order of 75-80% to have significant effect on Wnt signaling [212], as AKT would more easily alter the activity of GSK3β not sequestered by Axin due to quantity and availability within the cytoplasm.

4.2.2. Other Potential Candidates That Mediate Crosstalk between Wnt/β-Catenin and PI3K Pathways

4.2.2.1. AKT

There may be other components of the PI3K pathway which may be involved in changes in β-catenin and the Wnt pathway such as, AKT. AKT is a key effector of the PI3K system, canonically being phosphorylated in a PI3K-dependent fashion by PDK1 and PDK2. By phosphorylating GSK3β, AKT may induce inactivation of the destruction complex and thereby allowing β-catenin to accumulate in an AKT-dependent manner. Sharma et al. suggest an AKT-dependent increase in nuclear localization of β-catenin, which may operate through this type of direct mechanism [206]. Fukumoto et al. suggest that while AKT activity might not be sufficient to mimic a Wnt signal, it might prolong the duration of the signal to enhance the effect of the signal [213]. Thus increased phosphorylation of AKT by deregulated PI3K pathway might lead to longer periods of destruction complex inactivation and therein induce an increased accumulation of β-catenin. AKT has also been shown to directly modulate β-catenin interaction with E-cadherin, which comprises a central portion of the adherens junction [214]. He et al. [215] has shown that by phosphorylating Ser552 of β-catenin, AKT induces separation of β-catenin from E-cadherin and thereby frees it to accumulate unbound in the cell and subsequently promotes nuclear localization of β-catenin. AKT phosphorylation at additional sites of β-catenin increases its interaction with 14-3-3ζ, an oncogenic chaperone with implicated roles in signaling, cell cycle control and regulation of apoptosis [216]. Binding with 14-3-3ζ causes β-catenin to accumulate in the cytoplasm, sequestered away from E-cadherin. More importantly, this interaction inhibits β-catenin's binding with β-Trcp, inhibiting the proteosomal degradation of β-catenin and in turn increasing its stability. While binding to 14-3-3ζ reduces β-catenin's binding to B-Trcp, it actually increases β-catenin's affinity for its nuclear interactor Lef4. This may implicate 14-3-3ζ as playing a vital role as a chaperone in regulating β-catenin activity.

Dihlmann et al. show that β-catenin transcriptionally regulates AKT1, and Zhang et al. (2011) found similar regulation of AKT2 [217]. Additionally, Fukumoto et al. showed that Wnt signaling induces phosphorylation of AKT in the presence of Dvl [213]. This Dvl-dependent p-AKT binds the Axin destruction complex in the presence of Dvl, phosphorylating GSK3β and inducing accumulation of β-catenin. In this manner, AKT acts in a Dvl-dependent manner to transduce the canonical Wnt signal. The mechanism by which AKT is phosphorylated is not discussed, but its phosphorylation is measured at Thr308 and Ser473, its canonical PI3K dependent phosphorylation sites. If its phosphorylation is PI3K-dependent but is induced by Wnt signaling, a cyclic interaction between the PI3K and Wnt pathways may exist. To this end, Wnt signals would increase canonical AKT phosphorylation through PI3K, and newly phosphorylated AKT may bind in a Dvl-dependent manner to the axin destruction complex, wherein it phosphorylates and subsequently deactivates GSK3β. This deactivation of GSK3β would lead to increased stability of β-catenin, which would transcriptionally activate AKT and perpetuate the cycle. If this sort of system exists, deregulation of the PI3K pathway would lead to hypersensitivity of the destruction complex to regular Wnt signaling due to an abundance of activated AKT, thus inducing increased levels of β-catenin accumulation and subsequent translocation to the nucleus.

4.2.2.2. PI3K

PI3K itself is a candidate for crosstalk between PI3K and Wnt pathways. Espada et al. found that β-catenin binds to PI3Ks regulatory subunit p85α with a higher affinity than to its transcriptional partner Lefl [218]. β-catenin binding to p85α sequesters it away from the destruction complex by inhibiting its interaction with APC [218]. Since β-catenin is shielded from APC by p85α, binding to the catalytic domain of PI3K would inhibit its regular degradation pathway and thereby increase its stability. With sequestration from the destruction complex, β-catenin would be allowed to accumulate in the cytoplasm and translocate to the nucleus, where it can act transcriptionally. This may suggest an additional role for PI3K within the cell: its regulatory domain, p85α, may act as a chaperone for β-catenin, sequestering it from the destruction complex and thus inducting its stability. This could be accomplished by either solely sequestration or by inducing a conformational change that promotes some post-secondary modification of β-catenin.

4.2.2.3. mTOR

Some downstream targets of AKT could induce effects that become evident by alterations of AKT activity. One such target is mTOR. As discussed earlier, mTORC1 plays many roles in cellular regulation, translation and autophagy. On the other hand, mTORC2 acts as a PDK2 molecule, capable of phosphorylating molecules such as AKT, though its kinase functionality is not necessarily limited to AKT. As such, mTORC2 may play a role in transducing a signal to components of the Wnt cascade.

mTOR has been identified by Tanwar et al. as a therapeutic target for cancers characterized by deregulated PI3K activity and increased transcriptional activity of β-catenin [219]. Since this targeting is achieved via rapamycin treatment, mTORC1 is implicated. The mTORC1 complex plays roles in increasing protein synthesis through inhibition of 4EBP1, the negative regulator of elongation factor eIF4E [220]. When stimulated by insulin, mTORC1 is activated through PI3K, which downregulates its negative regulator, PRAS40, which specifically inhibits Raptor, a component of mTORC1 [220]. Along with promoting protein synthesis, mTORC1 differentially regulates phosphatase activity [221], which may be required to generate hypophosphorylated active β-catenin phosphorylated at Ser37/Thr41. In the study by Harwood et al., mTORC1 inhibited the phosphatase involved in maintaining the hypophosphorylataion of Thr202 on p44/42, while at the same time promoting the activity of the phosphatase involved in dephosphorylating Tyr204. Both sites require phosphorylation in order to activate p44/42, a key member of the MEK cascade. This suggests a complex role for mTORC1 in the regulation of phosphatase activity. Okadaic acid inhibited the activity of the phosphatase involved in Thr202 in the presence of rapamycin, suggesting that the phosphatase involved is PP2A. If mTORC1 is differentially promoting and inhibiting the activity of certain phosphatases, it may be involved in the generation of selectively hypophosphorylated active β-catenin. In support of this, a study by Liu et al. indicates that nuclear translocation of β-catenin occurs in a rapamycin-sensitive mTOR-dependent manner [222]. These effects may be as a result of mTORC1-induced generation of active β-catenin.

4.2.2.4. TGFβ1

Another downstream target of AKT is TGFβ. Walsh et al. showed that TGFβ1, an isoform of the known oncoprotein TGFB, regulates β-catenin localization in an insulin/PI3K-dependent manner [223]. Upon stimulation of insulin receptors, PI3K is stimulated and production of certain matrix metalloproteinases (MMPs) is promoted downstream. These MMPs cleave latent TGFβ1, activating it so that it can subsequently bind TGFβ1 receptors. This binding results in increased stabilization and nuclear translocation of β-catenin, according to results by Welsh et al. The mechanism for this is currently unknown. However, the binding of TGFβ to TGFβR is known to activate Smad proteins. Smad activates the Snail transcription factor, inhibiting production of E-cadherin [224]. In the absence of E-cadherin, β-catenin has no major interactor at the adherens junction and is allowed to accumulate in the cytoplasm, subsequently translocating to the nucleus. Interestingly, Snail is also modified by O-GlcNAcylation [225]. Since Snail has its transcriptional activity reduced by O-GlcNAcylation in a manner similar to β-catenin, the enzyme beta-N-acetlyglucosaminidase may be downstream of TGFβR, allowing the binding of its ligand to reduce the inhibition of Snail activity through removal of the sugar modification.

Section 5. Current Therapeutics of Melanoma and Concluding Remarks

Currently there are five different types of therapies for melanoma, depending on the stage of the cancer. Surgery, chemotherapy, radiation therapy, targeted therapy and biologic therapy are the treatments presented by the National Cancer Institute.

Surgery is the primary form of treatment as it excises the primary tumour or the lymph nodes to which the tumour cells have metastasized. Chemotherapy with Decarbazine or DTIC [5-(3,3-Dimethyl-1-triazenyl)imidazole-4-carboxamide] and radiation therapy are two other commonly used conventional cancer treatment regimens. Treating melanoma using chemotherapy has poor response rate and the effect is short lived. Biologic therapy targets the patient's immune system to fight the cancer. This therapy boosts the immune system by restoring the body's natural defences. An example is Interleukin -2 (IL-2), which promotes the growth and activity of lymphocytes, a group of cells used by the immune system in its defence against cancer cells. The adverse effects of such treatment are severe side effects at higher doses of these reagents. In light of this these drugs are used in low doses usually in combination with another form of therapy. Targeted therapy is focussed on signal transduction pathway components that are deregulated in melanoma [226]. This form of treatment is very specific compared to other conventional therapies. Some of the drugs that are commonly used in targeted therapy for melanoma are Vemurafenib, Sorafnib and Ipilimumab. Vemurafenib is a commonly used BRAF inhibiting drug which specifically targets BRAF substitution mutations. Sorafnib is a multikinase inhibitor that targets VEGF and Raf/MEK pathways at the level of RAF kinase. Ipilimumab, an antibody against cytotoxic T-lymphocyte (CTL) antigen, is a commonly used drug for stage IV melanoma. This drug removes inhibition of CTLs so they can target and destroy cancer cells [227]. Signaling pathways like the MAPK, PI3K, c-KIT and NFκB which are deregulated in melanoma are also targeted for treating melanoma progression. In this section we will discuss targeting of the components of the PI3K pathway, which is of primary focus in this review.

Perifosine is a novel alkyl phospholipid compound that inhibits AKT. It was shown to have cytotoxic effects in-vitro and in-vivo in human multiple myeloma cells [228]. Vyomesh Patel et al. showed Perifosine to cause cell cycle arrest in-vitro in squamous carcinoma cells by inducing $p21^{WAF1}$ in a p53 independent manner [229]. Sudhir et al. proposed the mechanism for induction of $p21^{WAF1}$ to be via PI3K pathway [230]. BI-69A11 is another inhibitor of AKT. Treatment of melanoma cells in-vitro with BI-69A11 led to reduced levels of AKT and intra-peritoneal injection of BI-69A11 caused primary tumour size regression in melanoma xenografts [231]. Isothiocyanates are naturally occurring compounds with anti-cancerous property. This compound targets AKT and lead to increased apoptosis in melanoma cells with low toxic effects [232]. Apart from these compounds which target AKT, some of the compounds that target mTOR are also found to be significant for melanoma therapy. Phase II study of Everolimus, an mTOR inhibitor in combination with Bevacizumab, an angiogenesis inhibitor has shown moderate efficacy in patients with metastatic melanoma. This combination treatment was also well tolerated by patients [233]. H. Niessner et al. tested the effect of Lonafarnib, an m-TOR inhibitor to cause apoptosis in melanoma cells. Lonafarnib significantly decreased cell growth in combination with sorafnib, a p-Raf inhibitor, whereas it had insufficient effect when used for treatment alone or in combination with other inhibitors of AKT. Hence suggests that lonafarnib inhibits mTOR signaling and potentiates sorafnib mediated apoptosis in melanoma cells [234].

Overall, co-targeting of pathways has proven to be more effective in treating melanoma compared to targeting a single pathway and hence an understanding of crosstalks among signal transduction pathways would be invaluable in increasing and improving the scope for melanoma therapy. Crosstalk between the PI3K and Wnt/β-Catenin pathways is a novel area of study, which will provide several targets of value in melanoma therapies, possibly intervening with metastasis.

References

[1] Carracedo, A., & Pandolfi, P. P. (2008). The PTEN-PI3K pathway: of feedbacks and cross-talks. *Oncogene,* 27, 5527-5541.
[2] Katso, R., Okkenhaug, K. et al. (2001). Cellular function of phosphoinositide 3-kinases: implications for development, homeostasis, and cancer. *Annu Rev Cell Dev Biol,* 17, 615–675.
[3] Petrocelli, T., & Slingerland, J. M. (2001). PTEN deficiency: a role in a mammary carcinogenesis. *Breast Cancer Res,* 3, 356-360.
[4] Fresno Vara, J. A., Casado, E. et al. (2004). PI3K/Akt signaling pathway and cancer. *Cancer Treat Reviews,* 30(2), 193-204.
[5] Paez, J., & Sellers, W. R. (2003). PI3K/PTEN/AKT Pathway. A critical mediator of oncogenic signaling. *Cancer Treat Res.,* 115, 145-67.
[6] Bader, A. G., Kang, S. et al. (2005). Oncogenic PI3K deregulates transcription and translation. *Nat Rev Cancer,* 5, 921–929.
[7] Engelman, J. A., Luo, J. et al. (2006). The evolution of phosphatidylinositol 3-kinases as regulators of growth and metabolism. *Nat Rev Genet,* 7, 606-619.
[8] Backer, J. M. (2008). The regulation and function of class II PI3Ks: novel roles for Vps34. *Biochem J,* 410, 1-17.
[9] Yuan, T. L., & Cantley, L. C. (2008). PI3K pathway alterations in cancer: variations on a theme. *Oncogene,* 27(41), 5497-510.
[10] Vivanco, I. & Sawyers, C. L. (2002). The phosphatidylinositol 3-kinase-akt pathway in human cancer. *Nature Review,* 2, 489-501.
[11] Chalhoub, N., & Baker, S. J. (2009). PTEN and the PI3-kinase pathway in cancer. *Annu Rev Pathol,* 4, 127-50.
[12] Brock,T. (2013). The PI3K Pathway: Fast Forward for Cancer. *Experimental Biology.*
[13] McCall, P. (2010). *The interaction between the PI3K/Akt cascade and the androgen receptor in the development and progression of castrate resistant prostate cancer.* PhD thesis. University of Glasgow.
[14] Ikenoue, T., Kanai, F., et al. (2005). Functional analysis of PIK3CA gene mutations in human colorectal cancer. *Cancer Res,* 65(11), 4562-4567.
[15] Samuels, Y. & Ericson, K. (2006). Oncogenic PI3K and its role in cancer. *Curr Opin Oncol,* 18(1), 77-82.
[16] Myers, M. P., & Tonk, N. K. (1997). PTEN: sometimes taking it off can be better than putting it on. *Am J Hum Genet,* 61(6), 1234-1238.

[17] Stambolic, V., Suzuki, A., et al. (1998). Negative regulation of PKB/Akt-dependent cell survival by the tumour suppressor PTEN. *Cell,* 95, 29–39.

[18] Maehama, T., Taylor, G. S., et al. (2001). PTEN and myotubularin: novel phosphoinositide phosphatases. *Annu Rev Biochem.* 70, 247-279.

[19] Li, D. M., & Sun, H. (1997). TEP1, encoded by a candidate tumour suppressor locus, is a novel protein tyrosine phosphatase regulated by transforming growth factor beta. *Cancer Res,* 57, 2124–2129.

[20] Ramaswamy, S., N. Nakamura., et al. (1999). Regulation of G1 progression by the PTEN suppressor protein is linked to inhibition of the phosphatidylinositol-3 kinase/Akt pathway. *Proc. Natl. Acad. Sci. USA,* 96, 2110–2115.

[21] Vasudvan, K. M., Guruurthy, S., et al. (2007). Suppression of PTEN expression by NF-kappa B prevents apoptosis. *Mol Cell Biol,* 24, 1007-1021.

[22] Papakonstanti, E. A., Ridley, A. J., et al. (2007). The p110delta isoform of PI 3-kinase negatively controls RhoA and PTEN. *EMBO J,* 26, 3050-3061.

[23] Wang, W., Trotman, L. C., et al. (2007). NEDD4-1 is a proto-oncogenic ubiquitin ligase for PTEN. *Cell,* 128, 129-139.

[24] Ahn, Y., Hwang, C. Y., et al. (2008). Tumour suppressor PTEN mediates a negative regulation of E3 ubiquitin-protein ligase Nedd4. *Biochem J,* 412, 331-338.

[25] Yang, Z. Z., Tschopp, O., et al. (2004). Physiological functions of protein kinase B/Akt. *Biochem Soc Trans,* 32(Pt 2), 350-354.

[26] Sarbassov, D. D., Guertin, D. A., et al. (2005). Phosphorylation and regulation of Akt/PKB by the Rictor-mTOR complex. *Science,* 307 (5712), 1098-1101.

[27] Stephens, L., Anderson, K., et al. (1998). Protein Kinase B kinases that mediate phosphatidylinositol 3,4,5-trisphosphate-dependent activation of protein kinase B. *Science,* 279 (5351), 710-714.

[28] Cully, M., You, H., et al. (2006). Beyond PTEN mutations: the PI3K pathway as an integrator of multiple inputs during tumourigenesis. *Nature Reviews,* 6, 184-192.

[29] Bader, A. G., Kang, S., et al. (2005). Oncogenic PI3K deregulates transcription and translation. *Nat Rev Cancer,* 5(12), 921–929.

[30] Vogt, P. K., Hart, J. R., et al. (2010). Phosphatidylinositol 3-Kinase: the oncoprotein. *Current Topics in Microbiology and Immunology,* 347, 79-104.

[31] Carpenter, C. L., Duckworth, B. C., et al. (1990). Purification and characterization of phosphoinositide 3-kinase from rat liver. *J Biol Chem,* 265, 19704-19711.

[32] Carnero, A., Blanco-Aparicio, C., et al. (2008). The PTEN/PI3K/Akt signaling pathway in cancer, therapeutic implications. *Curr. Cancer Drug Targets,* 8, 187–198.

[33] Cheng, G. Z., Park, S., et al. (2008). Advances of Akt pathway in human oncogenesis and as a target for anti-cancer drug discovery. *Curr. Cancer Drug Targets,* 8, 2–6.

[34] Gao, N., Zhang, Z., et al. (2003). Role of PI3K/Akt/mTOR signaling in the cell cycle progression of human prostate cancer. *Biochem. Biophys. Res. Commun,* 310, 1124–1132.

[35] de la Taille, A., Rubin, M. A., et al. (2003). β-Catenin-related anomalies in apoptosis-resistant and hormone-refractory prostate cancer cells. *Clin. Cancer Res,* 9, 1801–1807.

[36] Lee, H. K., Kwak, H. Y., et al. (2007). β-Catenin regulates multiple steps of RNA metabolism as revealed by the RNA aptamer in colon cancer cells. *Cancer Res,* 67, 9315–9321.

[37] Vignot, S., Faivre, S., et al. (2005). mTOR-targeted therapy of cancer with rapamycin derivatives. *Ann. Oncol,* 16, 525–537.

[38] Toker, A. (2008). mTOR and Akt signaling in cancer: SGK cycles in. Mol. *Cell,* 31, 6–8.

[39] Hanahan, D. & Weinberg, R. A. (2000). The hallmarks of cancer. The hallmarks of cancer. *Cell,* 100, 57-70.

[40] Manning, B. D. & Cantley, L. C. (2007). AKT/PKB signaling: navigating downstream. *Cell* 129, 1261–1274.

[41] Samuels, Y., Wang, Z., et al. (2004). High frequency of mutations of the PIK3CA gene in human cancers. *Science,* 304, 554.

[42] Zhao L. & Vogt P. K. (2008). Class I P13K in oncogenic cellular transformation. *Oncogene,* 27(41), 5486-96.

[43] Grossman, D. & Altieri, D. C. (2001). Drug resistance in melanoma: mechanisms, apoptosis, and new potential therapeutic targets. *Cancer Metastasis Rev,* 20, 3-11.

[44] Helmbach, H., Rossmann, E., et al. (2001). Drug-resistance in human melanoma. *Int J Cancer,* 93, 617-22.

[45] Soengas, M. S. & Lowe, S. W. (2003). Apoptosis and melanoma chemoresistance. *Oncogene,* 22, 3138-51.

[46] Kim, I. K., Lane, A. M., et al. (2010). Survival in patients with presymptomatic diagnosis of metastaic uveal melanoma. *Arch Ophtalmol,* 128, 871-5.

[47] Haass, N. K., Smalley, K. S., et al. (2004). The role of altered cell-cell communication in melanoma progression. *J. Mol. Histol,* 35, 309-18.

[48] Haass, N. K., Smalley, K. S., et al. (2005). Adhesion, migration and communication in melanocytes and melanoma. *Pigment Cell Res,* 18(3), 150-9.

[49] Hao, L., Ha, J. R., et al. (2012). Cadherin switch from E- to N- cadherin in melanoma progression is regulated by the PI3K/PTEN pathway through Twist and Snail. *Br J Dermatol,* 166(6), 1184-97.

[50] Hirohashi. S. (1998). Inactivation of the E-cadherin-mediated cell adhesion system in human cancers. *Am J Pathol,* 153, 333–9.

[51] Piris, A., Mihm, M. C Jr. et al. (2011). AJCC melanoma staging update: impact on dermatopathology practice and patient management. *J Cutan Pathol,* 38, 394-400.

[52] Sosman, J. A. (2013). *Patient Information: Melanoma treatment; advanced or metastatic melanoma* (Beyond the Basics). Upto Date.

[53] Padua, R. A., Barrass, N., et al. (1984). A novel transforming gene in a human malignant melanoma cell line. *Nature,* 311, 671–673.

[54] van't Veer, L. J., B, B. M. et al. (1989). N.-ras mutations in human cutaneous melanoma from sun-exposed body sites. *Mol. Cell. Biol,* 9, 3114–3116.

[55] Yang, G., Rajadurai, A., et al. (2005). Recurrent patterns of dual RB and p53 pathway inactivation in melanoma. *J. Invest. Dermatol,* 125, 1242–1251.

[56] Daniotti, M., Oggionni, M., et al. (2004). BRAF alterations are associated with complex mutational profiles in malignant melanoma. *Oncogene,* 23, 5968–5977.

[57] Curtin, J. A., Fridlyand, J. et al. (2005). Distinct sets of genetic alterations in melanoma. N. *Engl. J. Med,* 353, 2135–2147.

[58] Flaherty, K. T., Hodi, F. S., et al. (2012). From genes to drugs: targeted strategies for melanoma. *Nat Rev Cancer,* 12(5), 349-61.

[59] Smith, A. G., Beaumont, K. A. et al. (2009).PPARy agonists attenuate proliferation and modulate Wnt/ β-catenin signaling in melanoma cells. *Int J Biochem Cell Biol,* (41), 844-52.

[60] Rubinfeld, B., Robbins, P. et al. (1997). Stabilization of beta-catenin by genetic defects in melanoma cell lines. *Science,* 275, 1790-1792.

[61] Lucero, O. M., Dawson, D. W. et al. (2010). A re-evaluation of the "oncogenic" nature of Wnt/beta-catenin signaling in melanoma and other cancers. *Curr. Oncol. Rep,* (12), 314-318.

[62] Damsky, W. E., Curley, D. P. et al. (2011). β-Catenin Signaling Controls Metastasis in Braf-Activated Pten-Deficient Melanomas. *Cancer Cell,* 20(6), 741-754.

[63] Larue, L., Delmas, V. (2006). The WNT/Beta-catenin pathway in melanoma. *Front Biosci,* 11, 733-742.

[64] Lau, E. & Ronai, Z. A. (2011). *Chapter 7 Altered Signal Transduction Pathways in Melanoma.* In Bosserhoff, A., Melanoma Development (137-163). New York, New York: Springerwien.

[65] Sansal, I. & Sellers, W. R. (2004). The biology and clinical relevance of the PTEN tumour suppressor pathway. *J Clin Oncol,* 22, 2954–63.

[66] Guldberg, P., thor Straten, P. et al. (2007). Disruption of the MMAC1/PTEN gene by deletion or mutation is a frequent event in malignant melanoma. *Cancer Res,* 57, 3660–3.

[67] Tsao, H., Zhang, X. et al. (1998). Identification of PTEN/MMAC1 alterations in uncultured melanomas and melanoma cell lines. *Oncogene,* 16, 3397–402.

[68] Wu, H., Goel, V. et al. (2003). PTEN signaling pathways in melanoma. *Oncogene,* 22, 3113–22.

[69] Trotman, L. C., Niki, M. et al. *(2003).* PTEN dose dictates cancer progression in the prostate. *PLoS Biol,* 1(3), E59.

[70] Lopez-Bergami, P., Fitchman, Boris. et al. (2008). Understanding Signaling Cascades in Melanoma. *Photochem Photobiol,* 84(2), 289-306.

[71] Chudnovsky, Y., Adams, A. E. et al. (2005). Use of human tissue to assess the oncogenic activity of melanoma-associated mutations. *Nat Genet,* 37, 745–749.

[72] Dhawan, P., Singh, A. B. et al. (2002). Constitutive activation of Akt/protein kinase B in melanoma leads to upregulation of nuclear factor-kappaB and tumour progression. *Cancer Res,* 62, 7335–42.

[73] Govindarajan, B., Sligh, J. E. et al. (2007). Overexpression of Akt converts radial growth melanoma to vertical growth melanoma. *J Clin Invest,* 117, 719-29.

[74] Sauroja, I., Smeds, J., et al. (2000). Analysis of G(1)/S checkpoint regulators in metastatic melanoma. *Genes Chromosom Cancer,* 28, 404–414.

[75] Smalley, K. S., Haass, N. K. et al. (2006). Multiple signaling pathways must be targeted to overcome drug resistance in cell lines derived from melanoma metastases. *Br J Dermatol,* 156, 1204-13.

[76] Meister, M., Tomasovic, A., et al. (2013). Mitogen-Activated Protein (MAP) Kinase Scaffolding Proteins: A Recount. *Int. J. Mol.,* 14, 4854-4884.

[77] Krishna, M. & Narang, H. (2008). The complexity of mitogen-activated protein kinases (MAPKs) made simple. *Cell. Mol. Life Sci.,* 65, 3525 – 3544.

[78] Cargnello, M. & Philippe P. Roux. (2011). Activation and Function of the MAPKs and Their Substrates, the MAPK-Activated Protein Kinases. Microbiol. *Mol. Biol. Rev.,* 50–83.
[79] Duckworth, B. C. & Cantley, L. C. (1997). Conditional inhibition of the mitogen-activated protein kinase cascade by wortmannin.Dependence on signal strength. *J Biol Chem.* 272(44):27665-70.
[80] Aksamitiene, E., Kiyatkin, A. et al. (2012). Cross-talk between mitogenic Ras/MAPK and survival PI3K/Akt pathways: a fine balance. *Biochem Soc Trans.* 40(1):139-46.
[81] Castellano, E. & Downward, J. (2011). RAS Interaction with PI3K: More Than Just Another Effector Pathway. *Genes Cancer.* 2(3):261-74.
[82] Welch, H. C., Coadwell, W. J., et al. (2003). Phosphoinositide 3-kinase-dependent activation of Rac. *FEBS Lett.* 546(1):93-7.
[83] Ye, D. Z. & Field, J. (2012). PAK signaling in cancer. *Cell Logist.* 2(2):105-116.
[84] Chaudhary, A., King W. G., et al. (2000). Phosphatidylinositol 3-kinase regulates Raf1 through Pak phosphorylation of serine 338. *Curr Biol.* 10(9):551-4.
[85] Chiloeches, A., Mason, C. S., et al. (2001). S338 phosphorylation of Raf-1 is independent of phosphatidylinositol 3-kinase and Pak3. *Mol Cell Biol.* 21(7):2423-34.
[86] Zimmermann, S. & Moelling, K. (1999). Phosphorylation and regulation of Raf by Akt (protein kinase B). *Science.* 286(5445):1741-4.
[87] Moelling, K., Schad, K., et al. (2002). Regulation of Raf-Akt Cross-talk. *J Biol Chem.* 277(34):31099-106.
[88] Guan, K. L., Figueroa, C., et al. (2000). Negative regulation of the serine/threonine kinase B-Raf by Akt. *J Biol Chem.* 275(35):27354-9.
[89] Menges, C. W. & McCance, D. J. (2008). Constitutive activation of the Raf-MAPK pathway causes negative feedback inhibition of Ras-PI3K-AKT and cellular arrest through the EphA2 receptor. *Oncogene.* 27(20):2934-40.
[90] Sato, S., Fujita, N., et al. (2004). Involvement of 3-phosphoinositide-dependent Protein kinase-1 in the MEK/MAPK signal transduction pathway. *J Biol Chem.* 279(32):33759-67.
[91] Nasrazadani, A. & van den Berg C. L. (2011). c-Jun N-terminal Kinase 2 Regulates Multiple Receptor Tyrosine Kinase Pathways in Mouse Mammary Tumour Growth and Metastasis. *Genes Cancer.* 2(1):31-45.
[92] Logan, S. K., Falasca, M., et al. (1997). Phosphatidylinositol 3-kinase mediates epidermal growth factor-induced activation of the c-Jun N-terminal kinase signaling pathway. *Mol Cell Biol.* 17(10):5784-90.
[93] Zhou, H. Y., Wan, K. F., et al. (2008). Hepatocyte growth factor enhances proteolysis and invasiveness of human nasopharyngeal cancer cells through activation of PI3K and JNK. *FEBS Lett.* 582(23-24):3415-22.
[94] Merighi, S., Benini, A., et al. (2006). Modulation of the Akt/Ras/Raf/MEK/ERK pathway by A_3 adenosine receptor. *Purinergic Signal.* 2(4):627-32.
[95] Cheung, M., Sharma, A., et al. (2008). Akt3 and mutant V600E B-Raf cooperate to promote early melanoma development. *Cancer Res.* 68(9):3429-39.
[96] Chen, B., Tardell, C., et al. (2012). BRAFV600E negatively regulates the AKT pathway in melanoma cell lines. *PLoS One.* 7(8):e42598.
[97] Dankort, D., Curley, D. P., et al. (2009). Braf(V600E) cooperates with Pten loss to induce metastatic melanoma. *Nat Genet.* 41(5):544-52.

[98] Gilmore T. D. (2006). Introduction to NF-kappaB: players, pathways, perspectives. *Oncogene.* 25(51):6680-4.
[99] Ozes, O. N., Mayo L. D., et al. (1999). NF-kappaB activation by tumour necrosis factor requires the Akt serine-threonine kinase. *Nature.* 401(6748):82-5.
[100] Romashkova, J. A. & Makarov S. S. (1999). NF-kappaB is a target of AKT in anti-apoptotic PDGF signaling. *Nature.* 401(6748):86-90.
[101] Sizemore, N., Leung, S., et al. (1999). Activation of phosphatidylinositol 3-kinase in response to interleukin-1 leads to phosphorylation and activation of the NF-kappaB p65/RelA subunit. *Mol Cell Biol.* 19(7):4798-805.
[102] Madrid, L. V., Mayo, M. W., et al. (2001). Akt stimulates the transactivation potential of the RelA/p65 Subunit of NF-kappa B through utilization of the Ikappa B kinase and activation of the mitogen-activated protein kinase p38. *J Biol Chem.* 276(22):18934-40.
[103] Madrid, L. V., Wang, C. Y., et al. (2000). Akt suppresses apoptosis by stimulating the transactivation potential of the RelA/p65 subunit of NF-kappaB. *Mol Cell Biol.* 20(5): 1626-38.
[104] Burow, M. E., Weldon, C. B., et al. (2000). PI3-K/AKT regulation of NF-kappaB signaling events in suppression of TNF-induced apoptosis. *Biochem Biophys Res Commun.* 271(2):342-5.
[105] Hussain, A. R., Ahmed, S. O., et al. (2012). Cross-talk between NFkB and the PI3-kinase/AKT pathway can be targeted in primary effusion lymphoma (PEL) cell lines for efficient apoptosis. *PLoS One.* 7(6):e39945.
[106] Cuní, S., Pérez-Aciego, P., et al. (2004). A sustained activation of PI3K/NF-kappaB pathway is critical for the survival of chronic lymphocytic leukemia B cells. *Leukemia.* 18(8):1391-400.
[107] Li Y., Chinni, S. R., et al. (2005). Selective growth regulatory and pro-apoptotic effects of DIM is mediated by AKT and NF-kappaB pathways in prostate cancer cells. *Front Biosci.* 10:236-43.
[108] Julien, S., Puig, I., et al. (2007). Activation of NF-kappaB by Akt upregulates Snail expression and induces epithelium mesenchyme transition. *Oncogene.* (53):7445-56.
[109] Graham, T. R., Odero-Marah, V. A., et al. (2009). PI3K/Akt-dependent transcriptional regulation and activation of BMP-2-Smad signaling by NF-kappaB in metastatic prostate cancer cells. *Prostate.* 69(2):168-80.
[110] McNulty, S. E., del Rosario, R., et al. (2004). Comparative expression of NFkappaB proteins in melanocytes of normal skin vs. benign intradermal naevus and human metastatic melanoma biopsies. *Pigment Cell Res.* 17(2):173-80.
[111] Ueda, Y. & Richmond, A. (2006). NF-kappaB activation in melanoma. *Pigment Cell Res.* 19(2):112-24.
[112] Yang, J. & Richmond, A. (2001). Constitutive IkappaB kinase activity correlates with nuclear factor-kappaB activation in human melanoma cells. *Cancer Res.* 61(12):4901-9.
[113] McNulty, S. E., Tohidian, N. B et al. (2001). RelA, p50 and inhibitor of kappa B alpha are elevated in human metastatic melanoma cells and respond aberrantly to ultraviolet light B. *Pigment Cell* 14(6):456-65.
[114] Shattuck-Brandt, R. L., Richmond, A et al. (1997). Enhanced degradation of I-kappaB alpha contributes to endogenous activation of NF-kappaB in Hs294T melanoma cells. *Cancer Res.* 57(14):3032-9.

[115] Huang, S., de Guzman, A. et al. (2000). Nuclear factor-kappaB activity correlates with growth, angiogenesis, and metastasis of human melanoma cells in nude mice. *Clin Cancer Res.* 6(6):2573-81.
[116] Attisano, L & Wrana, J. L. (2002). Signal transduction by the TGF-beta superfamily. *Science.* 296(5573):1646-7.
[117] van Belle, P, Rodeck, U., et al. (1996). Melanoma-associated expression of transforming growth factor-beta isoforms. *Am J Pathol.* 148(6):1887-94.
[118] Krasagakis, K, Thölke, D., et al. (1998). Elevated plasma levels of transforming growth factor (TGF)-beta1 and TGF-beta2 in patients with disseminated malignant melanoma. *Br J Cancer.* 77(9):1492-4.
[119] Mohammad, K. S, Javelaud, D., et al. (2011). TGF-beta-RI kinase inhibitor SD-208 reduces the development and progression of melanoma bone metastases. *Cancer Res.* 71(1):175-84.
[120] Reed, J. A., McNutt, N. S., et al. (1994). Expression of transforming growth factor-beta 2 in malignant melanoma correlates with the depth of tumour invasion. Implications for tumour progression. *Am J Pathol.* 145(1):97-104.
[121] Javelaud, D., Delmas, V. et al. (2005). Stable overexpression of Smad7 in human melanoma cells inhibits their tumourigenicity *in vitro* and *in vivo*. *Oncogene.* 24(51): 7624-9.
[122] Javelaud, D., Mohammad, K. S., et al. (2007). Stable overexpression of Smad7 in human melanoma cells impairs bone metastasis. *Cancer Res.* 67(5):2317-24.
[123] di Vito, K. A., Trabosh, V. A., et al. (2010). Smad7 restricts melanoma invasion by restoring N-cadherin expression and establishing heterotypic cell-cell interactions *in vivo*. *Pigment Cell Melanoma Res.* 23(6):795-808.
[124] Fang, R, Zhang, G., et al. (2013). Nodal promotes aggressive phenotype via Snail-mediated epithelial-mesenchymal transition in murine melanoma. *Cancer Lett.* 333(1): 66-75.
[125] Fortini, M. E. (2009). Notch signaling: the core pathway and its posttranslational regulation. *Dev Cell.* 16(5):633-47.
[126] Hoek, K., Rimm, D. L., et al. (2004). Expression profiling reveals novel pathways in the transformation of melanocytes to melanomas. *Cancer Res.* 64(15):5270-82.
[127] Mauerer, A., Roesch, A., et al. (2011). Identification of new genes associated with melanoma. *Exp Dermatol.* 20(6):502-7.
[128] Massi, D., Tarantini, F., et al. (2006). Evidence for differential expression of Notch receptors and their ligands in melanocytic nevi and cutaneous malignant melanoma. *Mod Pathol.* 19(2):246-54.
[129] Pinnix, C. C., Lee, J. T., et al. (2009). Active Notch1 confers a transformed phenotype to primary human melanocytes. *Cancer Res.* 69(13):5312-20.
[130] Bedogni, B., Warneke, J. A., et al. (2008). Notch1 is an effector of Akt and hypoxia in melanoma development. *J Clin Invest.* 118(11):3660-70.
[131] Liu, Z. J., Xiao, M., et al. (2006). Notch1 signaling promotes primary melanoma progression by activating mitogen-activated protein kinase/phosphatidylinositol 3-kinase-Akt pathways and up-regulating N-cadherin expression. *M. Cancer Res.* 66(8): 4182-90.
[132] Heim, M. H. (1999). The Jak-STAT pathway: cytokine signaling from the receptor to the nucleus. *J Recept Signal Transduct Res.* 19(1-4):75-120.

[133] Aaronson, D. S. & Horvath, C. M. (2002). A road map for those who don't know JAK-STAT. *Science.* 296(5573):1653-5.
[134] Pansky, A., Hildebrand, P., et al. (2000). Defective Jak-STAT signal transduction pathway in melanoma cells resistant to growth inhibition by interferon-alpha. *Int J Cancer.* 85(5):720-5.
[135] Jackson, D. P, & Watling, D., et al. (2003). The JAK/STAT pathway is not sufficient to sustain the antiproliferative response in an interferon-resistant human melanoma cell line. *Melanoma Res.* 13(3):219-29.
[136] Guenterberg, K. D., Grignol, V. P., et al. (2010). Interleukin-29 binds to melanoma cells inducing Jak-STAT signal transduction and apoptosis. *Mol Cancer Ther.* 9(2):510-20.
[137] Krasilnikov, M., Ivanov V. N., et al. (2003). ERK and PI3K negatively regulate STAT-transcriptional activities in human melanoma cells: implications towards sensitization to apoptosis. *Oncogene.* 22(26):4092-101.
[138] Pópulo, H., Lopes, J. M., et al. (2012). The mTOR Signaling Pathway in Human Cancer. *Int J Mol Sci.* 13(2):1886-918.
[139] Laplante, M. & Sabatini, D. M. (2009). mTOR signaling at a glance. *J Cell Sci.* 122 (20):3589-94.
[140] Memmott, R. M. & Dennis, P. A. (2009). Akt-dependent and -independent mechanisms of mTOR regulation in cancer. *Cell Signal.* 21(5):656-64.
[141] Gulhati, P., Bowen, K. A. et al. (2011). mTORC1 and mTORC2 regulate EMT, motility, and metastasis of colorectal cancer via RhoA and Rac1 signaling pathways. *Cancer Res.* 71(9):3246-56.
[142] Guba, M., von Breitenbuch P., et al. (2002). Rapamycin inhibits primary and metastatic tumour growth by antiangiogenesis: involvement of vascular endothelial growth factor. *Nat Med.* 8(2):128-35.
[143] Guertin, D. A., Stevens, D. M., et al. (2009). mTOR complex 2 is required for the development of prostate cancer induced by Pten loss in mice. *Cancer Cell.* 15(2):148-59.
[144] Altomare, D. A., Wang, H. Q., et al. (2004). AKT and mTOR phosphorylation is frequently detected in ovarian cancer and can be targeted to disrupt ovarian tumour cell growth. *Oncogene.* 23(34):5853-7.
[145] Gao, N., Flynn, D.C., et al. (2004). G1 cell cycle progression and the expression of G1 cyclins are regulated by PI3K/AKT/mTOR/p70S6K1 signaling in human ovarian cancer cells. *Am J Physiol Cell Physiol.* 287(2):C281-91.
[146] Nishioka, C., Ikezoe, T., et al. (2008). Blockade of mTOR signaling potentiates the ability of histone deacetylase inhibitor to induce growth arrest and differentiation of acute myelogenous leukemia cells. *Leukemia.* 22(12):2159-68.
[147] Boulay, A., Rudloff, J., et al. (2005). Dual inhibition of mTOR and estrogen receptor signaling *in vitro* induces cell death in models of breast cancer. *Clin Cancer Res.* 11 (14): 5319-28.
[148] Zhang, Y. J., Dai, Q., et al. (2009). mTOR signaling pathway is a target for the treatment of colorectal cancer. *Ann Surg Oncol.* 16(9):2617-28.
[149] Panwalkar, A., Verstovsek, S. et al. (2004). Mammalian target of rapamycin inhibition as therapy for hematologic malignancies. *Cancer.* 100(4):657-66.

[150] Marinov, M., Fischer, B., et al. (2007). Targeting mTOR signaling in lung cancer. *Crit Rev Oncol Hematol.* 63(2):172-82.
[151] Chakraborty, S., Mohiyuddin, S. M., et al. (2008). Involvement of TSC genes and differential expression of other members of the mTOR signaling pathway in oral squamous cell carcinoma. *BMC Cancer.* 8:163.
[152] Karbowniczek, M., Spittle, C. S., et al. (2008). mTOR is activated in the majority of malignant melanomas. *J Invest Dermatol.* 128(4):980-7.
[153] Pópulo, H., Soares, P., et al. (2011). mTOR pathway activation in cutaneous melanoma is associated with poorer prognosis characteristics. *Pigment Cell Melanoma Res.* 24(1): 254-7.
[154] Aziz, S. A., Jilaveanu, L. B., et al. (2010). Vertical targeting of the phosphatidylinositol-3 kinase pathway as a strategy for treating melanoma. *Clin Cancer Res.* 16(24): 6029-39.
[155] Sinnberg, T., Lasithiotakis, K., et al. (2009). Inhibition of PI3K-AKT-mTOR signaling sensitizes melanoma cells to cisplatin and temozolomide. *J Invest Dermatol.* 129(6): 1500-15.
[156] Shapiro, L. & Weis, W. I. (2009). Structure and Biochemistry of Cadherins and Catenins. *Cold Spring Harb Perspectives in Biology.* 1(3), 1-21.
[157] Huber, A. H. & Nelson, W. J., et al. (1997). Three-Dimensional Structure of the Armadillo Repeat Region of β-Catenin. *Cell,* 90(5), 871-872.
[158] Xing, Y. & Takemaru, K., et al. (2008). Crystal Structure of a Full-Length β-Catenin, *Structure,* 16(3), 478-487.
[159] Huber, A. H., & Weis, W. I. (2001). The Structure of the B-Catenin/E-Cadherin Complex and the Molecular Basis of Diverse Ligand Recognition by B-Catenin. *Cell,* 105(3), 391-402.
[160] Maher, M. T. & Mo, R., et al. (2010). β-Catenin Phosphorylated at Serine 45 is Spatially Uncoupled from β-Catenin Phosphorylated in the GSK3 Domain: Implications for Signaling. *PLoS One,* 5(4), 1-12.
[161] Hecht, A. & Litterst, C. M., et al. (1999). Functional characterization of multiple transactivating elements in beta-catenin, some of which interact with the TATA-binding protein *in vitro*. *J Biol Chem,* 274, 18017-25.
[162] Piedra, J. & Martinez, D., et al. (2001). Regulation of B-Catenin Structure and Activity by Tyrosine Phosphorylation. *The Journ of Biol Chem,* 276(23), 20436-20443.
[163] Hecht, A. K. & Vleminckx, M. P., et al. (2000). The p300/CBP acetyltransferases function as transcriptional coactivators of β-catenin in vertebrates. *J EMBO,* 19, 1839-1850.
[164] Hülsken, J. & Birchmeier, W., et al. (1994). E-cadherin and APC complete for the interaction with beta-catenin and the cytoskeleton. *The Journ of Biol Chem,* 174, 2061-9.
[165] Roura, S. & Miravet, S., et al. (1999). Regulation of E-cadherin/Catenin association by tyrosine phosphorylation. *The Journ of Biol Chem,* 274,36734-40.
[166] Gumbiner, B. M. (2000). Regulation of cadherin adhesive activity. *J. Cell Biol,* 148, 399–404.
[167] Gottardi, C. J. & Wong, E., et al. (2001). E-Cadherin Suppresses Cellular Transformation by Inhibiting B-Catenin Signaling in an Adhesion-independent Manner. *The Journ of Cell Biol,* 153(5), 1049-1059.

[168] MacDonald, B. T. & Tamai, K., et al. (2009). Wnt/β-catenin signaling: components, mechanisms, and diseases. *Dev Cell,* 17(1), 9-26.

[169] Dajani, R. & Fraser, E., et al. (2003). Structural basis for recruitment of glycogen synthase kinase 3beta to the axin-APC scaffold complex. *EMBO J,* 22(3), 494-501.

[170] Amit, S. & Hatzubai, A., et al. (2002). Axin-mediated CKI phosphorylation of B-catenin at Ser 45: a molecular switch for the Wnt pathway. *Genes Dev,* 16, 1066–1076.

[171] Liu, J. & Xing, Y., et al. (2006). The third 20 amino acid repeat is the tightest binding site of APC for B-catenin. *J Mol Biol,* 360, 133–144.

[172] Kimelman, D., & Xu, W. (2006). beta-catenin destruction complex: insights and questions from a structural perspective. *Oncogene,* 25, 7482-91.

[173] http://www.stanford.edu/group/nusselab/cgi-bin/wnt/.

[174] Zeng, Y. A. & Rahnama, M. et al. (2008). Inhibition of Drosophila Wg Signaling Involves Competition between Mad and Armadillo/b-Catenin for dTcf Binding. *PLoS One,* 3(12), 1-9.

[175] Tamai K & Zeng X, et al. (2004). A mechanism for Wnt coreceptor activation. *Molecular cell,* 13(1), 149-156.

[176] Davidson, G. & Wu, W., et al. (2005). Casein kinase 1 gamma couples Wnt receptor activation to cytoplasmic signal transduction. *Nature,* 438(7069), 867-872.

[177] Mao, J. & Wang, J., et al. (2001). Low-density lipoprotein receptor-related protein-5 binds to Axin and regulates the canonical Wnt signaling pathway. *Molecular cell,* 4, 801-809.

[178] Bilic, J. & Huang, Y.L., et al. (2007). Wnt Induces LRP6 Signalosomes and Promotes Dishevelled-Dependent LRP6 Phosphorylation. *Science,* 316(5831), 1619-1622.

[179] Logan, C. Y., & Nusse, R. (2004). The Wnt Signaling Pathway in Development and Disease. Annu. Rev. *Cell Dev. Biol,* 20, 781-810.

[180] Xing, Y. & Clements, W. K. et al. (2003). Crystal structure of a beta-catenin/ axin complex suggest a mechanism for the beta-catenin destruction complex. *Genes Dev,* 17, 2753-64.

[181] Mo, R. & Chew, T., et al. (2000). The Terminal Region of B-Catenin Promotes Stability by Shiedling the Armadillo Repeats from the Axin-scaffold Destruction Complex. *The Journ of Biol Chem,* 284, 28222-28231.

[182] Staal, F. J. T. & Noort, Mv. M., et al. (2002). Wnt signals are transmitted through N-terminally dephosphorylated B-catenin. *EMBO reports,* 3(1), 63-68.

[183] Kielhorn, E. & Provost, E., et al. (2003). Tissue Microarray-Based Analysis Shows Phospho-Beta-Catenin Expression In Malignant Melanoma Is Associated With Poor Outcome. *Int J. Cancer,* 103, 652-656.

[184] Krieghoff, E. & Behrens, J., et al. (2006). Nucleo-cytoplasmic distribution of beta-catenin is regulated by retention. *J Cell Sci,* 119, 1453–1463.

[185] Behrens, J. & Jerchow, B. et al. (1998). Functional interaction of an axin homolog, conductin, with beta-catenin, APC, and GSK3-beta. *Science,* 280(5263), 596-599.

[186] Simcha, I. & Shtutman, M. et al. (1998). Differential Nuclear Translocation and Transactivation Potential of B-Catenin and Plakoglobin. *The Journ of Cell Biol,* 141(6), 1433-1448.

[187] Simcha, I. & Geiger, B., et al. (1996). Suppression of Tumourigenicity by Plankoglobin: An Augmenting Effect of N-Cadherin. *The Journ of Cell Biol,* 133(1), 199-209.

[188] Zhurinsky, J. & Shtutman, M., et al. (2000). Differential Mechanisms of LEF/TCF Family-Dependent Transcriptional Activation of B-Catenin and Plankoglobin. *Mol and Cell Biol,* 20(12), 4238-4252.

[189] Fagotto, F. & Gluck, U., et al. (1998). Nuclear localization signal-independent and importin/karyopherin-independent nuclear import of B-catenin. *Current Biology,* 8, 181-190.

[190] Yokoya, F. & Imamoto, N., et al. (1999). Beta-catenin can be transported into the nucleus in a Ran-unassisted manner. *Mol Biol Cell,* 10, 1119-1131.

[191] Polakis, P. (2000). Wnt Signaling and cancer. *Genes Dev,* 14, 1837-1851.

[192] Armengol, C. & Cairo, S., et al. (2009). Wnt signaling and hepatocarcinogenesis: the hepatoblastoma model. *Int J Biochem Cell Biol,* 43, 265–270.

[193] El Wakil, A. & Lalli, E. (2011). The Wnt/beta-catenin pathway in adrenocortical development and cancer. *Mol Cell Endocrinol,* 332, 32–37.

[194] Zardawi, S. J. & O'Toole, S. A., et al. (2009). Dysregulation of Hedgehog, Wnt and Notch signaling pathways in breast cancer. *Histol Histopathol,* 24, 385–398.

[195] Tycko, B. & Li, C. M., et al. (2007). The Wnt/beta-catenin pathway in Wilms tumours and prostate cancers. *Curr Mol Med,* 7, 479–489.

[196] Ge, X., & Wang, X. (2011). Role of Wnt canonical pathway in hematological malignancies. *J Hematol Oncol,* 3, 33.

[197] Laurent-Puig, P. & Zucman-Rossi, J. (2006). Genetics of hepatocellular tumours. *Oncogene,* 25, 3778–3786.

[198] Satoh, S. & Daigo, Y., et al. (2000). AXIN1 mutations in hepatocellular carcinomas, and growth suppression in cancer cells by virus-mediated transfer of AXIN1. *Nat Genet,* 24(3), 245-250.

[199] Neufeld, K.L. & Zhang, F., et al. (2000). APC-mediated downregulation of β-catenin activity involves nuclear sequestration and nuclear export. *EMBO Reports,* 1, 519-523.

[200] Morin, P. J. & Sparks, A.B., et al. (1997). Activation of β-catenin-Tcf signaling in colon cancer by mutations in β-catenin or APC. *Science,* 275, 1787-1790.

[201] Kageshita, T. & Hamby, C. V., et al. (2001). Loss of b-catenin expression associated with disease progression in malignant melanoma. *British Journal of Dermatology,* 145, 210-216.

[202] Demunter A. L. & Libbrecht, H. et al. (2002). Loss of membranous expression of beta-catenin is associated with tumour progression in cutaneous melanoma and rarely caused by exon 3 mutations. *Mod Pathol,* 15, 454-461.

[203] Persad, S. & Troussard, A. A., et al. (2001). Tumour Suppressor PTEN Inhibits Nuclear Accumulation of Beta-Catenin and T Cell/Lymphoid Enhancer Factor 1–mediated Transcriptional Activation. *J Cell Biol,* 153(6), 1161-1174.

[204] Pap, M., & Cooper, G. M. (1998). Role of Glycogen Synthase Kinase-3 in the Phosphatidylinositol 3-Kinase/ Akt Cell Survival Pathway. *The Journ of Biol Chem,* 273(32), 19929-19932.

[205] Ng, S. S. & Mahmoudi, T., et. al.(2009). Phosphatidylinositol 3-Kinase Signaling Does Not Activated the Wnt Cascade. *The Journ of Biol Chem,* 284(51), 35308-35313.

[206] Sharma, M. & Chuang, W. W., et al. (2002). Phosphatidylinositol 3-kinase/Akt stimulates androgen pathway through GSK3beta and inhibition and nuclear beta-catenin accumulation. *Journ of Biol Chem,* 277, 30935-41.

[207] Blume-Jensen, P., & Hunter, T. (2001). Oncogenic kinase signaling. *Nature,* 411, 355-365.

[208] Mulholland, D. J. & Dedhar, S. et al. (2006). PTEN and GSK3β: key regulators of progression to androgen-independent prostate cancer. *Oncogene,* 25, 329-337.

[209] Cross, D. A. & Alessi, D. R. et al. (1995). Inhibition of glycogen synthase kinase-3 by insulin mediated by protein kinase B. *Nature,* 378(6559), 785-9.

[210] Ding, V. W. & Chen, R. H., et al. (2000). Differential regulation of glycogen synthase kinase 3beta by insulin and Wnt signaling. *J Biol Chem,* 275(42), 32475-81.

[211] Patel, S. & Doble, B. W., et al. (2008). Tissue-Specific Role of Glycogen Synthase Kinase 3 β in Glucose Homeostasis and Insulin Action. *Molecular and Cellular Biology,* 28(20), 6314-6328.

[212] Doble, B. W. & Patel, S., et al. (2007). Functional Redundancy of GSK-3α and GSK-3β in Wnt/β-Catenin Signaling Shown by Using an Allelic Series of Embryonic Stem Cell Lines. *Developmental Cell,* 12, 951-971.

[213] Fukumoto, S. & Hsieh, C., et al. (2001). Akt Participation in the Wnt Signaling Pathway through Dishevelled. *J Biol Chem,* 276(20), 17479-83.

[214] Fang, D. & Hawke, D., et al. (2007). Phosphorulation of β-Catenin by AKT Promotes β-Catenin Transcriptional Activity. *J Biol Chem,* 282(15), 11221-11229.

[215] He, X. C. & Yin, T., et al. (2007). PTEN-deficient intestinal stem cells initiate intestinal polyposis. *Nature Genetic,* 39(2), 189-198.

[216] Tian, Q. & Feetham, M. C., et al. (2004). Proteomic analysis identifies that 14-3-3ζ interacts with β-catenin and facilitates its activation by Akt. *PNAS,* 101(43), 15370-15375.

[217] Ann, S. & Kloor, M. (2005). Regulation of AKT1 expression by beta-catenin/TCF/Lef signaling in colorectal cancer cells. *Carcinogenesis,* 26(9), 1503-1512.

[218] Espada, J. & Peinado, H., et al. (2005). Direct metabolic regulation of β-catenin activity by the p85α regulatory subunit of phosphorinosite 3-OH kinase. *Experimental Cell Research,* 305, 409-417.

[219] Tanwar, P. S. & Zhang, L., et al. (2011). Mammalian target of rapamycin is a therapeutic target for muring ovarian endometriod adenocarcinomas with dysregulated Wnt/β-catenin and PTEN. *PLoS One,* 6(6), e20715.

[220] Shen, W. H. & Boyle, D. W., et al. (2005). Insulin and IGF-I stimulate the formation of the eukaryotic initiation factor complex and protein synthesis in C2C12 myotubes independent of availability of external amino acids. *J Endocrinol,* 185(2), 275-89.

[221] Harwood, F. C. & Shu, L., et al. (2008). mTORC1 signaling can regulate growth factor activation of p44/42 mitogen-activated protein kinases through protein phosphatase 2A. *J Biol Chem,* 283(5), 2575-85.

[222] Liu, H. & Remedi, M. S., et al. (2009). Glycogen synthase kinase-3 and mammalian target of rapamycin pathways contribute to DNA synthesis, cell cycle progression, and proliferation in human islets. *Diabetes,* 58(3), 663-72.

[223] Walsh, L. A., & Damjanovski, S. (2011). IFG-1 increases invasive potential of MCF 7 breast cancer cells and induces activation of latent TGF-β1 resulting in epithelial to mesenchymal transition. *Cell Commun Signal,* 9(1), 1-11.

[224] Vincent, T. & Neve, E. P., et al. (2009). A SNAIL1-SMAD ¾ transcriptional repressor complex promotes TGF-beta mediated epithelial-mesenchymal transition. *Nat Cell Biol,* 11(8), 943-50.

[225] Sayat, R. & Leber, B., et al. (2008). O-GlcNAc-glycosylation of beta-catenin regulates its nuclear localization and transcriptional activity. *Exp Cell Res,* 314(15), 2774-87.

[226] http://www.cancer.gov/cancertopics/pdq/treatment/melanoma/ HealthProfessional.

[227] http://www.cancer.gov/cancertopics/pdq/treatment/melanoma/HealthProfessional/Page 9#Reference9.6.

[228] Hideshima, T., Catley, L., et al. (2006). Perifosine, an oral bioactive novel alkylphospholipid, inhibits Akt and induces *in vitro* and *in vivo* cytotoxicity in human multiple myeloma cells. *Blood.* 107(10), 4053-62.

[229] Patel, V., Lahusen, T., et al. (2002). Perifosine, a novel alkylphospholipid, induces p21(WAF1) expression in squamous carcinoma cells through a p53-independent pathway, leading to loss in cyclin-dependent kinase activity and cell cycle arrest. *Cancer Res.* 62(5), 1401-9.

[230] Kondapaka, S. B, Singh, S. S. et al. (2003). Perifosine, a novel alkylphospholipid, inhibits protein kinase B activation. *Mol Cancer Ther.* 2(11):1093-103.

[231] Gaitonde, S., De, S. K. et al. (2009). BI-69A11-mediated inhibition of AKT leads to effective regression of xenograft melanoma. *Pigment Cell Melanoma Res.* 22(2):187-95.

[232] Sharma, A., Sharma, A. K. et al. (2009). Targeting Akt3 signaling in malignant melanoma using isoselenocyanates. *Clin Cancer Res.* 15(5):1674-85.

[233] Hainsworth, J. D., Infante, J. R. et al. (2010). Bevacizumab and everolimus in the treatment of patients with metastatic melanoma: a phase 2 trial of the Sarah Cannon Oncology Research Consortium. *Cancer.* 116(17), 4122-9.

[234] Niessner, H., Beck, D. et al. (2011). The farnesyl transferase inhibitor lonafarnib inhibits mTOR signaling and enforces sorafenib-induced apoptosis in melanoma cells. *J Invest Dermatol.* 131(2), 468-79.

In: Horizons in Cancer Research. Volume 54
Editor: Hiroto S. Watanabe

ISBN: 978-1-63321-389-0

Chapter 5

Mushrooms: Proteins, Polysaccharide-Peptide Complexes and Polysaccharides with Antiproliferative and Anticancer Activities

***Tzi Bun Ng*[*], *Jack Ho Wong*[†], *Randy Chi Fai Cheung*[**], *Tak Fu Tse, Timothy Tam and Helen Chan*[‡]**
School of Biomedical Sciences, Faculty of Medicine, The Chinese University of Hong Kong, Shatin, New Territories, Hong Kong, China

Abstract

Proteins with antiproliferative activity toward cancer cells *in vitro* and/or anticancer activity *in vivo* are discussed in this review. Lectins, fungal immunomodulatory proteins, ribonucleases, ribosome-inactivating proteins, polysaccharide-peptide complexes, laccases, a hemolysin, a ubiquitin-like peptide, a protease, and a translation inhibiting protein are included in the discussion.The lectins comprise those from *Agaricus bisporus, Clitocybe nebularis, Cordyceps militaris, Flammulina velutipes, Ganoderma capense, Hericium erinaceum, Lactarius flavidulus, Pholiota adiposa, Pleurotus eous, Polyporus adusta, Russula delica, R.lepida, Schizophyllum commune, Tricholoma mongolicum, Xerocomus chrysenteron, Xylaria hypoxylon* and *Volvariella volvacea.* The fungal immunomodulatory proteins encompass those from *Flammulina velutipes, Ganoderma lucidum,* and *G. tsugae.* The ribonucleases comprise those from *Hypsizigus marmoreus, Pleurotus ostreatus, P. sajor-caju, Russula delica* and *Tuber indicum.*Ribosome-

[*] Corresponding author. School of Biomedical Sciences, Faculty of Medicine, The Chinese University of Hong Kong, Shatin, New Territories, Hong Kong, China. E-mail: b021770@mailserv.cuhk.edu.hk.
[†] Corresponding author. School of Biomedical Sciences, Faculty of Medicine, The Chinese University of Hong Kong, Shatin, New Territories, Hong Kong, China. E-mail: jack1993@yahoo.com.
[**] Corresponding author. School of Biomedical Sciences, Faculty of Medicine, The Chinese University of Hong Kong, Shatin, New Territories, Hong Kong, China. E-mail: chifaicheung@ cuhk.edu.hk.
[‡] Corresponding author. Vita Green Pharmaceutical (H.K.) Ltd., Ap Lei Chau, Hong Kong, China. E-mail: helen.chan@vitagreen.com.

inactivating proteins include hypsin and marmorin, both from *Hypsizigus marmoreus.*The polysaccharide-peptide complexes include those from *Agaricus blazei*, *Coriolus versicolor*, *Grifola frondosa, Pleurotus abalones* and *P.pulmonarius.* The polysaccharides comprise those from *Armillaria mellea, Grifola frondosa, Lentinula edodes, Pleurotus abalones* and *P. nebrodensis. Pleurotus eryngii* hemolysin, *Agaricus placomyces* laccase, *Agrocybe cylindracea* laccase, *Agrocybe cylindracea* ubiquitin-like peptide, *Amanita farinosa* protease, and *Calvatia caelata* translation-inhibiting protein also display antiproliferative activity.

Keywords: Antiproliferative, anticancer, mushroom proteins

Introduction

Mushrooms are rich in proteins and display a constellation of biological activities (Wasser, 2011). Among the bioactive mushroom proteins are DNases, RNases, lignolytic enzymes, proteases, protease inhibitors, lectins, antifungal proteins, antibacterial proteins, antiviral proteins, ribosome inactivating proteins (Wong et al., 2010; Wasser,2011;Xu et al., 2011). Low molecular weight compounds such as cattienoids and hispolon have been reported from mushrooms (Hien et al., 2013; Hsiao et al., 2013). The intent of this article is to review macromolecules from mushrooms encompassing proteins, polysaccharide-peptide complexes and polysaccharides with antiproliferative and anticancer activities.

Agaricus bisporus Lectin

The lectin has potently inhibited proliferation of human epithelial cancer cells, without obvious cytotoxic effects (Carrizo et al., 2005).

Agaricus blazei Glucan-Protein Complex

The glucan-protein complex exhibited a potent antitumor action on sarcoma 180 bearing mice but did not directly kill tumor cells *in vitro.* It alleviated leucopenia induced by 5-fluorouracil. It was devoid of toxic effects on the kidneys and the liver (Sde et al.,2009).

Agaricus Placomyces Laccase

The 68-kDa laccase suppressed proliferation of MCF 7 human breast cancer cells and Hep G2 hepatoma cells and inhibited human immunodeficiency virus type 1 (HIV-1) reverse transcriptase activity with an IC50 value of 1.8μM, 1.7μM, and 1.25μM, respectively (Sun et al., 2012).

Agrocybe cylindracea Ubiquitin-like Peptide

The 9.5-kDa poly C-specific peptide inhibited proliferation of M1leukemia cells and HepG2 hepatoma cells, and upregulated generation of nitric oxide in mouse peritoneal macrophages with a potency analogous to lipopolysaccharide (Ngai et al., 2004).

Agrocybe cylindracea Laccase

The 58-kDa laccase inhibited proliferation of HepG2 cells and MCF7 cells with an IC50 value of 5.6 μM and 6.5 μM, respectively (Hu et al., 2011).

Amanita farinosa Protease

The 15-kDa protease inhibited proliferation of human hepatoma HepG2 cells with an IC50 value of 25 μM (Sun et al., 2011).

Armillaria luteo-virens Lectin

The dimeric 29.4-kDa lectin demonstrated mitogenic activity on mouse spleen cells, and antiproliferative activity toward HeLa cells, L1210 cells and MBL2 cells with an IC50 value of, 5, 10 and 2.5μM, respectively. However, there was no effect on proliferation of HepG2 cells (Feng et al., 2006).

Armillaria mellea Polysaccharide

The polysaccharide brought about cell cycle disruption in the G0/G1 phase,. mitochondrial membrane potential disruption, mitochondrial cytochrome c release, caspase-3 and -9 activation, and apoptosis in A549 cells (Wu et al., 2012).

Calvatia caelata Ubiquitin-Like Peptide

The 8-kDa peptide exhibited antimitogenic splenocytes with an IC50 value of approximately 100 nM as shown by the attenuated incorporation of tritiated methylthymidine. At about 100 nM the peptide brought about a 50% reduction of viability of breast cancer cells (Lam et al., 2001).

Calvatia caelata Translation-Inhibiting Protein (Calcaelin)

It exhibited an antimitogenic activity toward mouse splenocytes, and it reduced the viability of MDA-MB-231breast cancer cells with an IC50 value of 2.3μM(Ng et al., 2003).

Clitocybe nebularis Ricin B-Like Lectin

A 15.9-kDa homodimeric lactose-specific immunomodulatory lectin bound to carbohydrate receptors on human leukemic T cells and exhibited antiproliferative activity (Pohleven et al., 2009).

Cordyceps militaris Haemagglutinin

The haemagglutinin exerted an antiproliferative action towards HepG2cells hepatoma and inhibited HIV-1 reverse transcriptase with an IC50 value of 10 μM. However, it was devoid of nitric oxide-inducing activity towards macrophages and mitogenic activity towards splenocytes (Wong et al., 2009).

Coriolus versicolor Protein-Bound Polysaccharide PSP

PSP possesses a molecular weight of approximately 100 kDa. Glutamic and aspartic acids are abundant in its polypeptide component, whereas its polysaccharide component is made up of monosaccharides with alpha-1,4 and beta-1,3 glucosidic linkages. The presence of fucose in PSK and rhamnose and arabinose in PSP distinguishes the two protein-bound polysaccharides, which are otherwise chemically similar. PSP is classified as a biological response modifier. It induces, in experimental animals, increased gamma-interferon production, interleukin-2 production, and T-cell proliferation. It also counteracts cyclophosphamide-induced depression of leukocyte count, interleukin-2 production and delayed-type hypersensitivity reaction. Its antiproliferative activity against tumor cell lines and *in vivo* antitumor activity have been demonstrated. A small peptide with a molecular weight of 16-18 kDa originating from PSP has been produced with antiproliferative and antitumor activities.. PSP administered to patients with esophageal cancer, gastric cancer and lung cancer, and who are undergoing radiotherapy or chemotherapy, helps alleviate symptoms and prevents the decline in immune status (Ng 1998).

Prior exposure of human promyelocytic leukemia HL-60 cells to PSP promoted the cell cycle perturbation and apoptotic activity of etoposide and doxorubicin. PSP upregulated the apoptotic machinery of doxorubicin and etoposide in a way dependent on the cell cycle. PSP modulated the regulatory checkpoints cyclin E and caspase 3 (Hui et al., 2005).PSP potentiated the apoptotic effect of Doxo and VP-16 on ZR-75-30 human breast cancer cells by producing a trap in theS-phase and by a reduced ratio of Bcl-xL/Bax protein expression of the cancer cells (Wan et al., 2008).

The inhibition of proliferation of pancreatic cancer cells can be preventted by neutralizing antibodies against TLR2 and TLR4. PSK enhanced the levels of cell cycle regulatory p21(WAF/Cip1) and pro-apoptotic protein Bax, leading ultimately to arrest of cell cycle and apoptotic cell death. Combined therapy with PSK and gemcitabine yielded an additive effect (Rosendahl. et al., 2012).

Flammulina velutipes Fungal Immunomodulatory Protein

FIP-fve exerted antiproliferative activity toward A549 lung cancer cells. FIP-fve brought about cell cycle arrest but did not trigger apoptosis as evidenced by results of flow cytometry. It upregulated the expression of p53 and its downstream gene p21 as revealed by Western blot. FIP-fve suppressed A549 cell migration in the wound healing assay and reduced filopodia fiber formation as shown by labeling with Texas Red-X phalloidin. FIP-fve attenuated activation of Rac1 by epidermal growth factor, and reduced RACGAP1 mRNA and protein levels and the reporter activity of RACGAP1. RacGAP1 silencing ensued in reduced cell migration, and RacGAP1 overexpression promoted cell migration in A549 lung cancer cells. In (Chang et al., 2013).

Flammulina velutipes Hemagglutinin

The 12-kDa hemagglutinin, with an N-terminal sequence distincnt from that of FIP-fve, enhanced tritiated methylthymidine incorporation by murine spleen cells. It exhibited antiproliferative activity on leukemia L1210 cells with an IC50 value of 13 μM (Ng et al., 2006).

Ganoderma capense Lectin

The 18-kDa lectin, with some N-terminal sequence homology to lectins and fungal immunomodulatory proteins, manifested a higher potency than the leguminous lectin concanavalin A in stimulating mitogenesis of murine spleen cells. suppressed proliferation of L1210 and M1 leukemia cells and HepG2 hepatoma cells (Ngai and Ng 2004).

Ganoderma lucidum Fungal Immunomodulatory Protein Lz-8

Recombinant Lz-8 induced caspase-independent autophagy in SGC-7901 human gastric cancer cells by aggregating in the endoplasmic reticulum(ER), evoking ER stress and the ATF4-CHOP pathway. It activated the ubiquitine/proteasome ER-associated degradation system whose autophagic arm was overstimulated by the accumulated recombinant Lz-8 (Liang et al., 2012).

Ganoderma tsugae Fungal Immunomodulatory Protein

The fungal immunomodulatory protein and its recombinant form produced a growth inhibiting effect on A549 cancer cells but not on normal MRC-5 fibroblasts. The recombinant protein downregulated telomerase activity and impeded transcriptional regulation of hTERT via a c-myc-responsive element-dependent mechanism (Liao et al., 2006).

Grifola frondosa Polysaccharide-Peptide

Crude polysaccharide-peptide, and three chemically modified polysaccharide-peptides including phosphorylated, acetylated and esterified polysaccharide-peptide produced a significant adjuvant effect to cyclophosphamide when administered to rats inoculated with C6 cancer cells. The native and chemically modified polysaccharide-peptides suppressed growth in C6 cancer cells but not normal brain cells. Only phosphorylated polysaccharide-peptide manifested a significant improvement in adjuvant and growth inhibitory activities over the crude polysaccharide-peptide (Chan et al., 2011).

Hericium erinaceum Lectin

The pH-stable and fairly thermostable lectin demonstrated antiproliferative activity toward HepG2 hepatoma and MCF7 breast cancer cells with an IC50 value of 56.1μM and 76.5μM, respectively. It manifested potent mitogenic action on mouse spleen cells (Li et al., 2010).

Hypsizigus marmoreus Ribosome-Inactivating Protein (Hypsin)

The 20-kDa ribosome-inactivating protein suppressed proliferation of mouse leukemia cells and human leukemia and hepatoma cells with an IC50 value of 5μM, 25μM, and 25μM, respectively. Translation in the cell-free rabbit reticulocyte lysate system was inhibited with an IC50 of 7 nM and HIV-1 reverse transcriptase activity was inhibited with an IC50 of 8μM (Lam and Ng, 2001).

Hypsizigus marmoreus Ribosome Inactivating Protein (Marmorin)

The 9,567-Da RIP inhibited proliferation of breast cancer MCF-7 cells and hepatoma Hep G2 cells, HIV-1 reverse transcriptase activity, and translation in the rabbit reticulocyte lysate system, more potently than RIPs from hairy gourd, bitter gourd, ridge gourd, garden pea, and the mushroom *Flammulina velutipes*(Wong et al.,2008).

Though marmorin adversely affected the survival of breast cancer *in vitro* as well as *in vivo,* it dispayed higher toxicity toward estrogen receptor (ER)-positive MCF7 breast cancer cells than the ER-negative counterpart MDA-MB-231 cells. The expression level of estrogen receptor α (ERα) was attenuated and 17β-estradiol -induced proliferation of MCF7 cells was suppressed. Knockdown of ERα in MCF7 cells impaired the antiproliferative action of marmorin, indicating the involvement of ERα-mediated pathway in the inhibitory effect of marmorin on ER-positive breast cancer cells. Marmorin elicited apoptosis in both MCF7 and MDA-MB-231 cells, causing arrest in G2/M-phase, depolarization of mitochondrial membrane potential and activation of caspase-9 in MCF7 cells, and to a lesser extent in MDA-MB-231 cells. Marmorin evoked the death receptor apoptotic pathway (e.g. caspase-8 activation) and endoplasmic reticulum stress (as witnessed by phosphorylation of IRE1α and

PERK, caspase-12 cleavage, and stimulation of CHOP expression) in both MCF7 and MDA-MB-231 cells (Pan et al., 2012).

Hypsizigus marmoreus Ribonuclease

The 18-kDa ribonuclease (RNase), with a novel N-terminal sequence and co-specificity for poly C and poly A, inhibited tritiated methylthymidine uptake by leukemia L1210 cells with an IC50 value of 60 μM (Guan et al., 2007).

Lactarius flavidulus Lectin

The dimeric 29.8-kDa lectin suppressed the proliferation of HepG2 hepatoma cells and L1210 leukemic cells with an IC50 value of 8.90 and 6.81 μM, respectively (Wu et al., 2011).

Lentinula edodes Polysaccharide (Lentinan)

The polysaccharide possesses a backbone of β-(1,3)-glucan with β-(1, 6) branches. It is an approved biological response modifier for gastric cancer therapy in Japan. Extended survival of advanced gastric cancer patients receiving both lentinan and chemotherapy compared to patients receiving only chemotherapy has been observed.

cytotoxic chemotherapeutic agents. Lentinan may synergize with anticancer monoclonal antibodies to activate complement systems via antibody-dependent cellular cytotoxicity and complement dependent cytotoxicity. (Ina et al., 2013).

Grifola frondosa Beta-Glucan

The beta-glucan induces apoptosis in prostatic cancer cells *in vitro* (Fullerton et al., 2000).

Lignosus rhinoceros Cold Water Extract either the Proteins or Protein-Carbohydrate Complex

The cold water extract inhibited proliferation of A549 human lung cancer cells and MCF-7 human breast cancer cells, with an IC50 value of 466.7μg/mL and 96.7μg/mL, respectively. By contrast, there was no cytotoxicity against normal human lung cells and human breast cells. Apoptosis of the treated cancer cells was disclosed by DNA fragmentation. The high-molecular-weight fraction of the cold water extract contained 68.7% carbohydrate and 3.6% protein. It was deduced that either the proteins or protein-carbohydrate complex contributed to the antiproliferative activity against cancer cells (Lee et al., 2012).

Pholiota adiposa Lectin

The16-kDa dimeric lectin inhibited proliferation of hepatoma Hep G2 cells and breast cancer MCF7 cells with an IC50 value of 2.1 μM and approximately 3.2 μM, respectively (Zhang et al., 2009)..

Pleurotus abalones Polysaccharide

The 120-kDa polysaccharide demonstrated antiproliferative activity against HepG2 human hepatoma cells, and also manifested antiproliferative activity toward MCF7 breast cancer cells with an IC50 of 3.7 μM (Wang et al., 2011).

Pleurotus abalones Polysaccharide-Peptide Complex

The ccomplex inhibited proliferation of breast cancer MCF7 cells and hepatoma HepG2 cells with an IC50 of 14μM, and 24μM, respectively. It lowered plasma glucose level in drug-induced diabetic mice and inhibited HIV-1 reverse transcriptase with an IC50 value of 12.5 μM. The complex possessed glucose, rhamnose, glucuronic acid and galactose in the molar ratio of 22.4:1:1.7:1.6 and demonstrated some N-terminal sequence homology to antioxidant enzymes(Li et al., 2012).

Pleurotus eous Lectin

The 16-kDa glycoprotein lectin demonstrated antiproliferative activity toward MCF-7, K562 and Hep2 cells lines at the lowest concentration of 2 μg/ml. and brought about a 50% reduction of proliferation of SK-N-MC cells at 50 μg/ml (Mahajan et al., 2002).

Pleurotus eryngii Hemolysin (Eryngeolysin)

The monomeric 17-kDa hemolysin exhibited cytotoxicity toward leukemia (L1210) cells with an IC50 value of 10 μM. It inhibited mitogenesis in ConA-stimulated as well as unstimulated mouse spleen cells. Its N-terminal sequence manifested pronounced resemblance to that of its counterparts ostreolysin from the oyster mushroom *Pleurotus ostreatus* and aegerolysin from the mushroom *Agrocybe cylindracea*. Eryngeolysin-induced hemolysis but not its anti-mitogenic and antiproliferative activities was protected by polyethylene glycol 10000 (Ngai and Ng, 2006).

Pleurotus nebrodensis Polysaccharide

Intraperitoneal injection with crude polysaccharides prolonged life span in sarcoma 180 bearing mice. Treatment with saline extract of the mushroom ensued in an increase in the splenocyte count numbers and greater production of nitric oxide, interleukin-1β, interleukin-6 and tumor necrosis factor-α. Treatment with hot water extract improved the immunopotentiating activity of B lymphocytes (Cha et al., 2012).

Pleurotus ostreatus Ribonuclease (Pleurostrin)

The 9 kDa ribonuclease, which exhibited preference for poly A among the various types of polyhomoribonucleotides, exerted antiproliferative activity toward leukemia L1210 cells with an IC50 value of 41 μM but was devoid of mitogenic activity (Xia et al., 2005).

Pleurotus pulmonarius Polysaccharide-Protein Complex

The polysaccharide suppressed liver cancer cell proliferation and invasion and also enhanced the sensitivity to cisplatin both *in vitro* and *in vivo*, by inhibiting the autocrine vascular endothelial growth factor-induced PI3K/AKT signaling pathway (Xu et al., 2012).

Pleurotus sajor-caju Ribonuclease

The 12-kDa ribonuclease, which demonstrated preference for poly U, suppressed incorporation of tritiated methylthymidine. by murine splenocytes with an IC50 of 65 nM. It reduced viability of HepG2 hepatoma cells and L1210 leukemia cells with an IC50 value of 0.22 and 0.1 μM, respectively (Ngai and Ng 2004).

Russula delica Lectin

The dimeric 60-kDa lectin suppressed proliferation of MCF 7 breast cancer cells and HepG2 hepatoma cells, with an IC50 value of 0.52 μM and 0.88 μM, respectively. There was no mitogenic activity toward mouse splenocytes (Zhao et al., 2010).

Russula delica Ribonuclease

The 14-kDa ribonuclease exhibited antiproliferative activity toward HepG2 and MCF-7 cancer cells with an IC50 value of 8.6 μM and 7.2 μM, respectively (Zhao et al., 2010).

Russula lepida Lectin

The 32-kDa lectin suppressed proliferation of hepatoma Hep G2 cells and human breast cancer MCF-7 cells with an IC50 value of 1.6 μM and 0.9 μM, respectively. The lectin when administered intraperitoneally (5.0 mg/kg body weight/day for 20 days) led to a decline in weight of the S-180 tumor by approximately two-thirds (Zhang et al., 2010).

Schizophyllum commune Lectin

The homodimeric 64-kDa lactose-binding lectin inhibited tritiated methylthymidine incorporation by L1210, MBL2, and HepG2 cells with an IC50 value of 0.5, 1.1, and 1.4 μM, respectively. It exhibited potent mitogenic activity toward mouse splenocytes, bringing about a maximal 15-fold stimulation at 4 μM concentration. It inhibited HIV-1 reverse transcriptase with an IC 50 value of 1.2 μM (Han et al., 2005).

Tricholoma mongolicum Lectins

The two 37-kDa dimeric nonglycoprotein lectins, TML-1 and TML-2, from *Tricholoma mongolicum* inhibited proliferation of mouse mastocytoma P815 cells and mouse monocyte-macrophage PU5-1.8 cells *in vitro* (Wang et al., 1995).

The two lectins upregulated nitrite production by macrophages in normal as well as tumor-bearing mice. The lectins had hardly any mitogenic activity toward T-cells from normal mice *in vitro* and T-cells from sarcoma-bearing mice *in vivo*. The lectins suppressed the growth of sarcoma 180 cells in the peritoneal cavity and prolonged survival of the mice (Wang et al.,1997).

Tuber indicum Ribonuclease

The 28-kDa RNase with high ribonucleolytic activity toward poly(A) inhibited the proliferation of HepG2 human hepatoma cells and MCF7 human breast cancer cells, with an IC50 value of 12.6 and 16.6 μM, respectively (Xiao et al., 2013).

Xerocomus chrysenteron Lectin

The lectin produced an antiproliferative effect on the adherent cell lines HeLa and NIH-3T3. Disruption of cell-substrate adhesion was the major contributing factor as the lectin did not produce a similar effect on SF9 cells which can grow without having to attach. The lectin affected cell adherence after suspension by trypsin treatment. It was found on the cell surface where it served as a coating agent, and elicited morphological alterations from well spread to rounded cells and destroyed the integrity of the actin cytoskeleton. It had no effect on the cell cycle, and did not trigger apoptosis (Marty-Detraves et al., 2004).

Xylaria hypoxylon Lectin

The lectin exhibited highly potent antiproliferative activity toward tumor cells.

IC50 values of 0.71, 0.73, 0.9 and 1.24μM in the case of M1 cells, and 0.31, 0.57, 0.68 and 0.74μM in the case of HepG2 cells were obtained for the lectin when incubation was performed in the presence of 0%, 2.5%, 5%, and 10% fetal bovine serum. The lectin exhibited a potent anti-mitogenic action on mouse splenocytes

(IC50 value=0.6 μM). It is a distinctive lectin in that it differs in molecular mass, N-terminal sequence and sugar specificity from previously reported ascomycete mushroom lectins (Liu et al., 2006).

Volvariella volvacea Lectin

S180 mouse sarcoma cells exposed to the lectin for 48 hr led to the appearance of surface bleb and cytoplasmic vacuoles, but not apoptotic bodies. The expression of cyclins A, D1, and E. was not affected. The expression of cyclin kinase inhibitors p21, p27, p53, and Rb was activated, Cell proliferation was arrested in the G2/M phase (Liu et al., 2001).

β-Glucans

Their *in vitro* and *in vivo* anticancer activities in experimental systems have been reported. They have been employed in the Far East as adjuvant therapy in clinical trials. Prolongation of patients' survival and improvement of the quality of life were observed, probably due to its immunoenhancing effect (Aleem, 2013).

Conclusion

A list of different mushroom proteins, polysaccharide-peptide complexes and polysaccharides with antiproliferative and anticancer activities is provided in the foregoing account. It has been demonstrated for some of the plant lectins that the activities of the lectins remained intact after passage through the gastrointestinal tract. The same may be true of mushroom lectins. Hence a diet containing ushrooms is beneficial to health. PSP and PSK from *Coriolus versicolor* have been used on cancer patients for a considerable number of years, and the results are gratifying. The bulk of research has so far been focused on polysaccharide-peptide complexes and polysaccharides although the fungal immunomodulatory proteins appear to be promising for further development. Further research on anticancer mushroom constituents may yield results that can be applied to the benefitan welfare of cancer patients.

Acknowledgments

The award of a research grant (number 81201270) from National Science Foundation of China is gratefully acknowledged.

References

Aleem E. β-Glucans and their applications in cancer therapy: focus on human studies. *Anticancer Agents Med Chem.* 2013;13(5):709-19.

Cha YJ, Alam N, Lee JS, Lee KR, Shim MJ, Lee MW, Kim HY, Shin PG, Cheong JC, Yoo YB, Lee TS. Anticancer and immunopotentiating activities of crude polysaccharides from *Pleurotus nebrodensis* on mouse sarcoma 180. *Mycobiology.* 2012;40(4):236-43.

Chan JY, Chan E, Chan SW, Sze SY, Chan MF, Tsui SH, Leung KY, Chan RY, Chung IY. Enhancement of *in vitro* and *in vivo* anticancer activities of polysaccharide peptide from *Grifola frondosa* by chemical modifications. *Pharm Biol.* 2011;49 (11):1114-20.

Chang YC, Hsiao YM, Wu MF, Ou CC, Lin YW, Lue KH, Ko JL. Interruption of lung cancer cell migration and proliferation by fungal immunomodulatory protein FIP-fve from *Flammulina velutipes. J Agric Food Chem.* 2013 Nov 22. Epub ahead of print

Feng K, Liu QH, Ng TB, Liu HZ, Li JQ, Chen G, Sheng HY, Xie ZL, Wang HX. Isolation and characterization of a novel lectin from the mushroom *Armillaria luteo-virens. Biochem Biophys Res Commun.* 2006;345(4):1573-8.

Gonzaga ML, Bezerra DP, Alves AP, de Alencar NM, Mesquita Rde O, Lima MW, Soares Sde A, Pessoa C, de Moraes MO, Costa-Lotufo LV. In vivo growth-inhibition of Sarcoma 180 by an alpha-(1-->4)-glucan-beta-(1-->6)-glucan-protein complex polysaccharide obtained from Agaricus blazei Murill. *J Nat Med.* 2009 ;63(1):32-40.

Guan GP, Wang HX, Ng TB. A novel ribonuclease with antiproliferative activity from fresh fruiting bodies of the edible mushroom *Hypsizigus marmoreus. Biochim Biophys Acta.* 2007;1770(12):1593-7.

Hien BT, Hoa le TP, Tham le X, Quang DN. Cattienoids A-C, three novel steroids from the mushroom *Tomophagus cattienensis. Fitoterapia.* 2013;91:125-7.

Hsiao PC, Hsieh YH, Chow JM, Yang SF, Hsiao M, Hua KT, Lin CH, Chen HY, Chien MH. Hispolon induces apoptosis through JNK1/2-mediated activation of a caspase-8, -9, and -3-dependent pathway in acute myeloid leukemia (AML) cells and inhibits AML xenograft tumor growth *in vivo. J Agric Food Chem.* 2013;61(42):10063-73.

Hu DD, Zhang RY, Zhang GQ, Wang HX, Ng TB. A laccase with antiproliferative activity against tumor cells from an edible mushroom, white common *Agrocybe cylindracea. Phytomedicine.* 2011;18(5):374-9.

Hui KP, Sit WH, Wan JM. Induction of S phase cell arrest and caspase activation by polysaccharide peptide isolated from *Coriolus versicolor* enhanced the cell cycle dependent activity and apoptotic cell death of doxorubicin and etoposide, but not cytarabine in HL-60 cells. *Oncol Rep* 2005:145-55.

Ina K, Kataoka T, Ando T. The use of lentinan for treating gastric cancer. *Anticancer Agents Med Chem.* 2013;13(5):681-8.

Lam SK, Ng TB. Hypsin, a novel thermostable ribosome-inactivating protein with antifungal and antiproliferative activities from fruiting bodies of the edible mushroom *Hypsizigus marmoreus. Biochem Biophys Res Commun.* 2001;285(4):1071-5.

Lam YW, Ng TB, Wang HX. Antiproliferative and antimitogenic activities in a peptide from puffball mushroom *Calvatia caelata. Biochem Biophys Res Commun.* 2001 ;289(3):744-9.

Lee ML, Tan NH, Fung SY, Tan CS, Ng ST. The Antiproliferative activity of sclerotia of *Lignosus rhinocerus* (Tiger Milk Mushroom). *Evid Based Complement Alternat Med.* 2012;2012:697603.

Li N, Li L, Fang JC, Wong JH, Ng TB, Jiang Y, Wang CR, Zhang NY, Wen TY, Qu LY, Lv PY, Zhao R, Shi B, Wang YP, Wang XY, Liu F. Isolation and identification of a novel polysaccharide-peptide complex with antioxidant, anti-proliferative and hypoglycaemic activities from the abalone mushroom. *Biosci Rep.* 2012 ;32(3):221-8.

Li Y, Zhang G, Ng TB, Wang H. A novel lectin with antiproliferative and HIV-1 reverse transcriptase inhibitory activities from dried fruiting bodies of the monkey head mushroom *Hericium erinaceum*. *J Biomed Biotechnol.* 2010;2010:716515.

Liang C, Li H, Zhou H, Zhang S, Liu Z, Zhou Q, Sun F. Recombinant Lz-8 from *Ganoderma lucidum* induces endoplasmic reticulum stress-mediated autophagic cell death in SGC-7901 human gastric cancer cells. *Oncol Rep.* 2012;27(4):1079-89.

Liao CH, Hsiao YM, Hsu CP, Lin MY, Wang JC, Huang YL, Ko JL. Transcriptionally mediated inhibition of telomerase of fungal immunomodulatory protein from *Ganoderma tsugae* in A549 human lung adenocarcinoma cell line. *Mol Carcinog.* 2006;45(4):220-9.

Liu Q, Wang H, Ng TB. First report of a xylose-specific lectin with potent hemagglutinating, antiproliferative and anti-mitogenic activities from a wild ascomycete mushroom. *Biochim Biophys Acta.* 2006;1760(12):1914-9.

Liu W, Ho JC, Ng T. Suppression of cell cycle progression by a fungal lectin: activation of cyclin-dependent kinase inhibitors. *Biochem Pharmacol.* 2001;61(1):33-7.

Ng TB. A review of research on the protein-bound polysaccharide (polysaccharopeptide, PSP) from the mushroom *Coriolus versicolor* (Basidiomycetes: Polyporaceae). *Gen Pharmacol.* 1998;30(1):1-4.

Ng TB, Lam YW, Wang H. Calcaelin, a new protein with translation-inhibiting, antiproliferative and antimitogenic activities from the mosaic puffball mushroom *Calvatia caelata*. *Planta Med.* 2003;69(3):212-7.

Ng TB, Ngai PH, Xia L. An agglutinin with mitogenic and antiproliferative activities from the mushroom *Flammulina velutipes*. *Mycologia.* 2006;98(2):167-71.

Ngai PH, Ng TB. A hemolysin from the mushroom *Pleurotus eryngii*. *Appl Microbiol Biotechnol.* 2006;72(6):1185-91.

Pan WL, Wong JH, Fang EF, Chan YS, Ye XJ, Ng TB. Differential inhibitory potencies and mechanisms of the type I ribosome inactivating protein marmorin on estrogen receptor (ER)-positive and ER-negative breast cancer cells. *Biochim Biophys Acta.* 2013;1833(5):987-96.

Pohleven J, Obermajer N, Sabotic J, Anzlovar S, Sepcić K, Kos J, Kralj B, Strukelj B, Brzin J. Purification, characterization and cloning of a ricin B-like lectin from mushroom *Clitocybe nebularis* with antiproliferative activity against human leukemic T cells. *Biochim Biophys Acta.* 2009; 1790(3):173-81.

Rosendahl AH, Sun C, Wu D, Andersson R. Polysaccharide-K (PSK) increases p21(WAF/Cip1) and promotes apoptosis in pancreatic cancer cells. *Pancreatology.* 2012;12(6):467-74.

Sun J, Chen QJ, Cao QQ, Wu YY, Xu LJ, Zhu MJ, Ng TB, Wang HX, Zhang GQ. A laccase with antiproliferative and HIV-I reverse transcriptase inhibitory activities from the mycorrhizal fungus *Agaricus placomyces*. *J Biomed Biotechnol.* 2012;2012:736472.

Sun J, Zhao Y, Chai H, Wang H, Ng TB. A novel alkaline protease with antiproliferative activity from fresh fruiting bodies of the toxic wild mushroom *Amanita farinosa. Acta Biochim Pol.* 2011;58(4):567-72.

Wan JM, Sit WH, Louie JC. Polysaccharopeptide enhances the anticancer activity of doxorubicin and etoposide on human breast cancer cells ZR-75-30. *Int J Oncol.* 2008 ;32(3):689-99.

Wang CR, Ng TB, Li L, Fang JC, Jiang Y, Wen TY, Qiao WT, Li N, Liu F. Isolation of a polysaccharide with antiproliferative, hypoglycemic, antioxidant and HIV-1 reverse transcriptase inhibitory activities from the fruiting bodies of the abalone mushroom *Pleurotus abalonus. J Pharm Pharmacol.* 2011 ;63(6):825-32.

Wang HX, Ng TB, Ooi VE, Liu WK, Chang ST. Actions of lectins from the mushroom *Tricholoma mongolicum* on macrophages, splenocytes and life-span in sarcoma-bearing mice. *Anticancer Res.* 1997;17(1A):419-24.

Wang HX, Ng TB. Isolation of pleuturegin, a novel ribosome-inactivating protein from fresh sclerotia of the edible mushroom *Pleurotus tuber-regium. Biochem Biophys Res Commun.* 2001;288(3):718-21.

Wang XM, Zhang J, Wu LH, Zhao YL, Li T, Li JQ, Wang YZ, Liu HG. A mini-review of chemical composition and nutritional value of edible wild-grown mushroom from China. Food Chem. 2014;151:279-85.

Wasser SP. Current findings, future trends, and unsolved problems in studies of medicinal mushrooms. *Appl Microbiol Biotechnol.* 2011;89(5):1323-32.

Wong JH, Ng TB, Cheung RC, Ye XJ, Wang HX, Lam SK, Lin P, Chan YS, Fang EF, Ngai PH, Xia LX, Ye XY, Jiang Y, Liu F. Proteins with antifungal properties and other medicinal applications from plants and mushrooms. *Appl Microbiol Biotechnol.* 2010;87(4):1221-35.

Wong JH, Wang HX, Ng TB. Marmorin, a new ribosome inactivating protein with antiproliferative and HIV-1 reverse transcriptase inhibitory activities from the mushroom *Hypsizigus marmoreus. Appl Microbiol Biotechnol.* 2008;81(4):669-74.

Wong JH, Wang H, Ng TB. A haemagglutinin from the medicinal fungus *Cordyceps militaris. Biosci Rep.* 2009;29(5):321-7.

Wu Y, Wang H, Ng TB. Purification and characterization of a lectin with antiproliferative activity toward cancer cells from the dried fruit bodies of *Lactarius flavidulus. Carbohydr Res.* 2011;346(16):2576-81.

Xiao C, Feng S, Wang H, Gong Z, Ng T. Purification and characterization of a ribonuclease with antiproliferative activity from the mystical wild mushroom *Tuber indicum. J Basic Microbiol.* 2013 Jun 21. [Epub ahead of print].

Xu X, Yan H, Chen J, Zhang X. Bioactive proteins from mushrooms. *Biotechnol Adv.* 2011;29(6):667-74.

Zhang G, Sun J, Wang H, Ng TB. First isolation and characterization of a novel lectin with potent antitumor activity from a *Russula* mushroom. *Phytomedicine.* 2010;17(10):775-81.

Zhang GQ, Sun J, Wang HX, Ng TB. A novel lectin with antiproliferative activity from the medicinal mushroom *Pholiota adiposa. Acta Biochim Pol.* 2009;56(3):415-21.

Zhao S, Zhao Y, Li S, Zhang G, Wang H, Ng TB. An antiproliferative ribonuclease from fruiting bodies of the wild mushroom *Russula delica. J Microbiol Biotechnol.* 2010;20(4):693-9.

Zhao S, Zhao Y, Li S, Zhao J, Zhang G, Wang H, Ng TB. A novel lectin with highly potent antiproliferative and HIV-1 reverse transcriptase inhibitory activities from the edible wild mushroom *Russula delica*. *Glycoconj J.* 2010;27(2):259-65.

In: Horizons in Cancer Research. Volume 54
Editor: Hiroto S. Watanabe
ISBN: 978-1-63321-389-0

Chapter 6

Low-Molecular-Weight Compounds with Anticancer Activity of Mushroom Origin

Tzi Bun Ng[*] and Charlene Cheuk Wing Ng
School of Biomedical Sciences, Faculty of Medicine,
The Chinese University of Hong Kong, Shatin,
New Territories, Hong Kong, China

Abstract

The following low-molecular-weight compounds of mushroom origins exhibit anticancer activity toward various cancer cells. The list of compounds include active hexose correlated compound, gamma-L-glutaminyl-4-hydroxybenzene derivatives from *Agaricus bisporus, Albatrellus confluens* grifolin, *Antrodia camphorata* ubiquinone derivative (antroquinonol), *Antrodia camphorata* sesquiterpene lactone (antrocin), *Astraeus odoratus* lanostane triterpenes (astraodoric acids A-D), *Boletus pseudocalopus* grifolin derivatives and phenolic compounds, *Chondrostereum sp.* hirsutane sesquiterpenoid (hirsutanol A), *Coprinus plicatilis* guanacastane-type diterpenoids, *Coprinus radians* diterpenoid (radianspene C), *Daedalea gibbosa* oleylamine-carbonyl-valinol, *Epicoccum sp* glycosylated tetramic acid derivative (epicoccamide D), ergosterol peroxide, *Fomitopsis nigra* lanostane triterpene glycoside (fomitoside-K), *Ganoderma lucidum* lanostanoid triterpene (ganodermanontriol), *Ganoderma lucidum* triterpene, *Ganoderma lucidum* ganoderic acids, *Ganoderma lucidum* ergosta-7,22-diene-2β,3α,9α-triol, *Hypholoma sublateritium* clavaric acid, *Inonotus obliquus* ergosterol peroxide and trametenolic acid, *Lentinus connatus* hirsutane sesquiterpenes (dihydrohypnophilin, panepoxydione, and panepoxydone), *Leucopaxillus gentianeus* cucurbitane triterpenoid (cucurbitacin B), L-glutamic acid dihydroxyanilide, *Naematoloma fasciculare* lanostane derivatives, *Naematoloma fasciculare* lanostane triterpenoids, *Omphalotus* illudin S derivative (Irofulven) and droxymethylacylfulvene, *Phellinus igniarius* phenolic (hispolon), *Phellinus linteus* phenolic (hispidin), *Poria cocos* triterpenes, *Thelephora*

[*] Corresponding author. School of Biomedical Sciences, Faculty of Medicine, The Chinese University of Hong Kong, Shatin, New Territories, Hong Kong, China. Email : b021770@mailserv.cuhk.edu.hk.

aurantiotincta thelephantin O and vialinin A, *Tomophagus cattienensis* steroids (cattienoids A-C), and *Tomophagus cattienensis* steroids (cattienoids A-C)

Keywords: Low-molecular-weight compounds, mushroom, anticancer activity

Introduction

Mushrooms have been employed in traditional oriental medicine. Mushrooms represent a source of pharmaceutical products and functional foods. There is a diversity of substances with antitumor activity identified in mushrooms. The low-molecular-weight compounds include amines, catechols, cerebrosides, isoflavones, organic germanium, quinones, selenium, sesquiterpenes, steroids, and triacylglycerols. High-molecular-weight compounds comprise homo glucans, heteroglucans, glycans, glycoproteins, glycopeptides, proteoglycans, proteins and RNA-protein complexes (Ferreira et al., 2010).

The purpose of the present article is to review the low-molecular-weight compounds with anticancer activity reported in the literature.

Active Hexose Correlated Compound

Active hexose correlated compound (AHCC) is an extract of a mushroom utilized as a supplement by some cancer patients undergoing chemotherapy to enhance the therapeutic efficacy and minimize the side effects of anticacer agents. AHCC potentiated the anticancer effects of cisplatin and mitigated its side effects in female BALB/cA mice inoculated with Colon-26 tumor cells.

AHCC supplementation to mice receiving monotherapy with paclitaxel, or multi-drug chemotherapy with paclitaxel plus cisplatin, 5-fluorouracil plus irinotecan, cisplatin plus5-fluorouracil, or doxorubicin plus cyclophosphamide. Bone marrow cell viability and white blood cell count were lowered after multi-drug treatments in all groups except for paclitaxel + cisplatin. These side effects, together with toxicity to the kidneys and the liver and mortality, were reduced by AHCC administration (Shigama et al., 2009)

Agaricus bisporus Gamma-L-Glutaminyl-4-Hydroxybenzene Derivatives

Synthesis of nucleic acid and protein in five types of murine ascites tumor cells was inhibited when these quinoids were added at millimolar concentrations to the tissue culture medium used to culture the tumor cells. Only a small percentage of the cells was killed immediately, as judged by trypan blue uptake. The survival times of histocompatible mice that received intraperitoneal injections of BP8 sarcoma and EL4 leukemic cells previously exposed to these quinoids were longer compared with animals that received tumor cells without prior treatment with the quinoids. Growth of thetumor cells was slowed by the quinoidtreatment (Vogel et al., 1975).

Albatrellus confluens Grifolin

The action of grifolin on CNE1 human nasopharyngeal carcinoma cells is mediated primarily by the ERK1/2 pathway. At high doses, both ERK1/2 and ERK5 pathways may be mplicated in the inhibitory action. Grifolin brought about cell-cycle arrest in G1 phase, and produced a suppression of expression of cyclin D1, cyclin E, and CDK4. There was an attenuation in pRB phosphorylation and upregulation of CKI (p19INK4D). The data indicate that inhibition of the ERK1/2 or the ERK5 pathway is responsible for grifolin-induced cell-cycle arrest in G1 phase (Ye et al., 2007).

Antrodia camphorata Ubiquinone Derivative (Antroquinonol)

Antroquinonol inhibited proliferation in PANC-1 and AsPC-1 pancreatic cancer cells. It arrested the cells in G1 phase of the cell cycle and subsequently elicited apoptosis. Antroquinonol suppressed Akt phosphorylation at Ser(473), the phosphorylation site pivotal to Akt kinase activity, and inhibited phosphorylation of mammalian target of rapamycin (mTOR) at Ser(2448), a site dependent on mTOR activity. Antroquinonol down-regulated cell cycle regulators and mitochondrial antiapoptotic proteins, and enhanced the expression of K-ras and its phosphorylation. It augmented the association of K-ras and Bcl-xL, signifying apoptotic cell death. Antroquinonol promoted cross-talk between apoptosis, autophagic cell death and expedited senescence, at least partly, explained by the up-regulation of p21(Waf1/Cip1) and K-ras. Antroquinonol induced anticancer activity in human pancreatic cancers through inhibition of PI3-kinase/Akt/mTOR pathways that downregulates cell cycle regulators. The inhibition brought about G1 arrest of the cell cycle and an ultimate mitochondria-dependent apoptosis. Moreover, autophagic cell death and accelerated senescence also explain antroquinonol-mediated anticancer effect (Yu et al., 2011).

Antrodia camphorata Sesquiterpene Lactone (Antrocin)

Antrocin exerted antiproliferative activity toward two non-small-cell lung cancer cells, H1975 (gefitnib-resistant mutant T790M, IC50 = 0.83 μM) and H441 (wild-type epidermal growth factor receptor, IC50 =0.75 μM). Antrocin inhibited colony formation and triggered apoptosis as witnessed by activated caspase-3 and an elevated Bax/Bcl2 ratio. Janus kinase/signal transducer and activator of transcription (JAK/STAT) signaling pathway was downregulated. antrocin suppressed Antrocin downregulated both constitutively activated and interleukin 6-induced STAT3 phosphorylation and its subsequent nuclear translocation through the inhibition of JAK2 and interaction between STAT3 and extracellular signal-regulated kinase. MicroRNA let-7c expression was augmented and STAT signaling was attenuated. Together antrocin and JAK2/STAT3 gene silencing stimulated apoptosis in H441 cells.

This dual intervention of JAK2 and STAT3 pathways suppressed antiapoptotic protein mcl-1 and enhanced caspase-3 expression. Intraperitoneally administered antrocin inhibited the growth of lung cancer tumor xenografts (Yeh et al., 2013).

Astraeus odoratus Lanostane Triterpenes (Astraodoric Acids A-D)

Astraodoric acids A and B exhibited cytotoxic activities (IC50 values of 19.99 and 48.35 μg/mL against NCI-H187, and 34.69 and 18.57 μg/mL against KB, respectively) (Arpha et al., 2012).

Boletus pseudocalopus Grifolin Derivatives and Phenolic Compounds

All of the compounds displayed anticancer activity (IC50 values of 3.5-11.0 microg/ml against A549 human lung carcinoma cells and B16F1 mouse melanoma cells (Song et al., 2009).

Chondrostereum Sp. Hirsutane Sesquiterpenoid (Hirsutanol A)

Hirsutanol A demonstrated a highly potent cytotoxic action against various cancer cell lines including human colon cancer cell line (SW620, SW480, and LoVo), human hepatic cancer cell lines (Hep3B, HepG2, and Bel-7402) Human lung cancer cell line A549, human nasopharyngeal carcinoma cell lines (CNE1, CNE2, and SUNE1), human breast cancer cell lines (MCF 7 MDA-MB-231, MDA-MB-435 and MDA-MB-453), and human cervical cancer cell line HeLa (Li et al., 2011).

Coprinus plicatilis Guanacastane-Type Diterpenoids

The diterpenoids exhibited a cytotoxic action against BGC-823 human stomach adenocarcinoma cells; HCT 116 human colon cancer cells; HeLa human cervical cancer cells; HepG2 human hepatocellular carcinoma cells; MDA-MB-231 human metastatic breast adenocarcinoma cells; and U2OS human osteosarcoma cells with IC50 values ranging from 1.2 to 6.0 μM (Liu et al., 2012).

Coprinus radians Diterpenoid (Radianspene C)

Radianspene C inhibited MDA-MB-435 human breast carcinoma cells with IC50 of 0.91 μM (Ou et al., 2012).

Daedalea gibbosa Oleylamine-Carbonyl-Valinol

Chronic myeloid leukemia is accompanied by the presence of p210(Bcr-Abl) with an abnormal kinase activity. In spite of availability of selective Abl kinase inhibitors for the treatment of chronic myeloid leukemia and high clinical response rates, resistance has developed against these kinase inhibitors primarily because of point mutations within the Abl protein kinase domain. Oleic acid in the mushroom *Daedalea gibbosa* is a Bcr-Abl kinase inhibitor. The oleyl amine derivatives, S-1-(1-Hydroxymethyl-2-methyl-propyl)-3-octadec-9-enyl-urea[oleylaminocarbonyl-L-N-valinol, oroleylaminocarbonyl-S-2-isopropyl-N-ethanol-amine, oleylamine-carbonyl-L-valinol] and R-1-(1-Hydroxymethyl-2-methyl-propyl)-3-octadec-9-enyl-urea oleylamineocarbonyl-D-N-valinol, oleylaminocarbonyl-R-2-isopropyl-N-ethanolamine, or oleylamine-carbonyl-D-valinol] (cpd 7), inhibited the activity of the native and T315I mutated Bcr-Abl. Furthermore, the compounds displayed more potent activity toward the oncogenic Bcr-Abl compared to native c-Abl in SupB15 Ph-positive ALL cell line (Najajreh et al., 2013).

Epicoccum Sp Glycosylated Tetramic Acid Derivative (Epicoccamide D)

Epicoccamide D exhibited weak to moderate cytotoxicity on HeLa cells (IC50 17.0 microM). It suppressed proliferation of K-562 human leukemia cells and L-929 mouse fibroblasts with IC50 of 33.3 and 50.5 microM, respectively (Wangun et al., 2007).

Ergosterol Peroxide

Ergosterol peroxide from an edible mushroom inhibited growth of HT29 colon adenocarcinoma cells, increased intracellular reactive oxygen species, upregulated the expression of oxidative stress-inducible genes, and the cyclin-dependent kinase inhibitor CDKN1A, and downregulated STAT1 and interferon-inducible genes. (Kobori et al., 2007)..

Fomitopsis nigra Lanostane Triterpene Glycoside (Fomitoside-K)

Fomitoside-K triggered apoptosis in YD-10B human oral squamous cell carcinomas cells as characterized by cell morphology, cell cycle arrest, downregulation of survivin, activation of poly(ADP-ribose) polymerase (PARP), caspase-3, -9 and an elevated expression ratio of Bax/Bcl-2. Loss of mitochondria membrane potential and release of cytochrome c from mitochondria to cytosol, elevation of intracellular reactive oxygen species level and increased phosphorylation of c-Jun N-terminal kinase and extracellular signal-regulated kinase in YD-10B cells occurred. Reactive oxygen species level was lowered by N-acetyl-L-cysteine NAC, extracellular signal-regulated kinase (PD98059) and c-Jun N-terminal kinase inhibitor (SP600125). Fomitoside-K synergized with adriamycin in retarding the growth of YD-10B cells. (Bhattarai et al., 2012).

Ganoderma lucidum Lanostanoid Triterpene (Ganodermanontriol)

Ganodermanontriol repressed proliferation (anchorage-dependent growth) and colony production (anchorage-independent growth) of highly invasive MDA-MB-231 human breast cancer cells. Expression of the cell cycle regulatory protein CDC20 overexpressed in precancerous and breast cancer cells was attenuated compared to normal mammary epithelial cells. CDC20 is over-expressed in tumors when compared to the tissue surrounding the tumor in specimens from breast cancer patients. Ganodermanontriol downregulated invasive behavior (cell adhesion, cell migration, and cell invasion) by inhibiting the secretion of urokinase-plasminogen activator and expression of its receptor (Jiang et al., 2011).

Ganodermanontriol inhibited proliferation of HCT-116 and HT-29 colon cancer cells without affecting cell viability. Transcriptional activity of ß-catenin and protein expression of its target gene cyclin D1 was attenuated. Pronounced suppression of Cdk-4 and PCNA expression was observed, but there was no effect on expression of Cdk-2, cyclin E and p21. Protein expression of E-cadherin and ß-catenin in HT-29 cells was augmented. Tumor growth in a xenograft model of HT-29 human colon adenocarcinoma cells implanted in nude mice and cyclin D1 expression in tumors were inhibited (Jedinak et al., 2011).

Ganoderma lucidum Triterpene

The triterpene-enriched fraction WEES-G6 inhibited growth of human hepatoma Huh-7 cells. WEES-G6 rapidly attenuated the activity of cell growth regulative protein, protein kinase C, and the activation of JNK and p38 mitogen activating protein kinases. The G2 phase of the cell cycle was extended. There were no similar effects on normal human Chang liver cells. The authors concluded that the triterpenes in WEES-G6 were responsible for the observed anticancer effects (Lin et al., 2003).

Ganoderma lucidum Ganoderic Acids

The antitumor compounds, ganoderic acids, are produced by *G. lucidum* (Zhao et al., 2011).

Ganoderma lucidum Ergosta-7,22-Diene-2β,3α,9α-Triol

Ergosta-7,22-diene-2β,3α,9α-triol triggered apoptosis in HL-60 human premyelocytic leukemia cells. The triol promoted fragmentation and caspase-3 activity, and cleavage of procaspase-3 and poly(ADP-ribose) polymerase (PARP) into active forms. Treatment of to Lewis lung carcinoma -bearing mice with the triol brought about a significant suppression of tumor growth (Lee et al., 2011).

Hypholoma sublateritium Clavaric Acid

Squalene epoxidase is involved in antitumor clavaric acid formation and in ergosterol biosynthesis (Godio et al., 2007).

Inonotus obliquus Ergosterol Peroxide And Trametenolic Acid

Ergosterol peroxide and trametenolic acid manifested a cytotoxic action on MDA-MB-231breast carcinoma cells and PC3 human prostatic carcinoma cells (Ma et al., 2013).

Lentinus connatus Hirsutane Sesquiterpenes (Dihydrohypnophilin, Panepoxydione, and Panepoxydone)

The sesquiterpenes manifested a cytotoxic action on human breast cancer (BC), human epidermoid carcinoma (KB), and human small cell lung cancer (NCI-H187) cells (Rukachaisirikul et al., 2005).

Leucopaxillus gentianeus Cucurbitane Triterpenoid (Cucurbitacin B)

Cucurbitacin B inhibited proliferation of A549, CAKI-1, HepG2, and MCF-7 human tumor cells (Clericuzio et al., 2004).

L-Glutamic Acid Dihydroxyanilide

L-glutamic acid, gamma-(p-hydroxyanilide), inhibited the growth of B-16 melanoma in vivo. The 2,5-dihydroxy derivative has a higher activity with a 5-fold decline in IC50 for both human and B-16 melanoma cells in vitro. The 3,4-dihydroxy derivative exerted inhibitory effects on thymidine incorporation into melanoma cells in vitro while the 2,5-dihydroxy derivative also inhibited uridine and leucine incorporation (Wick et al., 1980).

Naematoloma fasciculare Lanostane Derivatives

The petroleum ether fraction of *Naematoloma fasciculare* suppressed proliferation of breast cancer MCF-7 cells and tumor growth H22 bearing mice due to the activity of unsaturated aliphatic acids, ergosterol peroxide and ergosterol (Yan et al., 2009).

Naematoloma fasciculare Lanostane Triterpenoids

The triterpenoids inhibited the proliferation of the human cancer cell lines A549, HCT-15, SK-MEL-2, and SK-OV-3 (Kim et al., 2013).

Omphalotus illudin S Derivative (Irofulven) and Droxymethylacylfulvene

MGI 114 (6-hydroxymethylacylfulvene, HMAF) is a semisynthetic antitumor compound derived from the sesquiterpene mushroom toxin illudin S. MGI 114 displayed activity against both adult and pediatric primary tumor colony-forming units. The *in vitro* activity of MGI 114 at concentrations attainable in clinical trials, together with activity against drug-resistant tumors had been oberved (Hidalgo et al., 1999).

Concurrent exposure to irofulven and cisplatin is at least additive for most cell lines examined including HT-29 and HCT-116 colorectal and A2780 ovarian carcinoma cells whereas simultaneous exposure to irofulven and 5-fluorouracil is additive to synergistic for all the cell lines studied, including the cisplatin-resistant and irofulven- resistant cell lines. The enhanced cytotoxicity of irofulven in conjunction with 5-fluorouracil and cisplatin advocated their clinical application (Poindessous et al., 2003).

Irofulven, activates the ATM-CHK2 DNA damage-signaling pathway, and CHK2 activation contributes to S phase cell cycle arrest in ovarian cancer cell lines induced by irofulven(Wang et al., 2004).

Mutation of the tumor suppressor gene BRCA1, which is vital to the maintenance of genomic stability by interaction with proteins regulating the cell cycle and DNA repair, is often detected in familial breast and ovarian cancer. Irofulven activates ATM and its targets, NBS1, SMC1, CHK2, and p53. Irofulven induces DNA double-strand breaks and radical formation and the activation and foci formation of gamma-H2AX, BRCA1, and RAD51. BRCA1 contributes to the control of S and G(2)/M cell cycle arrest and of paramount importance for repair of DNA double-strand breaks and for RAD51-dependent homologous recombination. BRCA1 deficiency leads to increased chromosomal damage and chemosensitivity after irofulven treatment (Wiltshire et al., 2007).

Phellinus igniarius Phenolic (Hispolon)

Hispolon manifested antiproliferative activity toward a variety of acute myeloid leukemia cell lines. It triggered apoptosis of HL-60 acute myeloid leukemia cells through activation of caspases -3, -8, and -9 and PARP cleavage. Hispolon activated JNK1/2, and inhibited JNK by JNK1/2 inhibitor or JNK1/2-specific siRNA abolished the activation of the caspase-3/-9/-8 hispolon. In vivo, hispolon significantly reduced tumor growth in mice with HL-60 tumor xenografts. In hispolon-treated tumors, activation of caspase-3 and a decrease in Ki67-positive cells were observed (Hsiao et al., 2013).

Hispolon inhibited growth of human hepatocellular carcinoma Hep3B cells by bringing about cell cycle arrest and apoptotic cell death. Hispolon-induced S-phase arrest was accompanied with a striking decline in the protein expression of cyclins A and E and cyclin dependent kinase 2, with simultaneous stimulation of p27Kip1 and. p21waf1/Cip1 Exposure of Hep3B cells to hispolon resulted in apoptosis as evidenced by caspase activation, PARP cleavage, and DNA fragmentation. Hispolon activated ERK, JNK, and p38 MAPK expression. Inhibitors of ERK (PB98095), but not those of JNK (SP600125) and p38 MAPK (SB203580), suppressed hispolon-induced S-phase arrest and apoptosis in Hep3B cells. (Huang et al., 2011).

Phellinus linteus Phenolic (Hispidin)

Hispidin manifested potent anticancer, antioxidant, and antidiabetic activities (Chen et al., 2012).

Poria cocos Triterpenes

The triterpenes dehydropachymic acid, pachymic acid and polyporenic acid inhibited the proliferation of AsPc-1, BxPc-3, MiaPaca-2, and Panc-1 human pancreatic cancer cells without affecting proliferation of HPDE-6 normal pancreatic duct epithelial cells to any major extent. Pachymic acid downregulated the protein level of matrix metalloproteinase-7 and thus inhibited the invasiveness of BxPc-3 cells (Cheng et al., 2013).

Thelephora aurantiotincta Thelephantin O And Vialinin A

Vialinin A and thelephantin O adversely affected cell viability in HepG2 human hepatocellular carcinoma cells and Caco2 human colonic carcinoma cells, but had no effect on noncancerous human hepatocytes (Norikura et al., 2011).

Tomophagus cattienensis Steroids (Cattienoids A-C)

The cattienoids exerted a cytotoxic action on KB (a human epidermal carcinoma) cells with an IC50 value below 100 μM (Hien et al., 2013).

Tomophagus cattienensis Steroids (Cattienoids A-C)

Terreumols A, C and D 3, and 4 demonstrated an inhibitory action against MCF-7 breast cancer cells, SMMC-7721 hepatocellular carcinoma cells, SW480 colon cancer cells, A-549 lung cancer cells and HL-60 human myeloid cells, with IC50 values similar to those of cisplatin (Yin et al., 2013).

Conclusion

A spectrum of low-molecular-weight mushroom compounds demonstrate anticancer activity toward a diversity of cancer cells. The mechanism of anticancer action including the apoptotic pathways induced has been elucidated in a few cases. Yet the molecular details await clarification in many other cases. The safety and bioavailability of these potentially exploitable also remain to be ascertained. The presence of both low-molecular-weight compounds and high-molecular-weight substances, very often in the same mushroom, attests to the ability of mushrooms to promote health when included in the diet.

References

Arpha K, Phosri C, Suwannasai N, Mongkolthanaruk W, Sodngam S. Astraodoric acids A-D: new lanostane triterpenes from edible mushroom *Astraeus odoratus* and their anti-*Mycobacterium tuberculosis* H37Ra and cytotoxic activity. *J. Agric. Food Chem.* 2012 60(39):9834-41.

Bhattarai G, Lee YH, Lee NH, Lee IK, Yun BS, Hwang PH, Yi HK. Fomitoside-K from *Fomitopsis nigra* induces apoptosis of human oral squamous cell carcinomas (YD-10B) via mitochondrial signaling pathway. *Biol. Pharm. Bull.* 2012;35(10):1711-9.

Chen W, Feng L, Huang Z, Su H. Hispidin produced from *Phellinus linteus* protects against peroxynitrite-mediated DNA damage and hydroxyl radical generation. *Chem. Biol. Interact.* 2012; 199(3):137-42.

Cheng S, Eliaz I, Lin J, Sliva D. Triterpenes from *Poria cocos* suppress growth and invasiveness of pancreatic cancer cells through the downregulation of MMP-7. *Int. J. Oncol.* 2013; 42(6):1869-74.

Clericuzio M, Mella M, Vita-Finzi P, Zema M, Vidari G. Cucurbitane triterpenoids from *Leucopaxillus gentianeus*. *J. Nat. Prod.* 2004;67(11):1823-8.

Ferreira IC, Vaz JA, Vasconcelos MH, Martins A. Compounds from wild mushrooms with antitumor potential. *Anticancer Agents Med. Chem.* 2010; 10(5):424-36.

Godio RP, Fouces R, Martín JF. A squalene epoxidase is involved in biosynthesis of both the antitumor compound clavaric acid and sterols in the basidiomycete *H. sublateritium*. *Chem. Biol.* 2007;14(12):1334-46.

Hidalgo M, Izbicka E, Eckhardt SG, MacDonald JR, Cerna C, Gomez L, Rowinsky EK, Weitman SD, Von Hoff DD. Antitumor activity of MGI 114 (6-hydroxymethylacylfulvene, HMAF), a semisynthetic derivative of illudin S, against adult and pediatric human tumor colony-forming units. *Anticancer Drugs.* 1999;10(9):837-44.

Hien BT, Hoa le TP, Tham le X, Quang DN. Cattienoids A-C, three novel steroids from the mushroom *Tomophagus cattienensis*. *Fitoterapia*. 2013; 91:125-7.

Hsiao PC, Hsieh YH, Chow JM, Yang SF, Hsiao M, Hua KT, Lin CH, Chen HY, Chien MH. Hispolon induces apoptosis through JNK1/2-mediated activation of a caspase-8, -9, and -3-dependent pathway in acute myeloid leukemia (AML) cells and inhibits AML xenograft tumor growth *in vivo*. *J. Agric. Food Chem.* 2013; 61(42):10063-73.

Huang GJ, Deng JS, Huang SS, Hu ML. Hispolon induces apoptosis and cell cycle arrest of human hepatocellular carcinoma Hep3B cells by modulating ERK phosphorylation. *J. Agric. Food Chem.* 2011; 59(13):7104-13.

Jedinak A, Thyagarajan-Sahu A, Jiang J, Sliva D. Ganodermanontriol, a lanostanoid triterpene from *Ganoderma lucidum*, suppresses growth of colon cancer cells through ß-catenin signaling. *Int. J. Oncol.* 2011; 38(3):761-7.

Jiang J, Jedinak A, Sliva D. Ganodermanontriol (GDNT) exerts its effect on growth and invasiveness of breast cancer cells through the down-regulation of CDC20 and uPA. *Biochem. Biophys. Res. Commun.* 2011;415(2):325-9.

Kim KH, Moon E, Choi SU, Kim SY, Lee KR. Lanostane triterpenoids from the mushroom *Naematoloma fasciculare*. *J. Nat. Prod.* 2013;76(5):845-51.

Kobori M, Yoshida M, Ohnishi-Kameyama M, Shinmoto H. Ergosterol peroxide from an edible mushroom suppresses inflammatory responses in RAW264.7 macrophages and growth of HT29 colon adenocarcinoma cells. *Br. J. Pharmacol.* 2007 ;150(2):209-19.

Lee MK, Hung TM, Cuong TD, Na M, Kim JC, Kim EJ, Park HS, Choi JS, Lee I, Bae K, Hattori M, Min BS. Ergosta-7,22-diene-2β,3α,9α-triol from the fruit bodies of *Ganoderma lucidum* induces apoptosis in human myelocytic HL-60 cells. *Phytother Res.* 2011;25(11):1579-85.

Li HJ, Lan WJ, Lam CK, Yang F, Zhu XF. Hirsutane sesquiterpenoids from the marine-derived fungus *Chondrostereum* sp. *Chem. Biodivers.* 2011; 8(2):317-24.

Lin SB, Li CH, Lee SS, Kan LS. Triterpene-enriched extracts from *Ganoderma lucidum* inhibit growth of hepatoma cells via suppressing protein kinase C, activating mitogen-activated protein kinases and G2-phase cell cycle arrest. *Life Sci.* 2003;72(21):2381-90.

Liu Y, Li Y, Ou Y, Xiao S, Lu C, Zheng Z, Shen Y. Guanacastane-type diterpenoids with cytotoxic activity from *Coprinus plicatilis*. *Bioorg. Med. Chem. Lett.* 2012;22(15):5059-62.

Ma L, Chen H, Dong P, Lu X. Anti-inflammatory and anticancer activities of extracts and compounds from the mushroom *Inonotus obliquus*. *Food Chem.* 2013; 139(1-4):503-8.

Najajreh Y, Khamaisie H, Ruimi N, Khatib S, Katzhendler J, Ruthardt M, Mahajna J. Oleylamine-carbonyl-valinol inhibits auto-phosphorylation activity of native and T315I mutated Bcr-Abl, and exhibits selectivity towards oncogenic Bcr-Abl in Sup B15 ALL cell lines. *Mol Biol Rep.* 2013;40(3):2205-13.

Norikura T, Fujiwara K, Narita T, Yamaguchi S, Morinaga Y, Iwai K, Matsue H. Anticancer activities of thelephantin O and vialinin A isolated from *Thelephora aurantiotincta*. *J Agric. Food Chem.* 2011; 59(13):6974-9.

Ou YX, Li YY, Qian XM, Shen YM. Guanacastane-type diterpenoids from *Coprinus radians*. *Phytochemistry.* 2012;78:190-6.

Poindessous V, Koeppel F, Raymond E, Cvitkovic E, Waters SJ, Larsen AK. Enhanced antitumor activity of irofulven in combination with 5-fluorouracil and cisplatin in human colon and ovarian carcinoma cells. *Int. J. Oncol.* 2003;23(5):1347-55.

Rukachaisirikul V, Tansakul C, Saithong S, Pakawatchai C, Isaka M, Suvannakad R. Hirsutane sesquiterpenes from the fungus *Lentinus connatus* BCC 8996. *J. Nat. Prod.* 2005;68(11):1674-6.

Shigama K, Nakaya A, Wakame K, Nishioka H, Fujii H. Alleviating effect of active hexose correlated compound (AHCC) for anticancer drug-induced side effects in non-tumor-bearing mice. *J. Exp. Ther. Oncol.* 2009; 8(1):43-51.

Shi XW, Li XJ, Gao JM, Zhang XC. Fasciculols H and I, two lanostane derivatives from Chinese mushroom *Naematoloma fasciculare*. *Chem. Biodivers.* 2011;8(10):1864-70.

Song J, Manir MM, Moon SS. Cytotoxic grifolin derivatives isolated from the wild mushroom *Boletus pseudocalopus* (Basidiomycetes). *Chem. Biodivers.* 2009;6(9):1435-42.

Vogel FS, Kemper LA, McGarry SJ, Graham DG. Cytostatic, cytocidal and potential antitumor properties of a class of quinoid compounds, initiators of the dormant state in the spores of *Agaricus bisporus*. *Am. J. Pathol.* 1975;78(1):33-48.

Wang HM, Chen CY, Wu PF. Isophilippinolide a arrests cell cycle progression and induces apoptosis for anticancer inhibitory agents in human melanoma cells. *J. Agric. Food Chem.* 2014; 62(5):1057-65.

Wang J, Wiltshire T, Wang Y, Mikell C, Burks J, Cunningham C, Van Laar ES, Waters SJ, Reed E, Wang W. ATM-dependent CHK2 activation induced by anticancer agent, irofulven. *J. Biol. Chem.* 2004;279(38):39584-92.

Wangun HV, Dahse HM, Hertweck C. Epicoccamides B-D, glycosylated tetramic acid derivatives from an *Epicoccum* sp. associated with the tree fungus *Pholiota squarrosa*. *J. Nat. Prod.* 2007 ;70(11):1800-3.

Wick MM, Rosowsky A, Ratliff J. Antitumor effects of L-glutamic acid dihydroxyanilides against experimental melanoma. *J. Invest. Dermatol.* 1980;74(2):112-4.

Wiltshire T, Senft J, Wang Y, Konat GW, Wenger SL, Reed E, Wang W. BRCA1 contributes to cell cycle arrest and chemoresistance in response to the anticancer agent irofulven. *Mol. Pharmacol.* 2007;71(4):1051-60.

Yan D, Bao HY, Bau T, Li Y, Kim YH. Antitumor components from *Naematoloma fasciculare*. *J. Microbiol. Biotechnol.* 2009;19(10):1135-8.

Ye M, Luo X, Li L, Shi Y, Tan M, Weng X, Li W, Liu J, Cao Y. Grifolin, a potential antitumor natural product from the mushroom *Albatrellus confluens*, induces cell-cycle arrest in G1 phase via the ERK1/2 pathway. *Cancer Lett.* 2007;258(2):199-207.

Yeh CT, Huang WC, Rao YK, Ye M, Lee WH, Wang LS, Tzeng DT, Wu CH, Shieh YS, Huang CY, Chen YJ, Hsiao M, Wu AT, Yang Z, Tzeng YM. A sesquiterpene lactone antrocin from *Antrodia camphorata* negatively modulates JAK2/STAT3 signaling via microRNA let-7c and induces apoptosis in lung cancer cells. *Carcinogenesis.* 2013 ; 34(12):2918-28.

Yin X, Feng T, Li ZH, Dong ZJ, Li Y, Liu JK. Highly oxygenated meroterpenoids from fruiting bodies of the mushroom *Tricholoma terreum*. *J. Nat. Prod.* 2013 ;76(7):1365-8.

Yu CC, Chiang PC, Lu PH, Kuo MT, Wen WC, Chen P, Guh JH. Antroquinonol, a natural ubiquinone derivative, induces a cross talk between apoptosis, autophagy and senescence in human pancreatic carcinoma cells. *J. Nutr. Biochem.* 2012 ;23(8):900-7.

Zhao W, Xu JW, Zhong JJ. Enhanced production of ganoderic acids in static liquid culture of *Ganoderma lucidum* under nitrogen-limiting conditions. *Bioresour. Technol.* 2011;102(17):8185-90.

In: Horizons in Cancer Research. Volume 54
Editor: Hiroto S. Watanabe
ISBN: 978-1-63321-389-0

Chapter 7

Lifestyle and Cancer Prevention

Hirokazu Takahashi*
Gastroenterology Division, Yokohama City University Graduate School of Medicine,
Yokohama, Japan

Abstract

The burden of modern lifestyle diseases is enormous and the true unifying factor for most cancers seems to be lifestyle. The intervention with the modification of lifestyle factors seems to be a physiological and safe approach for the prevention and management of modern lifestyle diseases including cancer. Defining the precise role of diet and other lifestyle factors in cancer may require the elucidation of genetic susceptibility and genetic-environmental interactions. The modifications in the diet along with secondary prevention measures may have a major impact on reducing the mortality from cancer. Lifestyle modifications offer an important strategy for cancer prevention. However, a change in only one lifestyle factor is unlikely to reduce the risk of cancer or other diseases. Environmental exposures by themselves do not cause cancer. Cancer is complex and involves many gene-gene interactions that occur inside you and are not well understood. Over your lifetime, random gene changes are passed along as your body cells grow and divide, so they accumulate. The unique patterns that evolve over time may make some people more likely than others to increase their risk for cancer after exposure to a particular chemical or after choosing a particular behavior. Whether a future obesity-related cancer burden is realized will depend greatly on competing risks and survival from other affected chronic diseases—cardiovascular disease and diabetes in particular. Similarly for alcohol, multiple competing risks of mortality from, for instance, accidents and violence, alcohol poisoning, and acute ischemic heart disease will affect whether individuals survive to be at risk for cancer.

---

* Corresponding author: Hirokazu Takahashi, M.D. Gastroenterology Division, Yokohama City University Graduate School of Medicine, 3-9 Fuku-ura, Kanazawa-ku, Yokohama, 236-0004 Japan, Email: hirokazu@med.yokohama-cu.ac.jp Tel; +81-45-787-2640, Fax; +81-45-784-3546.

Introduction

Cancer is the leading cause of death in developed countries and the second leading cause of death in developing countries. Despite improvements in the treatment of various common cancers, providing a growing incentive to address this problem by a preventive approach. Although eliminating exposure to carcinogens, such as tobacco, is a well-established approach to prevention, active intervention with agents that are expected to reduce the risk of cancer is becoming increasingly accepted [1, 2].

Almost 1.5 million people in the USA are diagnosed with cancer every year and due to the substantial effect of the modifiable lifestyle factors, it has been estimated that 50% of cancers are preventable [3]. The burden of modern lifestyle diseases is enormous as the true unifying factor for most cancers seems to be lifestyle. The intervention with the modification of lifestyle factors seems to be a physiological and safe approach for the prevention and management of modern lifestyle diseases including cancer. Defining the precise role of diet and other lifestyle factors in cancer may require the elucidation of genetic susceptibility and genetic-environmental interactions. The balance between genetic predisposition and environmental factors, including nutritional components and lifestyle behaviors, determines individual susceptibility to develop cancer. The modifications in the diet along with secondary prevention measures may have a major impact on reducing the mortality from cancer. Continued focus on primary prevention of cancer, in combination with efforts aimed at screening and surveillance, will be vital in attaining the greatest possible progress against cancer.

Lifestyle modifications offer an important strategy for cancer prevention. Evidence that has accumulated since the 1980s strongly suggests that better dietary choices, increasing physical activity, maintaining a healthy weight, stopping the use of tobacco, moderating alcohol intake and other lifestyle factors can reduce cancer risk [4, 5]. However, a change in only one lifestyle factor is unlikely to reduce the risk of cancer or other diseases. The exception is stopping tobacco use, which decreases the risk of several diseases, including cardiovascular, lung and kidney diseases, as well as cancer. Of course, environmental exposures by themselves do not cause cancer. Cancer is complex and involves many gene-gene interactions that occur inside you and are not well understood. Over your lifetime, random gene changes are passed along as your body cells grow and divide, so they accumulate. The unique patterns that evolve over time may make some people more likely than others to increase their risk for cancer after exposure to a particular chemical or after choosing a particular behavior.

International Variations and Trends

Cancer, already the leading cause of death in many high-income countries, is set to become a major cause of morbidity and mortality in the next few decades in every region of the world, irrespective of level of income [6-8]. The effect of population ageing and growth will be greatest in low-income and middle-income countries. These changes translate to a predicted global burden of 20.3 million new cancer cases by 2030 compared with an estimated 12.7 million cases in 2008, and a predicted 13.2 million cancer-related deaths worldwide by 2030, up from 7.6 million in 2008 [7]. Such a demographic transition and the resulting upsurge in cancer incidence and mortality are contingent on population projections that assume decreases in human fertility and population growth as a result of continuous social and economic development [9], and on incidence and mortality rates of all cancer types combined remaining unaltered over the next few decades. Cancer is a heterogeneous mix of diseases with different types of cancer more common in some populations than in others, sometimes substantially so [4]. Cancers have very different causes, some of which are well understood and some of which are poorly understood, and differences in the regional and temporal distribution of risk factors will determine the geographical and secular patterns of cancer. Therefore, many barriers exist to the understanding of global patterns of cancer—the availability of information about disease incidence and mortality, an understanding of the underlying causes and how these can change, and knowledge of the demographics of populations in terms of size and age structure [10].

Forecasts are dependent not only on demographics and risk factors, but also on the extent and modalities of early detection and screening for cancer, which vary from country to country. Increasing levels of screening at the population level have the potential to independently increase the future cancer incidence burden in many settings, especially for those cancers in which a precursor lesion is not the target of the intervention. This would include prostate and breast cancer, for which incidence is already increasing in many populations. In the theory of epidemiological transition [11], the shift from infections to degenerative diseases in Europe was not associated with progress in medical science but rather with improved socioeconomic conditions [12]. Medical progress became more important at a later stage in high-income countries, but was seen to have a great effect in low-income countries, causing accelerated epidemiological transitions. Public health programs should include campaigns for immunization [13], tobacco control, reduction in alcohol consumption and obesity [14], and the implementation of cancer-screening programs that have been shown to reduce mortality effectively [15]. In high-income countries, there is strong evidence of the simultaneous start of decline of lung cancer incidence [16], at least in men, and the rise and increasing relative importance of other cancer types, often with unknown cause or known risk factors that explain only a small fraction of cases.

The forces that bring about altered population structures often go hand in hand with broader lifestyle changes associated with urbanization, increased income and car ownership, altered social and family structures, and more sedentary daily activities and occupations. Lifestyle risk factors for cancer likely to undergo changes include smoking, alcohol consumption, and excess body weight, via changes in diet and physical activity, all of which are established carcinogens [17-20]. The major contribution of these five factors, as well as four others (unsafe sex, air pollution, indoor smoke, and contaminated injections), in 2001 accounted for 35% of cancer deaths worldwide [21]. Changes in cancer incidence rates that occurred among international migrants from low- to high-risk areas can be viewed to some degree as examples of what might occur on a much larger scale with Westernization of lifestyles, i.e. a gradual convergence of cancer incidence rates towards that of the host population [22]. Migrants from Japan to Hawaii had higher rates of colon, breast, and prostate cancer than their counterparts in Japan. Furthermore, time trends are already apparent in societies in transition. A 56% increase in incidence of cancers occurred in the rural Qigong province of China between 1978 and 2002, being predominantly a demographic effect, as age-standardized incidence rates for all cancers combined showed a slight decline. However, there were heterogeneous patterns by cancer site with increases for colorectal, liver, lung, and breast cancers counterbalanced by decreases for stomach, esophagus, and cervical cancers [23]. Similarly in India, rapid industrialization and consequent socioeconomic transition over the past few decades have been accompanied by increased incidence rates for breast, ovarian, and uterine cancers and decreases for cervical, stomach, and oral cavity cancers [24-26].

Risk Factors

Common, adult, epithelial cancers represent the final step in a multi-year progression from normal tissue, through increasingly abnormal-looking stages of pre-malignancy to invasion of the basement membrane, which constitutes overt cancer. Once a histological boundary has been penetrated, invasive cancer has the potential to metastasize, and metastases generally lead to cancer-related mortality. The evolution of these adult malignancies involves the gradual accumulation of genetic and epigenetic cancer-promoting changes. The affected genes, oncogenes, as well as tumor suppressor genes, are mutated in a manner that subverts their normal function, thereby contributing to the multiple processes that are considered to be the hallmarks of cancer [27, 28]. Additional modifications, such as epigenetic silencing of tumor suppressor genes also contribute to the relentless progression to invasive cancer, as can aspects of the immune response, such as immunoediting [29]. The good news is that the major environmental factors that are linked to cancer deaths can be modified, because most of them involve lifestyle choices. Almost half of all cancer deaths could be prevented by eliminating the use of tobacco products, for example, and making better dietary choices could prevent many more premature deaths from this disease. Our knowledge and certainty about diet is much less firm than it is for tobacco. Diets are very complex and we need to know what people ate in the past that impacted their cancer diagnoses today.

Research shows that certain risk factors increase the chance that a person will develop cancer. These are the most common risk factors for cancer:

1. Growing older
2. Tobacco
3. Sunlight
4. Ionizing radiation
5. Environmental Pollution
6. Occupational Carcinogens
7. Viruses and bacteria
8. Certain hormones
9. Family history of cancer
10. Alcohol
11. Poor diet
12. Lack of physical activity, or being overweight

Many of these risk factors can be avoided. Others, such as family history, cannot be avoided. People can help protect themselves by staying away from known risk factors whenever possible.

Over time, several factors may act together to cause normal cells to become cancerous.

1. Growing Older

The most significant risk factor for cancer is growing older. Most cancers occur in people over the age of 65. However people of all ages, including children, can get cancer, too.

2. Tobacco

Tobacco use is the most preventable cause of death. Using tobacco products or regularly being around tobacco smoke increases the risk of cancer. Smokers are more likely than nonsmokers to develop cancer of the lung, larynx, mouth, esophagus, bladder, kidney, throat, stomach, pancreas, or cervix. They also are more likely to develop acute myeloid leukemia. Quitting is important for anyone who uses tobacco, even people who have used it for many years. The risk of cancer for people who quit is lower than the risk for people who continue to use tobacco. Also, for people who have already had cancer, quitting may reduce the chance of getting another cancer.

3. Sunlight

Ultraviolet radiation, which comes from natural sunlight, sunlamps, or tanning beds, can lead to melanoma and other forms of skin cancer. While some sun exposure is good for health, excessive exposure during childhood seems a particularly important factor that increases skin cancer risk, and repeated exposure as an adult can increase risk as well. Wear long sleeves, long pants, a hat with a wide brim, and sunglasses with lenses that absorb UV. Sunscreen may help prevent skin cancer, especially sunscreen with a sun protection factor (SPF) of at least 15. But sunscreens cannot replace avoiding the sun and wearing clothing to protect the skin.

4. Ionizing Radiation

Ionizing radiation can cause cell damage that leads to cancer. This kind of radiation comes from rays that enter the Earth's atmosphere from outer space, *radioactive fallout, radon* gas, *x-rays*, and other sources. Radioactive fallout can come from accidents at nuclear power plants or from the production, testing, or use of atomic weapons. People exposed to fallout may have an increased risk of cancer, especially leukemia and cancers of the *thyroid*, breast, lung, and stomach. Radon is a *radioactive* gas that you cannot see, smell, or taste. It forms in soil and rocks. People who work in mines may be exposed to radon. In some parts of the country, radon is found in houses. People exposed to radon are at increased risk of lung cancer. The risk of cancer from low-dose x-rays is extremely small. The risk from radiation therapy is slightly higher. For both, the benefit nearly always outweighs the small risk.

5. Environmental Pollution

Environmental pollution of air, water and soil with carcinogenic chemicals accounts for 1–4% of all cancers [19]. Exposure to carcinogenic chemicals in the environment can occur through drinking water or pollution of indoor and ambient air. In an arsenic-contaminated region in Bangladesh, 5–10% of all cancer deaths were attributable to arsenic exposure [30]. Exposure to carcinogens also occurs via the contamination of food by chemicals, such as aflatoxins or dioxins. Indoor air pollution from coal fires doubles the risk of lung cancer, particularly among non-smoking women. Worldwide, indoor air pollution from domestic coal fires is responsible for approximately 1.5% of all lung cancer deaths. Coal use in households is particularly widespread in Asia.

6. Occupational Carcinogens

More than 40 agents, mixtures and exposure circumstances in the working environment are carcinogenic to humans and are classified as occupational carcinogens [31]. People who have certain jobs (such as painters, construction workers, and those in the chemical industry) have an increased risk of cancer. Many studies have shown that exposure to asbestos, benzene, benzidine, cadmium, nickel, or vinyl chloride in the workplace can cause cancer. Those occupational carcinogens are causally related to cancer of the lung, bladder, larynx and skin, leukemia and nasopharyngeal cancer is well documented. Mesothelioma (cancer of the outer lining of the lung or chest cavity) is to a large extent caused by work-related exposure to asbestos. Occupational cancers are concentrated among specific groups of the working population, for whom the risk of developing a particular form of cancer may be much higher than for the general population. About 20–30% of the male and 5–20% of the female working-age population (people aged 15–64 years) may have been exposed to lung carcinogens during their working lives, accounting for about 10% of lung cancers worldwide. About 2% of leukemia cases worldwide are attributable to occupational exposures.

7. Viruses and Bacteria

Being infected with certain viruses or bacteria may increase the risk of developing cancer:

1) Human Papillomavirus (HPV)

Certain strains of HPV, which are sexually transmitted, are the primary causes of cervical and anal cancer. Women who begin having sexual intercourse before age 17, or who have multiple sexual partners, are at the greatest risk of HPV infection. HPV may also be responsible for some cancers of the head and neck. It's important to note that most people infected with HPV will not get cancer. Also, a vaccine is now available that can prevent infection with the strains of HPV that cause cervical cancer.

2) Hepatitis B and C

The hepatitis B and hepatitis C viruses are major causes of liver cancer worldwide. The viruses are transmitted through blood transfusions, injectable drug use, and unprotected sex. Vaccinations can protect against hepatitis B, but there is not yet a vaccine for hepatitis C.

3) Human T-cell leukemia/lymphoma Virus (HTLV-1)

Infection with HTLV-1 increases a person's risk of lymphoma and leukemia.

4) Human Immunodeficiency Virus (HIV)

HIV is the virus that causes *AIDS*. People who have HIV infection are at greater risk of cancer, such as lymphoma and a rare cancer called *Kaposi sarcoma*.

5) Epstein-Barr Virus (EBV)

Epstein-Barr virus causes mononucleosis. In people with weakened immune systems, it can also lead to some types of lymphoma.

6) Human Herpesvirus 8 (HHV8)

This virus is a risk factor for Kaposi's sarcoma.

7) Helicobacter pylori (H. pylori)

H. pylori is the primary cause of stomach ulcers and inflammation of the stomach. *H. pylori* can contribute to the development of stomach cancer, but most infections lead to neither symptoms nor cancer.

Do not have unprotected sex or share needles. You can get an HPV infection by having sex with someone who is infected. You can get hepatitis B, hepatitis C, or HIV infection from having unprotected sex or sharing needles with someone who is infected. You may want to consider getting the vaccine that prevents hepatitis B infection. Health care workers and others who come into contact with other people's blood should ask their doctor about this vaccine. If you think you may be at risk for HIV or hepatitis infection, ask your doctor about being tested. These infections may not cause *symptoms*, but blood tests can show whether the virus is present.

8. Certain Hormones

Doctors may recommend hormones (*estrogen* alone or estrogen along with *progestin*) to help control problems (such as hot flashes, vaginal dryness, and thinning bones) that may occur during *menopause*. However, studies show that *menopausal hormone therapy* can cause serious *side effects*. Hormones may increase the risk of breast cancer, heart attack, stroke, or blood clots.

9. Family History of Cancer

Most cancers develop because of *mutations* in *genes*. A normal cell may become a cancer cell after a series of gene changes occur. Tobacco use, certain viruses, or other factors in a person's lifestyle or environment can cause such changes in certain types of cells. Some gene changes that increase the risk of cancer are passed from parent to child. These changes are present at birth in all cells of the body. It is uncommon for cancer to run in a family. However, certain types of cancer do occur more often in some families than in the rest of the population. For example, *melanoma* and cancers of the breast, ovary, prostate, and colon sometimes run in families. Several cases of the same cancer type in a family may be linked to inherited gene changes, which may increase the chance of developing cancers. However, environmental factors may also be involved. Most of the time, multiple cases of cancer in a family are just a matter of chance.

10. Alcohol

The risk of cancer for alcohol drinkers may be modulated by genetic factors, such as variants in genes for alcohol metabolism, folate and methionine metabolism and DNA repair [32, 33]. Acetaldehyde, a toxic metabolite of alcohol that damages DNA, is considered a major cause of the observed carcinogenic effect on the upper aerodigestive tract. Ingested ethanol is oxidized by the enzymes alcohol dehydrogenase (ADH), cytochrome P-450 2E1 (CYP2E1) and catalase to form acetaldehyde, which is subsequently oxidized by aldehyde dehydrogenase 2 (ALDH2) to produce acetate, not toxic to the body. Polymorphisms of the genes that encode enzymes for ethanol metabolism affect the ethanol/acetaldehyde oxidizing capacity, and are responsible for the limited action of the enzyme that converts acetaldehyde to acetate [34]. As a confirmation to this, the risk of cancers of the upper aerodigestive tract associated with alcohol is highest in East Asia, where 28%–45% of the population has a variation of the gene ALDH2 [35, 36]. Alcohol increases the risk of cancer of the oral cavity and pharynx, squamous cell carcinoma of the esophagus and breast even at low doses. Given the high proportion of light drinkers in the population there is a high prevalence of these tumors, especially breast cancer [7].

11. Poor Diet

The federal report on carcinogens doesn't discuss specific foods and cancer risk. However, studies show that consuming large quantities of red meat, preserved meats, salt-preserved meats, and salt probably increases the risk of stomach and colorectal cancers. Research also shows that a diet high in fruits and vegetables may decrease the risks of these cancers. And calorie restriction has been shown to reduce cancer risk for several cancer types. Eat a healthy calorie-restricted diet rich in whole grains, fruits, and vegetables. Avoid consuming large amounts of fatty foods, red meats, salt, or salt-preserved food. Large population studies have revealed associations between certain dietary patterns and cancer risk, thus setting the stage for nutritional intervention programs that encourage healthier diets and clinical trials that include cancer risk reduction as an end point [37, 38]. Going beyond studies of overall diets, laboratory-based investigations are progressively identifying specific cancer-preventive nutrients and the molecular mechanisms by which they exert this property [39]. Among the biologically active food components that seem to be somewhat promising for cancer prevention are soy isoflavones for breast cancer, lycopene (found in tomatoes) for prostate cancer, as well as resveratrol (from grapes and red wine), omega-3-fatty acids (found in fish oil), pomegranate, curcumin and antioxidants such as selenium and vitamin E, for other cancers [40].

12. Lack of Physical Activity and Obesity

Being overweight is an important lifestyle factor related to cancer risk. There are links between obesity and the risks of breast cancer (in older women), endometrial cancer, and cancers of the kidney, colon, and esophagus. Not being physically active increases the risk of colorectal and breast cancers. Together, obesity and physical inactivity are linked to about 30 percent of the cases of colon, endometrial, kidney, and esophageal cancers, as well as 30 percent of breast cancers in older women. Losing weight and exercising can help reduce your risk. Exercise at least 30 minutes a day, most days of the week. Exercise alone can decrease the risk of colon cancer and breast cancer. The goal should be for adults age 20 or older to keep their Body Mass Index (BMI) below 25. The BMI is a number that shows your body weight adjusted for your height. A parallel increase in the levels of aromatase expression or activity with obesity (in adipose and breast tissue) has suggested a possible mechanism for the increased incidence of hormone receptor-positive breast cancer in obese, postmenopausal women [41]. The obesity–inflammation–aromatase axis was investigated in a small trial using breast tissue samples from obese women who had undergone breast surgery [42]. Of these patient samples, 50% contained crown-like structures, a marker of inflammation, and the severity of breast inflammation significantly correlated with body mass index (BMI) and adipocyte size, increased nuclear factor-κB (NF-κB)-binding activity and increased aromatase expression. This suggests that the crown-like structures, with BMI and adipocyte size, may serve as a potential biomarker for increased breast cancer risk or poor prognosis, especially in obese and overweight women [42].

The relationship between obesity and cancer can also be viewed through the lens of metabolism, the reprogramming of which has increasingly been addressed as a feature of carcinogenesis and as a potential target of therapeutic intervention [43]. Cancer cells generally use aerobic glycolysis to generate the energy needed for cell proliferation [44]. This phenomenon, known since its description in the 1920s as the Warburg effect [45], distinguishes malignant cells from normal differentiated cells, which rely on mitochondrial oxidative phosphorylation to generate energy. Metabolic syndrome, which encompasses abdominal obesity, hypertension, dyslipidemia and hyperglycemia [46], offers another look at the connection between the deregulation of metabolism and cancer [47]. Energy balance is a term that describes the relationship between the following three factors: energy consumed (food), energy expended (physical activity and basal metabolism), and energy stored (adipose tissue). Observational studies have linked each of these factors to cancer risk and prognosis, especially in patients with breast, colon, and prostate cancers [48], but there have been limited data from randomized trials that tested the impact of changes in energy balance after diagnosis (i.e., weight loss, increased physical activity, and improvements in dietary quality) on risk of cancer recurrence and mortality.

Much less evidence exists regarding the relationship between weight change after diagnosis and cancer prognosis. A few older studies suggested that weight gain after breast cancer diagnosis was associated with increased risk of recurrence [49-51], but most modern reports, which focused on patients treated with shorter, modern chemotherapy regimens, have not shown a relationship between weight change after diagnosis and breast cancer outcomes [52]. One notable exception is the Nurses' Health Study, in which investigators showed that non-smoking women who gained 0.5 to 2 kg/m^2, as well as women who gained greater than 2 kg/m^2, had a significantly increased risk of breast cancer death compared with women who maintained a stable weight [53]. The relationship between weight change and cancer outcomes has also been studied in colon cancer, in which there was no relationship between weight gain or loss and risk of colon cancer recurrence [54]. Thus, the available evidence does not suggest an effect of weight gain after cancer diagnosis on outcomes. However, relatively few participants included in these reports lost weight, and it is not possible to separate purposeful from involuntary weight loss in these studies.

Despite the observational studies that demonstrated an association between obesity and poor prognosis in patients with breast, prostate, and, perhaps, colorectal cancer, there is no direct evidence from randomized trials that purposeful weight loss after diagnosis improves outcomes. Several small studies have looked at the feasibility and benefits of weight-loss interventions in cancer survivors [55-57]. Most of these studies enrolled fewer than 100 patients, focused exclusively on breast cancer survivors, and evaluated weight loss or quality of life as a primary end point.

Recommendations for Cancer Prevention

Here's a list of 10 diet and activity recommendations of the American Dietetic Association.

1. Be as lean as possible without becoming underweight.
2. Be physically active for at least 30 minutes every day.
3. Avoid sugary drinks, and limit consumption of high-calorie foods, especially those low in fiber and rich in fat or added sugar.
4. Eat a variety of vegetables, fruits, whole grains, and legumes (such as beans).
5. Limit consumption of red meats (including beef, pork, and lamb) and avoid processed meats.
6. If you drink alcohol, limit your daily intake to two drinks for men and one drink for women.
7. Limit consumption of salty foods and food processed with salt (sodium).
8. Don't use supplements to try to protect against cancer.
9. It's best for mothers to exclusively breastfeed their babies for up to six months and then add other liquids and foods.
10. After treatment, cancer survivors should follow the recommendations for cancer prevention.

Discussion

Whether a future obesity-related cancer burden is realized will depend greatly on competing risks and survival from other affected chronic diseases—cardiovascular disease and diabetes in particular. Similarly for alcohol, multiple competing risks of mortality from, for instance, accidents and violence, alcohol poisoning, and acute ischemic heart disease will affect whether individuals survive to be at risk for cancer. Risk factors may have different magnitudes of effects across settings if, for instance, the nature of the exposure itself differs (different chemical constituent of exposure, e.g. types of tobacco smoked), there are different patterns of use (intensity, duration of use, and age at commencement of exposure) or interactions with other environmental or genetic factors. As lifestyles change, if multiple changes occur in the same people, then the precise nature of the effect of joint exposures needs to be well characterized. For example, the effect of alcohol consumption on liver cancer is stronger in overweight individuals than in those within the normal BMI range [58].

A focus on the lifestyles of the younger adult generation—the current population from which future cancer cases will arise—is useful not only to project cancer trends but also to gain information on priority risk factors that need to be tackled today at the forefront of cancer control and research agendas for both prevention and resource planning purposes. Prevention, the ideal target in reducing the cancer burden, comprises reversal or halting of time trends in populations, protection of groups that have not experienced them, and encouragement of risk factor modifications in individuals with raised risks, if such modifications lead to risk reduction. Quitting smoking reduces risk with benefits realized immediately [59]. Cessation of alcohol drinking has beneficial effects for risk of cancers of the upper aerodigestive tract, and risk returns to that of non-drinkers after several decades [60, 61]. For BMI, diet, and physical activity, most studies relate adult status to subsequent cancer risk, but fewer studies have examined changes along the life course to identify critical periods of exposure and to examine whether reducing an individual's BMI later in life can lead to a real risk reduction, or alternatively, whether it is too late for such changes to be beneficial. Greater insight into the stage of the carcinogenic process affected by these factors, insights possibly gained through the use of intermediate biomarkers along the disease process, will help determine their effects. Repeated measures of relevant lifestyle factors at different points in a lifetime, ideally obtained prospectively, are needed to assess the potential reversal of increased risks. With obesity currently impacting young ages, early-life lifestyles affecting growth and development are also crucial [62], and evidenced by the higher overall cancer rates in people of taller stature [63].

References

[1] Lippman, S. M. & Hawk, E. T. (2009). Cancer prevention: from 1727 to milestones of the past 100 years. *Cancer Res*, *69*, 5269–5284.

[2] Greenwald, P. & Dunn, B. K. (2009). Landmarks in the history of cancer epidemiology. *Cancer Res*, *69*, 2151–2162.

[3] Buc, E., Kwiatkowski, F., Alves, A., Panis, Y., Mantion, G. & Slim, K. (2006). Tobacco smoking: a factor of early onset of colorectal cancer. *Dis. Colon Rectum*, *49*, 1893–1896.

[4] Doll, R. & Peto, R. (1981). The causes of cancer: quantitative estimates of avoidable risks of cancer in the United States today. *J. Natl Cancer Inst*, *66*, 1191–1308.

[5] Willett, W. C. (2001). Diet and cancer: one view at the start of the millennium. *Cancer Epidemiol. Biomarkers Prev*, *10*, 3–8.

[6] WHO. Global Status Report on Non-Communicable Diseases (2010). http://www.who.int/nmh/publications/ncd_report2010/en/

[7] Ferlay, J., Shin, H. R., Bray, F., Forman, D., Mathers, C. & Parkin, D. M. (2010). Estimates of worldwide burden of cancer in 2008. *Int J Cancer*, *127*, 2893–2917.

[8] Jemal, A., Bray, F., Center, M. M., Ferlay, J., Ward, E. & Forman, D. (2011). Global cancer statistics. *Cancer J Clin*, *61*, 69–90.

[9] Myrskyla, M., Kohler, H. P. & Billari, F. C. (2009). Advances in development reverse fertility declines. *Nature*, *460*, 741–743.

[10] Bray, F. & Moller, B. (2006). Predicting the future burden of cancer. *Nat Rev Cancer*, *6*, 63–74.

[11] Omran, A. R. (1971). The epidemiologic transition. A theory of the epidemiology of population change. *Milbank Mem Fund Q*, *49*, 509–538.

[12] McKeown, T. & Brown, R. G. (1955). Medical evidence related to English population change in the eighteenth century. *Population Studies*, *9*, 119–141.

[13] Sylla, B. S. & Wild, C. P. (2011). A million Africans a year dying from cancer by 2030: what can cancer research and control offer to the continent? *Int J Cancer*, *130*, 245–250.

[14] Beaglehole, R., Bonita, R., Horton, R., Adams, C., Alleyne, G., Asaria, P., Baugh, V., Bekedam, H., Billo, N., Casswell, S., Cecchini, M., Colagiuri, R., Colagiuri, S,, Collins, T., Ebrahim, S., Engelgau, M., Galea, G., Gaziano, T., Geneau, R., Haines, A., Hospedales, J., Jha, P., Keeling, A., Leeder, S., Lincoln, P., McKee, M., Mackay, J., Magnusson, R., Moodie, R., Mwatsama, M., Nishtar, S., Norrving, B., Patterson, D., Piot, P., Ralston, J., Rani, M., Reddy, K. S., Sassi, F., Sheron, N., Stuckler, D., Suh, I., Torode, J., Varghese, C., Watt, J., Lancet NCD Action Group & NCD Alliance. (2011). Priority actions for the non-communicable disease crisis. *Lancet*, *377*, 1438–1447.

[15] Peto, J., Gilham, C., Fletcher, O. & Matthews, F. E. (2004). The cervical cancer epidemic that screening has prevented in the UK. *Lancet*, *364*, 249–256.

[16] Kohler, B. A., Ward, E., McCarthy, B. J., Schymura, M. J., Ries, L. A., Eheman, C., Jemal, A., Anderson, R. N., Ajani, U. A. & Edwards, B. K. (2011). Annual report to the nation on the status of cancer, 1975–2007, featuring tumors of the brain and other parts of the nervous system. *J Natl Cancer Inst*, *103*, 714–736.

[17] Baan, R., Straif, K., Grosse, Y., Secretan, B., El Ghissassi, F., Bouvard, V., Altieri, A., Cogliano, V. & WHO International Agency for Research on Cancer Monograph Working Group. (2007). Carcinogenicity of alcoholic beverages. *Lancet Oncol*, *8*, 292–293.

[18] Key, T. J., Allen, N. E., Spencer, E. A. & Travis, R. C. (2002). The effect of diet on risk of cancer. *Lancet*, *360*, 861–868.

[19] ARC Working Group on the Evaluation of Carcinogenic Risks to Humans. (2004). Tobacco smoke and involuntary smoking. *IARC Monogr Eval Carcinog Risks Hum*, *83*, 1–1438.

[20] Vainio, H., Kaaks, R. & Bianchini, F. (2002) Weight control and physical activity in cancer prevention: international evaluation of the evidence. *Eur J Cancer Prev*, *11*, (Suppl 2): S94–S100.
[21] Danaei, G., Vander Hoorn, S., Lopez, A. D., Murray, C. J., Ezzati, M. & Comparative Risk Assessment collaborating group (Cancers). (2005). Causes of cancer in the world: comparative risk assessment of nine behavioural and environmental risk factors. *Lancet*, *366*, 1784–1793.
[22] Stirbu, I., Kunst, A. E., Vlems, F. A., Visser, O., Bos, V., Deville, W., Nijhuis, H. G. & Coebergh, J. W. (2006). Cancer mortality rates among first and second generation migrants in the Netherlands: convergence toward the rates of the native Dutch population. *Int J Cancer*, *119*, 2665–2672.
[23] Chen, J. G., Zhu, J., Parkin, D. M., Zhang, Y. H., Lu, J. H., Zhu, Y. R. & Chen, T. Y. (2006). Trends in the incidence of cancer in Qidong, China, 1978-2002. *Int J Cancer*, *119*, 1447–1454.
[24] Sunny, L., Yeole, B. B., Hakama, M., Shiri, R., Sastry, P. S., Mathews, S. & Advani, S. H. (2004). Oral cancers in Mumbai, India: a fifteen years perspective with respect to incidence trend and cumulative risk. *Asian Pac J Cancer Prev*, *5*, 294–300.
[25] Yeole, B. B. (2008). Trends in cancer incidence in female breast, cervix uteri, corpus uteri, and ovary in India. *Asian Pac J Cancer Prev*, *9*, 119–122.
[26] Sunny, L., Yeole, B. B., Hakama, M., Shiri, R., Mathews, S., Falah Hassani, K. & Advani, S. H. (2004). Decreasing trend in the incidence of stomach cancer in Mumbai, India, during 1988 to 1999. *Asian Pac J Cancer Prev*, *5*, 169–174.
[27] Hanahan, D. & Weinberg, R. A. (2000). The hallmarks of cancer. *Cell*, *100*, 57–70.
[28] Hanahan, D. & Weinberg, R. A. (2011). Hallmarks of cancer: the next generation. *Cell*, *144*, 646–674.
[29] Schreiber, R. D., Old, L. J. & Smyth, M. J. (2011). Cancer immunoediting: integrating immunity's roles in cancer suppression and promotion. *Science*, *331*, 1565–1570.
[30] Smith, A. H., Lingas, E. O. & Rahman, M. (2000). Contamination of drinking-water by arsenic in Bangladesh: a public health emergency. *Bull World Health Organ*, *78*, 1093-1103.
[31] Siemiatycki, J., Richardson, L., Straif, K., Latreille, B., Lakhani, R., Campbell, S., Rousseau, M. C. & Boffetta, P. (2004). Listing occupational carcinogens. *Environ Health Perspect*, *112*, 1447-1459.
[32] Giovannucci, E. (2004). Alcohol, one-carbon metabolism, and colorectal cancer: recent insights from molecular studies. *J Nutr*, *134*, 2475S–2481S.
[33] Boffetta, P. & Hashibe, M. (2006). Alcohol and cancer. *Lancet Oncol*, *7*, 149–156.
[34] Yu, H. S., Oyama, T., Isse, T., Kitagawa, K., Pham, T. T., Tanaka, M. & Kawamoto, T. (2010). Formation of acetaldehyde-derived DNA adducts due to alcohol exposure. *Chem Biol Interact*, *188*, 367–375.
[35] Goedde, H. W., Agarwal, D. P., Fritze, G., Meier-Tackmann, D., Singh, S., Beckmann, G., Bhatia, K., Chen, L. Z., Fang, B., Lisker, R., et al. (1992). Distribution of ADH2 and ALDH2 genotypes in different populations. *Hum Genet*, *88*, 344–346.
[36] Oze, I., Matsuo, K., Wakai, K., Nagata, C., Mizoue, T., Tanaka, K., Tsuji, I., Sasazuki, S., Inoue, M., Tsugane, S. & Research Group for the Development and Evaluation of Cancer Prevention Strategies in Japan. (2011). Alcohol drinking and esophageal cancer

risk: an evaluation based on a systematic review of epidemiologic evidence among the Japanese population. *Jpn J Clin Oncol*, *41*, 677–692.

[37] Prentice, R. L., Thomson, C. A., Caan, B., Hubbell, F. A., Anderson, G. L., Beresford, S. A., Pettinger, M., Lane, D. S., Lessin, L., Yasmeen, S., Singh, B., Khandekar, J., Shikany, J. M., Satterfield, S. & Chlebowski, R. T. (2007). Low-fat dietary pattern and cancer incidence in the Women's Health Initiative Dietary Modification Randomized Controlled Trial. *J. Natl Cancer Inst*, *99*, 1534–1543.

[38] World Cancer Research Fund/American Institute for Cancer Research. Food, Nutrition, Physical Activity, and the Prevention of Cancer: a Global Perspective. (American Institute for Cancer Research, 2007).

[39] Davis, C. D., Emenaker, N. J. & Milner, J. A. (2010). Cellular proliferation, apoptosis and angiogenesis: molecular targets for nutritional preemption of cancer. *Semin. Oncol*, *37*, 243–257.

[40] Gullett, N. P., Ruhul Amin, A. R., Bayraktar, S., Pezzuto, J. M., Shin, D. M., Khuri, F. R., Aggarwal, B. B., Surh, Y. J. & Kucuk, O. (2010). Cancer prevention with natural compounds. *Semin. Oncol*, *37*, 258–281.

[41] Subbaramaiah, K., Howe, L. R., Bhardwaj, P., Du, B., Gravaghi, C., Yantiss, R. K., Zhou, X. K., Blaho, V. A., Hla, T., Yang, P., Kopelovich, L., Hudis, C. A. & Dannenberg, A. J. (2011). Obesity is associated with inflammation and elevated aromatase expression in the mouse mammary gland. *Cancer Prev. Res*, *4*, 329–346.

[42] Morris, P. G., Hudis, C. A., Giri, D., Morrow, M., Falcone, D. J., Zhou, X. K., Du, B., Brogi, E., Crawford, C. B., Kopelovich, L., Subbaramaiah, K. & Dannenberg, A. J. (2011). Inflammation and increased aromatase expression occur in the breast tissue of obese women with breast cancer. *Cancer Prev. Res*, *4*, 1021–1029.

[43] Hanahan, D. & Weinberg, R. A. (2011). Hallmarks of cancer: the next generation. *Cell*, *144*, 646–674.

[44] Vander Heiden, M. G., Cantley, L. C. & Thompson, C. B. (2009). Understanding the Warburg effect: the metabolic requirements of cell proliferation. *Science*, *324*, 1029–1033.

[45] Hamanaka, R. B. & Chandel, N. S. (2011). Cell biology. Warburg effect and redox balance. *Science*, *334*, 1219–1220.

[46] Braun, S., Bitton-Worms, K. & LeRoith, D. (2011). The link between the metabolic syndrome and cancer. *Int. J. Biol. Sci*, *7*, 1003–1015.

[47] Lazar, M. A. & Birnbaum, M. J. (2012). Physiology. De-meaning of metabolism. *Science*, *336*, 1651–1652.

[48] Davies, N. J., Batehup, L. & Thomas, R. (2011). The role of diet and physical activity in breast, colorectal, and prostate cancer survivorship: a review of the literature. *Br J Cancer*, *105*, Suppl 1, S52-73.

[49] Chlebowski, R. T., Weiner, J. M., Reynolds, R., Luce, J., Bulcavage, L. & Bateman, J. R. (1986). Long-term survival following relapse after 5-FU but not CMF chemotherapy. *Breast Cancer Research and Treatment*, *7*, 23-29, 1986

[50] Levine, E. G., Raczynski, J. M. & Carpenter, J. T. (1991). Weight gain with breast cancer adjuvant treatment. *Cancer*, *67*, 1954-1959.

[51] Bonomi, P., Bunting, N. & Fishman, D. (1984) Weight gain during adjuvant chemotherapy or hormonochemotherapy for stage II breast cancer in relation to disease free survival. *Breast Cancer Research and Treatment 4*, 339.

[52] Caan, B. J., Emond, J. A., Natarajan, L., Castillo, A., Gunderson, E. P., Habel, L., Jones, L., Newman, V. A., Rock, C. L., Slattery, M. L., Stefanick, M. L., Sternfeld, B., Thomson, C. A. & Pierce, J. P. (2006). Postdiagnosis weight gain and breast cancer recurrence in women with early stage breast cancer. *Breast Cancer Research and Treatment*, *99*, 47-57.

[53] Kroenke, C. H., Chen, W. Y., Rosner, B. & Holmes, M. D. (2005). Weight, weight gain, and survival after breast cancer diagnosis. *J Clin Oncol.*, *23*, 1370-1378.

[54] Meyerhardt, J. A., Catalano, P. J., Haller, D. G., Mayer, R. J., Benson, A. B. 3rd, Macdonald, J. S. & Fuchs, C. S. (2003). Influence of body mass index on outcomes and treatment-related toxicity in patients with colon carcinoma. *Cancer*, *98*, 484-495.

[55] Goodwin, P., Esplen, M., Butler, K., Winocur, J., Pritchard, K., Brazel, S., Gao, J. & Miller, A. (1998). Multidisciplinary weight management in locoregional breast cancer: results of a phase II study. *Breast Cancer Res Treat*, *48*, 53-64.

[56] Shaw, C., Mortimer, P. & Judd, P. (2007). Randomized controlled trial comparing a low-fat diet with a weight-reduction diet in breast cancer lymphedema. *Cancer*, *109*, 1949-1956.

[57] Dujuric, Z., DuLaura, N., Jenkins, I., Darga, L., Jen, C. K., Mood, D., Bradley, E. & Hryniuk, W. M. (2002). Combining weight-loss counseling with the Weight Watchers plan for obese breast cancer survivors. *Obesity Research 10*, 657-665.

[58] Hart, C. L., Morrison, D. S., Batty, G. D., Mitchell, R. J. & Davey Smith, G. (2010). Effect of body mass index and alcohol consumption on liver disease: analysis of data from two prospective cohort studies. *BMJ*, *340*, c1240.

[59] Peto, R., Darby, S., Deo, H., Silcocks, P., Whitley, E. & Doll, R. (2000). Smoking, smoking cessation, and lung cancer in the UK since 1950: combination of national statistics with two case-control studies. *BMJ*, *321*, 323–329.

[60] Marron, M., Boffetta, P., Zhang, Z. F., Zaridze, D., Wünsch-Filho, V., Winn, D. M., Wei, Q., Talamini, R., Szeszenia-Dabrowska, N., Sturgis, E. M., Smith, E., Schwartz, S. M., Rudnai, P., Purdue, M. P., Olshan, A. F., Eluf-Neto, J., Muscat, J., Morgenstern, H., Menezes, A., McClean, M., Matos, E., Mates, I. N., Lissowska, J., Levi, F., Lazarus, P., La Vecchia, C., Koifman, S., Kelsey, K., Herrero, R., Hayes, R. B., Franceschi, S., Fernandez, L., Fabianova, E., Daudt, A. W., Dal Maso, L., Curado, M. P., Cadoni, G., Chen, C., Castellsague, X., Boccia, S., Benhamou, S., Ferro, G., Berthiller, J., Brennan, P., Møller, H. & Hashibe, M. (2010). Cessation of alcohol drinking, tobacco smoking and the reversal of head and neck cancer risk. *Int J Epidemiol*, *39*, 182–196.

[61] Franceschi, S., Levi, F., Dal Maso, L., Talamini, R., Conti, E., Negri, E. & La Vecchia, C. (2000). Cessation of alcohol drinking and risk of cancer of the oral cavity and pharynx. *Int J Cancer*, *85*, 787–790.

[62] Uauy, R. & Solomons, N. (2005). Diet, nutrition, and the life-course approach to cancer prevention. *J Nutr*, *135*, 2934S–2945S.

[63] Batty, G. D., Barzi, F., Woodward, M., Jamrozik, K., Woo, J., Kim, H. C., Ueshima, H., Huxley, R. R. & Asia Pacific Cohort Studies Collaboration. (2010). Adult height and cancer mortality in Asia: the Asia Pacific Cohort Studies Collaboration. *Ann Oncol*, *21*, 646–654.

In: Horizons in Cancer Research. Volume 54
Editor: Hiroto S. Watanabe
ISBN: 978-1-63321-389-0

Chapter 8

Pathology and Pathogenesis of Hodgkin's Lymphoma: Analysis of Its Status over a Period of Five Decades

Dilip K. Das*
Department of Pathology, Faculty of Medicine,
Kuwait University, Kuwait

Abstract

The histopathological and fine-needle aspiration (FNA) cytologic diagnosis of Hodgkin's lymphoma (HL) is based on demonstration of the so called pathognomonic mononucleated Hodgkin's and bi- to multinucleated Reed-Sternberg (HRS) cells among reactive cellular component composed of lymphocytes, benign histiocytes, neutrophils and eosinophils. Hodgkin's lymphoma (HL) is one of the most common lymphomas in the developed world with an incidence of approximately three per 100,000 person-years but it is uncommon in the Far-East countries as compared to rest of the world and relatively uncommon in Sub-Saharan African countries. When the reported frequency in the Far-East countries was compared with the rest of the world, it exceeded 20% in none of the reports from the Far-East countries, as opposed to 15 (68.2%) from rest of the world (p=0.00002). When Sub-Saharan African countries were compared with rest of the non-Far-East countries of the world, it was observed that the frequency of HL exceeded 20% in 2 (28.6%) of the Sub-Saharan African countries and in13 (86.7%) of the 15 other counties (p=0.01355). Nearly five decades ago Hodgkin's lymphoma, then known as Hodgkin's disease (HD) was categorized under Rye classification into lymphocytic predominant (LP), nodular sclerosis (NS), mixed cellularity (MC) and lymphocytic depletion (LD) sub-types. Analysis of 33 reports on Rye classification from various countries revealed that the median percentages for LP, NS, MC and LD subtypes were 10.0%, 58.5%, 26.0% and 2.6%, respectively, from the developed economies and the corresponding figures from the developing countries were 9.5%, 29.4%, 44.1% and 8.9%,

* Address for Correspondence: Dr. Dilip K. Das, MBBS, MD, PhD, DSc, FRCPath. Department of Pathology, Faculty of Medicine, Kuwait University, P.O. Box: 24923, Safat 13110. Kuwait. Tel: 00965-25319476, Fax: 00965-25338905, E-mail: dilip76@hotmail.com.

respectively. In NS subtype, the frequency exceeded 50% in significantly higher number of reports from the developed (9 of 13, 69.2%) than developing countries (3 of 20, 15.0%, p= 0.00281). A reverse trend was observed in MC subtype wherein frequency exceeding 30% of cases were compared (23.1% of the reports in developed vs. 90.0% in the developing world, p=0.00016). However, there was no significant difference between the developed and developing countries in respect of LP and LD subtypes when the number of reports with frequency exceeding 10% were compared (p=1.0000, and =0.70059, respectively).

The sub-classification of HL into LP, MC, and LD in histology as well as cytology depends on relative proportion of neoplastic HRS cells and reactive cellular components. In nodular sclerosis type of HL, islands of neoplastic cells including a special type of R-S cells called lacunar cells and reactive cell components are surrounded by collagenous bands, which are not appreciated in cytologic preparations leading to limitation of cytology in the diagnosis of NS subtype. HL is an unusual malignancy in which the malignant cells are much less (about 1% cells in tumor tissue) compared to reactive cell components. In the past, various possibilities put forth regarding nature of Hodgkin's disease were inflammatory, neoplastic, autoimmune reaction and an intermediate stage between inflammatory & neoplastic lesions. HRS cells were traditionally believed to be abnormal reticulum cells. With the advent of immunological markers in 1970s, three candidates emerged as possible sources of HRS cells: T-lymphocytes, B-lymphocytes and macrophages; interdigitating reticulm cells and early progenitor myeloid cells subsequently joined the membership club of progenitor cells. Based on observation of R-S cell and T-lymphocyte interaction, and stepwise cytolysis of R-S cells in scanning electron microscopic study, it was proposed that Hodgkin's disease was a war between T-lymphocytes and transformed macrophages; the various histological subtypes depended upon the outcome of this war. During this period, the understanding of nature of cells in the formation of non-Hodgkin's lymphoma (NHL) led to the emergence of a number of classifications and wide range of controversies was associated with it. Unlike non-Hodgkin's lymphoma, the fortress of Hodgkin's lymphoma seemed invincible in seventies through eighties into early nineties. But gradually notes of dissent started to appear. In earlier reports, Reed-Sternberg-like cells were reported not only in benign lymphoproliferative conditions like reactive lymphoid hyperplasia and infectious mononucleosis, but some of nonHodgkin lymphoma subtypes, e.g., chronic lymphocytic leukemia, mycosis fungoides, Burkitt's lymphoma, lymphoepithelioid lymphoma and immunoblastic lymphoma, and non-lymphoid malignancies like metastatic carcinoma, melanoma, sarcomas and germ cell tumors revealed presence of RS-like cells. It was subsequently found that some subtypes of non-Hodgkin lymphoma like anaplastic large cell lymphoma (ALCL), T-cell-histiocytic-rich B-cell lymphoma (TCHRBCL), and pleomorphic peripheral T-cell lymphoma were most commonly misdiagnosed as Hodgkin's disease. The immunocytochemical markers like CD15, CD30, CD45, CD3 and CD20 were of help in differentiating these entities. The immunocytochemical markers for HL were CD15+, CD30+, CD45-, B-, T-, and EMA-. ALCL were CD15-, CD30+, CD45+, B±, T±, EMA± and Alk1 ±; later B+ cases were excluded from ALCL pool. The neoplastic cells in TCHRBCL were CD15-, CD30-, CD45+, CD3-, CD20+, EMA-; the accompanying rich lymphoid cell population was CD3+ and histiocytes were CD68+. With the separation of these entities, the empire of Hodgkin's disease started disintegrating. New immunohistochemical and molecular studies proved that the neoplastic cells in Hodgkin's disease was of B-cell origin and it was renamed as Hodgkin's lymphoma. In the WHO classification of Tumors of Hematopoietic and Lymphoid Tissue, Hodgkin's lymphoma was classified as nodular lymphocytic predominant HL and classical HL which was in turn classified into lymphocyte-rich, mixed cellular, lymphocytic depleted and nodular sclerosis subtypes. At present there is compelling evidence that HRS cells are clonal B-cells that have lost their B-cell phenotype. Whereas, classical HL is associated with crippling mutation of immunoglobulin genes, which prevents the production of a functional immunoglobulin molecule, the nodular lymphocytic predominance HL is associated with ongoing immunoglobulin gene hypermutation but absence of crippling mutation in their immunoglobulin genes. Mature B-cells lacking B-cell receptors would normally die by apoptosis. The rescue of Hodgkin cells and R-S cells from apoptosis is a key event in HL pathogenesis. Hodgkin cells and R-S cells express a number of receptors (at least six receptors that belong to TNF receptor family) that regulate tumor cell survival. Epstein-Barr virus (EBV), which was initially implicated in the pathogenesis of Burkitt's lymphoma, was found to be associated with other nonlymphoid malignancies (e.g., nasoparyngeal carcinoma and gastric carcinoma) and lymphoid neoplasms (B- and T-cell NHL). HL in varying proportions (ranged 26.1%to 93.8%, with a median 46.8%) was found to be associated with EBV in different studies. The escape from apoptosis and transcriptional reprogramming of HRS cells are interlinked and appear central to pathogenesis of HL. It is likely that EBV plays a role in reprogramming and survival through dysregulation of several signaling networks and transcription factors. As regards the reactive cellular infiltrate in HL, there is increased number of T-cells (CD4 and NKT subsets), decreased B-cells, and increased regulatory T-cells in comparision with reactive hyperplasia of lymph node; the tumor associated macrophages in HL are of prognostic importance. As it stands today, most of the cases of NHL and HL cases can be diagnosed based on cyto/histomorphology, immunocytochemistry, cytogenetic and molecular studies. However, there were some grey zone lymphomas, which do not exactly fall into either HL or NHL sub-types like ALCL and TCHRBCL. It appears that Hodgkin lymphoma and its pathogenesis is still in a stage of evolution and only future will tell when this turbulent phase will settle down.

Introduction

Hodgkin's disease (HD) is characterized by the presence of the typical, clonal malignant Hodgkin and Reed-Sternberg (HRS) cells in a hyperplastic background of normal reactive lymphocytes, plasma cells, histiocytes, neutrophils, eosinophils and stromal cells. [1] One hundred and eighty years have passed since the publication of an article in 1832 by Thomas Hodgkin (1798-1866) entitled "On some morbid appearances of the adsorbent glands and spleen," describing the post-mortem appearance of seven patients who had enlargements of these organs. [2] Thirty three years later, based on some 15 additional cases, Wilks published his article entitled "Cases of enlargement of the lymphatic glands and spleen, or, Hodgkin's disease with remarks," which ultimately named the disease after Thomas Hodgkin. [3] Carl von Sternberg in 1898 [4] and Dorothy Reed in 1902 [5] independently described the pathognomonic cell of Hodgkin's disease, presently called Hodgkin cell and Reed-Sternberg cell (HRS cells). The microenvironment of Hodgkin's disease is dominated by an extensive mixed and potentially inflammatory cellular infiltrate, and the HRS cells have several characteristics that are unusual for lymphoid tumor cells. [6] According to Cozen et al., [7] the histopathology and symptomatology of HD were reminiscent of chronic infectious granulomatous disease, but the untreated clinical course was that of a malignancy. However, molecular analysis has put all the speculations to rest and revealed that almost all cases of this disease are clonal B cell neoplasms; therefore the term Hodgkin's lymphoma instead of Hodgkin's disease was proposed in the new WHO classification [8] and in 2001, the World Health Organization (WHO) lymphoma classification system re-designated Hodgkin's disease to Hodgkin's lymphoma. [9] The present chapter is going to cover four and half decades, which accounts for exactly 25% of the entire history of Hodgkin's lymphoma and a period since the publication of the most widely used Rye classification [10] to the year 2011.

Incidence and Frequency of HL

As per a report one and half decade ago, the incidence of HD varied from about 0.5 per 100,000 person-years in parts of Asia to over 3 in parts of North America. [11] A recent publication also shows that Hodgkin's lymphoma (HL) is one of the most common lymphomas in the developed world, with an incidence of approximately three per 100,000 person-years. [12] Hodgkin's lymphoma comprises about 11% of all lymphomas in western countries and has a unique bimodal age-incidence shape. [13] During 1992-2001, the incidence of HL in USA was 2.67 per 100,000. [14] The crude incidence of HL in the European Union is 2.2 and mortality is 0.7 cases per 100,000 per year. [15] In Taiwan, the crude and age-adjusted rates of HL were 0.19-0.62 and 0.21-0.60 per 100,000 per year respectively, from year 1979 to 2002. [16] When the reported frequency of HL among all lymphoma cases from different countries of the world was analyzed (Table 1), [17-53] it ranged from 3.0% to 57.3% with a median of 17.8%. It was found that the frequency exceeded 10% in 5 (33.3%) among the 15 reports from Far-East countries [20-23, 30, 31, 34, 35, 39, 40, 43, 45, 47, 49, 53] and in 21 (95.5%) among 22 reports from the rest of the world [17-19, 24-29, 32, 33, 36-38, 41, 42, 44, 46, 48, 50-52] the difference being highly significant ($p=0.00008$). When the two groups were compared in respect of frequency exceeding 20%, none of reports from the Far-East countries had this feature as opposed to 15 (68.2%) from rest of the world ($p=0.00002$). When Sub-Saharan African countries were compared with rest of the non-Far-East countries of the world, it was observed that the frequency of HL exceeded 20% in 2 (28.6%) of the seven Sub-Saharan African countries [25, 26, 28, 29, 33, 37, 48] and 13 (86.7%) of the 15 among the other counties ($p=0.01355$). Thus, whereas Hodgkin's lymphoma is uncommon in the Far-East countries as compared to rest of the world, it is relatively uncommon in Sub-Saharan African countries.

Table 1. Frequency of Hodgkin's lymphoma versus of non-Hodgkin lymphoma in reports from various countries of the world [17-53]

Authors (year)	Country	No of lymphomas	Frequency of HL versus NHL in %		
			HL	NHL	NOS
Bastien et al. (1979) [17]	France	246	38.6	61.4	-
Radaszkiewicz (1980) [18]	Germany	800	22.9	77.1	-
Kelényi and Várbiró (1980) [19]	Hungary	383	18.0	78.9	3.1
Shimizu et al. (1982) [20]	Japan	118	7.6	92.4	-
Ho et al. (1984) [21]	China	294	9.2	90.8	-
Su et al. (1985) [22]	Taiwan	104	8.7	86.5	4.8*

Authors (year)	Country	No of lymphomas	Frequency of HL versus NHL in %		
			HL	NHL	NOS
Calderon et al. (1986) [23]	Philippines	434	18.0	82.0	-
Burla et al. (1990) [24]	Germany	168	33.9	66.1	-
Okpala et al. (1991) [25]	Nigeria	508	18.7	81.3	-
Walter et al. (1991) [26]	Gabon	72	6.9	93.1	-
Ramani et al. (1991) [27]	India	103	30.1	69.9	-
Obafunwa et and Akinsete (1992) [28]	Nigeria	167	32.3	67.7	-
Ngendahayo and Schmauz (1992) [29]	Rawnda	115	16.5	83.5	-
Ji and Li (1992) [30]	China	1082	9.4	90.4	-
Yang et al. (1993) [31]	China	209	12.0	88.0	-
Dasgupta et al. (1993) [32]	India	192	57.3	42.7	-
Cool and Bitter (1997) [33]	Kenya	73	17.8	82.2	-
Chai et al. (1999) [34]	Malaysia	107	10.3	89.7	-
Chuang et al. (2000) [35]	Taiwan	205	3.9	96.1	-
Castella et al. (2001) [36]	UAE	208	40.9	59.1	-
Getachew (2001) [37]	Malawi	83	25.3	73.5	1.2
Naresh et al. (2002) [38]	India	562	31.3	68.7	-
He et al. (2003) [39]	China	370	3.0	97.0	-
Sukpanichnant (2004) [40]	Thailand	1983	7.9	92.1	-
Haddadin (2005) [41]	Jordan	347	21.6	78.4	-
Shivarov et al. (2005) [42]	Bulgaria	790	24.6	73.3	2.2
Wang et al. (2006) [43]	China	447	13.9	86.1	-
Hashemi-Bahremani et al. (2007) [44]	Iran	385	28.1	71.9	-
Jeong et al. (2007) [45]	Korea	507	6.7	93.3	-
Akhtar et al. (2009) [46]	Saudi Arabia	385	30.4	65.2	4.4
Yoon et al. (2010) [47]	Korea	5318	4.1	95.9	-
Mwakigonja et al. (2010) [48]	Tanzania	158	15.2	84.8	-
Chen et al. (2010) [49]	Taiwan	303	8.3	91.7	-
Chakrabarti et al. (2010) [50]	India	124	38.7	61.3	-
Jayasekara et al. (2010) [51]	Australia	28709	8.4	86.3	5.2
Yago et al. (2011) [52]	Iraq	270	24.1	75.9	-
Yang et al. (2011) [53]	China	6382	13.1	86.9	-

* Histiocytic malignancies.

Classifications of Hodgkin's Lymphoma

Hodgkin's lymphoma (HL), which was earlier known as Hodgkin disease (HD), is a malignant lymphoma whose unusual heterogeneous clinical, histologic, and epidemiologic features have suggested either a single disease entity with a complex host response or more than one possible distinct entity. [54] A comprehensive classification of HD was first proposed by Jackson and Parker in 1943, [55] which classified Hodgkin's disease into paragranuloma, granuloma and sarcoma subtypes; this classification was subsequently found to be clinically irrelevant because most of the patients belonged to ganuloma subtype with a huge variation in response to therapy and outcome. Lukes and Butler [56] suggested a histologic classification distinguishing 6 types of HD, viz., lymphocytic and/or histiocytic nodular, lymphocytic and/or histiocytic diffuse, nodular sclerosis, mixed cellularity, diffuse fibrosis and reticular based on a varying degrees of lymphocytic infiltration; this classification was simplified at the Rye symposium in 1965 and the number of histologic groups was reduced from 6 to 4 [10]: lymphoytic predominance, nodular sclerosis, mixed cellularity and lymphocytic depletion. The Rye classification was applied to routine histopathological and cytological diagnoses from mid-sixties to mid-nineties because of good clinicopathologic correlation and high reproducibility. In the mean time along with morphologic and clinical findings, studies on phenotypic, genotypic and molecular parameters threw new lights into the natural history of Hodgkin's disease. In view of these findings, HL was listed in the Revised European-American Lymphoma (REAL) classification, and subdivided into 2 main types [57]: nodular lymphocytic predominant nodular/diffuse HL and classic HL, the latter in turn was further divided into four subtypes: nodular sclerosis, mixed cellularity, lymphocyte rich diffuse (provisional) and lymphocyte depleted. This approach has been adopted by WHO classification of lymphomas, which promoted lymphocyte-rich classic HL from a provisional to an accepted entity. [9] Thus, the WHO classifications [9, 58] classified HL into nodular lymphocytic predominant HL (NLPHL) and classic HL (CHL), which in turn was divided into nodular sclerosis HL (grades 1 and 2), lymphocyte-rich HL (nodular and diffuse), mixed cellularity, lymphocytic depleted and unclassifiable HL.

Rye Classification

Nearly five decades ago Hodgkin's lymphoma, then known as Hodgkin's disease (HD), was classified into lymphocytic predominant (LP), mixed cellularity (MC), lymphocytic depletion (LD) and nodular sclerosis (NS) type. [10] Classification of Hodgkin's disease in FNA cytologic material was performed with satisfactory results following histologic criteria but nodular sclerosis type of HL, which is characterized by islands of neoplastic cells including a special type of R-S cells called lacunar cells and reactive cell components being surround by collagenous bands, was rarely sub-classified in cytologic preparations due to inherent difficulty in identifying these characteristics. [59] The sub-classification into LP, MC, and LD in histology as well as cytology depended on relative proportion of neoplastic HRS cells and reactive cellular components. Differential counts of HRS cells and reactive components in Hodgkin's disease by Das and Gupta [60] revealed significantly lower number of LP cases (6/26) with $\geq$1.5% HRS cells as compared to MC (32/39) and LD (9/9) subtypes

($p<0.0001$); and significantly lower number of MC (3/39) with ≥7.5% HRS cell compared to LD (7/9) subtypes ($p<0.0001$). Lymphocyte content exceeded 95% in 18 of 28 LP subtype, which was significantly higher than MC (8/39) and LD (0/9) subtypes ($p<0.0001$). In another report by Fuggle et al., [61] a significant difference was found between the mean percentages of eosinophil polymorphs between the subtypes of HD: LP (range 0-0.9%, mean 0.24%), NS (range 0-34.2%, mean 13.2%), MC (range 0-20.8%, mean 5.35%) and LD (range 8.2-31.9%, mean 22.6%). Crocker et al. [62] observed that the number of macrophage and macrophage-like cells as determined by α-naphthyl acetate esterase (ANAE)-positive staining in subtypes of HD was as follows: LP (1.8%-16%), NS (13.6%-22.1%), MC (6.5%-14.6%), and LD (39.8%-47.7%). Analysis of 33 reports on Rye classification from various countries (Table 2) [6, 7, 16, 25, 32, 44, 56, 63-88] revealed that the use of this classification continued well after the introduction of WHO classification. [6, 16, 44, 84-88] The range and median of the percentages of the four major subtypes of HL, viz., LP, NS, MC and LD were as follows: LP (range 3.1% to 27.3%, median10.0%), NS (range 2.6% to 74.4%, median 45.1%), MC (range 14.5% to 80.7%, median 35.0%) and LD (range 0% to 36%, median 6.2%), respectively. From the developed economies, [7, 56, 63-65, 69, 72, 73, 75, 81, 82, 84, 86] the median percentages for LP, NS, MC and LD subtypes were 10%, 58.5%, 26.0% and 2.6%, respectively. From the developing countries, [6, 16, 25, 32, 44, 66-68, 70, 71, 74, 76-80, 83, 85, 87, 88] the median percentages for LP, NS, MC and LD subtypes were 9.5%, 29.4%, 44.1% and 8.9%, respectively. In NS subtype, the frequency exceeded 50% in significantly higher number of reports from the developed (9 of 13, 69.2%) than developing countries (3 of 20, 15.0%, $p= 0.00281$). A reverse trend was observed when the reports with MC subtype exceeding 30% of cases were compared (23.1% of the reports in developed vs. 90.0% in the developing world, $p=0.00016$). However, there was no significant difference between the developed and developing countries in respect of LP and LD subtypes when the number of reports with frequency exceeding 10% were compared ($p=1.0000$, and $=0.26346$, respectively).

Application of immunohistochemical as well as other ancillary studies involving molecular parameters in HD in 1980s onwards threw light on true nature of HRS cell and nature of HL. Based on new findings, REAL/WHO classifications of HL were proposed. Not only difference between NLPHL and CHL started to become clear, NHL subtypes like ALCL and TCRBCL, which were earlier confused with HL could be separated from HL; and finally there was useful information on etiology of HL and the pathogenesis of HL could be understood with greater clarity.

Nature of HRS Cells

The histologic hallmark of Hodgkin's lymphoma is the presence of characteristic Hodgkin and Reed-Sternberg (HRS) cells in classical HL and so-called lymphocyte-predominant (LP) cells in nodular lymphocyte-predominant HL. [89]During 1950s and 1960s, Hodgkin cells and Reed-Sternberg (R-S) cells were traditionally believed to be abnormal reticulum cells. [90, 91] Rappaport [92] considered them to be of histiocytic origin on morphologic ground, although Dorfman [93] had failed to demonstrate lysosomal enzymes characteristic of macrophages in Reed-Sternberg cells. With the advent of immunological markers in 1970s, three candidates emerged as possible sources of HRS cells: T-lymphocytes, B-lymphocytes and macrophages; interdigitating reticulm cells and early progenitor myeloid cells subsequently joined the membership club of progenitor cells. A T-lymphocyte origin was proposed in a few studies. [94-96] In one of these reports, Binaminov and Ramot [95] demonstrated a T-cell abnormality rather than T-cell transformation. Payne et al. [97] also found that the T-cells cluster around the atypical cells but are not identical with them. Based on demonstration of cytoplasmic immunoglobulin (Ig) in R-S cells, a B-lymphocyte origin was also proposed. [98-100] However, some contemporary studies based on immunology and electron microscopy provided evidence against B-cell origin of R-S cells. Papadimitrou et al. [101] found that the intracytoplasmic immunoglobulin was polyclonal and the R-S cells contained both lysozyme and alpha-1-antitrypsin. Kadin et al. [102]concluded from their study that R-S cells did not synthesize immunoglobulin but ingested them from the extracellular environment. Along with Kadin and associates, [102] investigators in two other earlier studies favored macrophage as the malignant cell in Hodgkin's disease. [103, 104] According to Kaplan, [105] the capacity of Hodgkin cell and R-S cell for sustained proliferation in vitro, their aneuploidy and hetero-transplantability established their neoplastic character; further, the cell marker studies, phagocytic activity, positive staining reaction for nonspecific esterase and capacity to excrete lysozyme identify them as being derived from macrophages or other closely related cell of mononuclear phagocytic system, rather than from lymphocytes. In addition, the leaky membrane theory of Poppema et al. [106] and the theory of selective ingestion of Ig by Kadin et al. [102] supported the macrophage histogenesis. According to Maksem et al., [107] Hodgkin's disease was a malignant neoplasm that shared many histologic features with granulomatous disease; ultrastructurally, a close parallelism existed between the cells that typify granulomatous inflammation and Reed-Sternberg cells. It was the authors' contention [107] that the heterogeneity among R-S cells in all types of HD paralleled the diversity of the monocyte-macrophage system. However, during this period a report by Diehl et al. [108] based on long term cultures from tumor material revealed that in vitro, the cells have malignant characteristics that represent the in vivo H- and Rs cells but common immunological, functional and morphological assays did not characterize the in vitro cells to be a known cell type of lymphoid, myeloid or monocytoid tissue.

Experimental evidences suggested that multinucleated Reed-Sternberg cells with limited clonal growth capacity arose from mononuclear Hodgkin's cells by endomitosis. [109, 110] According to Drexler, [111] the mononuclear and polynuclear HRS cells are capable of DNA synthesis and nuclear division; the lack of cellular division leads to multinuclearity through the process of endomitosis. Farrell and Jarrett [12] showed that the HRS cells classically express the tumor necrosis factor receptor (TNFR) family member CD30 and the myeloid marker CD15; there may be aberrant expression of T-cell markers such as CD3, CD4 and granzyme B, and dendritic cell markers such as fascin and TARC (thymus activation-regulated chemokine, also known as CCL17) by HRS cells but the phenotype of HRS cell does not reveal B-cell origin. Markers of B lineage, such as CD20, CD19, CD79 and surface Ig, and transcription factors OCT2, BOB1 and PU1 are generally down-regulated in HRS cells, but B-cell specific transcription factor PAX5 is usually retained, albeit at low levels, and can be helpful in distinguishing CHL from T-cell lymphomas. On the other hand, LP cells express B-cell markers including CD20, CD79, PAX5, OCT2 and BOB1.

Table 2. Histological classification of Hodgkin's disease (HD) following Rye Classification [6, 7, 16, 25, 32, 44, 56, 63-88]

Authors (year)	Country	No of cases	Subtype of HD in percentages				
			LP	NS	MC	LD	UC
Lukes & Butler (1966) [56]	USA	377	16	40	26	18	-
Kadin et al. (1971) [63]	USA	117	11	73	16	10	-
Gough (1970) [64]	UK	96	20	15	29	36	-
Farrer Brown et al. (1971) [65]	UK	50	14	56	30	0	-
Wright (1973) [66]	Uganda	128	18	12	50	20	-
Mehrotra et al. (1977) [67]	India	300	8	2.6	80.7	8.7	-
Das et al. (1983) [68]	India	102	26.5	16.7	40.2	13.8	2.9
Petrella et al. (1989) [69]	France	108	10.2	71.3	15.7	0.0	2.8
Liang et al. (1989) [70]	Hong Kong	92	9.8	37.0	31.5	9.8	12
Soriano Rosas et al. (1990) [71]	Mexico	422	5.9	19.7	41.5	6.2	26.8
Okpala et al. (1991) [25]	Nigeria	95	18.9	17.9	45.3	17.9	-
Carde (1992) [72]	France	5096	6.3	63.9	24.6	1.9	3.2
Bernhards et al. (1992) [73]	Germany	1045	3.0	63.2	18.9	0.8	14.2
Cozen et al. (1992) [7]	USA	2492	10.0	50.0	32.0	8.0	-
Chang et al. (1993) [74]	Peru	32	3.1	21.9	62.5	12.5	-
Dasgupta et al. (1993) [32]	India	110	27.3	10.0	44.5	18.2	-
Medeiros and Greiner (1995) [75]	USA	9418	6.0	57.7	23.4	3.8	9.1
Rana et al. (1995) [76]	India	104	16.3	16.3	57.7	9.7	-
De Souza et al. (1997) [77]	Brazil	134	5.2	50.7	34.3	9.0	0.7
Peh et al. (1997) [78]	Malaysia	100	15.0	41.0	40.0	3.0	1.0
Liu et al. (1998) [79]	Taiwan	70	8.6	51.4	37.1	2.9	-
Monterroso et al. (1998) [80]	Costa Rica	40	12.5	50.0	35.0	2.5	-
Mourad et al. (1998) [81]	Canada	62	12.9	72.6	14.5	0	-
Enblad et al. (1999) [82]	Sweden	117	4.3	74.4	17.9	2.6	0.9
Macák et al. (2000) [83]	Czech Rep	142	9.2	45.1	43.7	2.1	-
Glavina-Durdov et al. (2001) [84]	UK	100	8.0	48.0	37.0	7.0	-
De Oliveira et al. (2002) [85]	Brazil	96	4.2	28.1	58.3	4.2	5.2
Krugmann et al. (2003) [86]	Austria	119	5.9	58.8	32.8	2.5	-
Almasri and Khalidi (2004) [87]	Jordan	64	3.1	43.8	53.1	0.0	-
Vassalo et al. (2005) [88]	Brazil	1025	4.9	69.3	21.2	4.7	-
Hashemi-Bahremani et al. (2007) [44]	Iran	108	11.1	30.6	48.1	10.2	-
Wu et al. (2008) [16]	Taiwan	133	12.8	45.1	28.6	2.3	11.3
Olu-Eddo and Omoti (2011) [6]	Nigeria	56	5.4	10.7	64.3	19.6	-

In an immunohistochemical study of 20 HD cases (5 NS, 12 MC, 3 LD), Wachi et al. [112] observed that majority of RS-cells expressed CD30 and CD15, and some RS-cells could be of B-cell lineage since 7/20 cases consisting of 1 NS, 5 MC and 1 LD were CD20+. Schmid et al. [113] performed immunohistochemistical and molecular analysis 55 patients with pre-treatment HD (45 NS, 10 MC) to determine the phenotype of H-RS cells; the H-RS cells were CD45- (100%), CD 30+ (100%), CD15+ (78%) and were reactive for at least one B-cell marker (CD19, CD20, CD22, CDw75, MB2) in 87% and a subpopulation of HRS cells were positive for T-cell marker (CD3, betaF1); all cases that expressed T-cell antigen were also reactive with at least one B-cell marker. The authors [113] were unable to confirm the previous reports of bcl-2 gene rearrangements in HD but the results strongly supported B-cell origin of H-RS cells. Zukerberg et al. [114] also demonstrated co-expression of B-cell marker CD20 and the granulocyte associated antigen CD15 by Reed-Sternberg cells, with some expressing CD20, some CD15, and others expressing both antigens. According to these authors, [114] cells co-expressing both CD15 and CD20 may represent an unstable intermediate in the process of antigen switching, and the possibility that antigen expression by neoplastic cells in a given case may modulate depending on the background infiltrate could explain the heterogeneity of immune-phenotype among cases of Hodgkin's disease. Immune-phenotypic analysis of H-RS cells by Drexler [111] also suggested a lymphoid cell expressing T- and/or B-cell associated markers and certain activated antigens while lacking immunological features of monocytes-macrophages or other lineages. In an immune-histochemical study of 92 CHL cases, the neoplastic cells were CD20+ in 12/84 (14.3%), CD15+ in 67/75 (89.3%), CD30+ in 75/77 (97.4%), and CD45RO in 0/75 (0.0%). [85] According to Chang et al., [115] there was no significant difference between Hodgkin's cells and R-S cells in respect of CD15 staining (82.8% vs. 74.6%), the common staining sites in the cell being Golgi region (71.1% vs. 61.9%) and cytoplasm (8.2% vs. 8.5%); similarly there was no significant difference between Hodgkin's and R-S cells in respect of CD30 staining (99.9% vs. 98.7%); the common sites in the cell being cytoplasm (69.2% vs. 63.6%) and ER-Golgi/cytoplasm (17.3% vs. 18.8%). According to Papadimitrou et al., [101] H-RS cells in 20% HD cases were CD57 positive, which were not of B-cell origin but may be related to natural killer (NK) or T-cells expressing CD57 antigens.

With the hypothesis that viral proteins may induce aberrant expression of cyclin A and lead to multinucleation in virus infected cells, Chang et al. [115] investigated whether Epstein-Barr virus (EBV) latent membrane protein-1 (LMP1) and cyclin A are involved in the morphogenesis of R-S cells, which represents the histologic hallmark for Hodgkin's lymphoma. These investigators [115]found that in LMP1+ and LMP1- HLs, multinucleated R-S cells aberrantly expressed cyclin A in cytoplasm, while the mononuclear Hodgkin cells expressed cyclin A predominantly in nuclei ($p<0.001$). No difference in expression of CD15, CD30 or CD99 in HL cells was found between the two groups. In vitro, EBV-LMP1 increased cytoplasmic cyclin A expression and multinucleation in an HL cell line. Therefore, the aberrant expression of cyclin A was thought to be commonly associated with RS cell morphologic features in HL, probably through LMP1 signaling or other similar mechanisms in EBV- cases. Bai, et al. [116] observed that EBV-positive cases, as demonstrated by the presence of EBER-1 and-2 RNA and LMP-1 protein expression, showed a significant reduction in expression on H-RS cells of T-cell lineage (CD3, $p<0.02$), B-cell lineage (CD20, $p<0.005$) and activation markers (EMA, $p<0.002$ and the 115D8 antigen, $p<0.001$) as compared to EBV-negative cases but no differences were found in the expression of CD15,

CD30, CD45RO, CD45RB, CDW75, or the MB2 antigen on H-RS cells in these two groups; these data suggested that EBV in H-RS cells was able to down regulate the expression of T-(CD3) and B-(CD20) cell lineage markers and lymphoid activation markers EMA and the 115D8 antigen.

The cellular origin of Hodgkin and Reed-Sternberg (HRS) cells, the neoplastic cells of classic Hodgkin's lymphoma (HL), resisted clarification until the second half 1990s. Siebert et al. [117]reported a case of HD (mixed cellularity) in which the H-RS cells expressed the characteristic markers CD15 and CD30; in addition they expressed CD19, CD20 and CD45/LCA and clonal rearrangement for Ig heavy chain gene was detected by Southern blot analysis. During the recent years, not only extensive phenotypical characterization HRS cells were performed, clonality of these cases has been demonstrated by cytogenetics and molecular genetics parameters. Immunophenotypical studies demonstrated frequent expression of "lymphoid activation markers" including CD15, CD25, CD30, CD40, CD54, CD70, CD71, CD80, CD86, and MHC class II and less frequent expression of T- or B-cell associated antigens by the neoplastic H-RS cells; the clonality of H-RS cells has been demonstrated by clonal EBV integration, clonal cytogenetic abnormalities including p53 mutations and clonal immunoglobulin rearrangements in some HD cases. [1]

According to Stein and Hummel, [118] one major obstacle to successful experimental investigations was the rarity of HRS cells in the tissue affected by HL; although the immunophenotypic studies pointed towards a B-cell origin of HRS cells in early 1980s, they were not definitive because of variable expression B-cell and/or T-cell antigens and the additional expression of markers typical for other lineages, especially dendritic cells, attempts to elucidate the cellular derivation by demonstrating the clonal rearrangements of the Ig gene or TCR genes in whole tissue extracts also remained inconclusive due inconsistent results. The extraction of single CD30+ HRS cells from immunostained frozen sections by means of hydraulic micromanipulation proved to be most suitable answer to these problems; using this method, monoclonal Ig gene rearrangements were detected in HRS cells in 95% of HL cases by Stein and Hummel [118] and their findings were summarized as follows: (1) Approximately 95% of classic HLs originate from B-cells; (2) the direct precursors of the HRS cells are germinal center B-cells; (3) the transforming event that causes HL leads to complete morphologic and immunophenotypical change of the HRS cell precursors; and (4) the HRS cell population of a given case exclusively arises from a single transformed cell and expands by clonal growth. The finding of Ig gene rearrangements in HRS cells in most cases of HD identified B cells as the precursors of HRS cells in most, if not all cases; furthermore, the presence and pattern of somatic mutations within the rearranged Ig genes showed that the HRS cells in classical (i.e. nodular sclerosis, mixed cellularity, and lymphocyte depletion HD) as well as lymphocyte predominant (LP) HD originated from germinal center (GC) B cells. [119] By molecular single cell analysis of Hodgkin and Reed-Sternberg (HRS) cells in Hodgkin's disease (HD), it could not only be shown that the HRS cells in classical as well as lymphocyte predominant (LP) HD represent clonal populations of mature B-cells but further information was obtained on their phenotypical differences; whereas HRS cells in classical HD appear to derive from crippled G B cells that lost the capacity to express antigen receptor, the precursors of the HRS cells in LP HD are mutating, antigen-selected GC B cells. [120] These findings were confirmed by many other studies in the years that followed. [110, 121, 122] According to Schmitz et al., [122] HRS cells have largely lost their B-cell phenotype and aberrantly express markers and transcriptional regulators of other hematolymphoid cell types; deregulation of multiple signaling pathways and downstream transcription factors, including receptor tyrosine kinases, nuclear factor-kappa B (NF-kappaB), and Janus kinase/signal transducer and activator of transcription (JAK/STAT) was a further hallmark of HRS cells.

Table 3. Histological classification of Hodgkin's disease (HD) following WHO classification [38, 42, 47, 48, 52, 53, 115, 138-147]

Authors (year)	Country	No of cases	Subtype of HL in percentages					
			NLPHL	CHLLR	CHLNS	CHLMC	CHLLD	CHLUC
LSGJP (2000) [138]	Japan	141	3.5	5.7	40.4	36.9	5.7	7.8
Naresh et al. (2002) [38]	India	176	6.8	1.1	46.0	36.9	2.3	6.8 [†]
Makar et al. (2003) [139]	Kuwait	134	6.7	3.0	37.3	45.5	3.0	4.5
De Matteo et al. (2003) [140]	Argen-tina	173	2.9	6.9	38.7	48.6	2.9	-
Shivarov et al. (2005) [42]	Bulgaria	194	1.0	1.0	64.4	23.2	5.7	4.6
Zhang et al. (2006) [141]*	USA	42	0.0	6.1	39.4	36.4	12.1	6.1
Lee et al. (2006) [142]	Taiwan	42	7.1	4.8	69.0	4.8	0.0	14.3
Keresztes et al. (2006) [143]	Hungary	109	1.8	4.6	21.1	65.1	5.5	1.8
Al-Salam et al. (2008) [144]	U.A.E.	88	10.2	1.1	45.5	31.8	4.5	6.8
Hudnall et al. (2008) [145]	USA	59	8.5	3.4	69.5	15.3	3.4	-
Fong et al. (2009) [146]	Austria	158	6.3	2.5	60.1	27.8	-	3.2
Chang et al. (2009) [115]	Taiwan	34	2.9	11.8	67.6	14.7	0.0	2.9
Trankov e al (2010) [147]	Switze-rland	105**	-	2.9	57.1	30.5	1.9	7.6
Mwakigonja et al. (2010) [48]	Tanzania	24	8.3	12.5	25.0	45.8	8.3	-
Yoon et al. (2010) [47]	Korea	219	3.7	3.2	55.7	25.6	4.1	7.8
Yago et al. (2011) [52]	Iraq	65	4.6	1.5	47.7	36.9	9.2	-
Yang et al. (2011) [53]	China	833	4.2	4.2	17.4	72.7	1.4	-

* FNA-based study.** Only CHL cases included. [†]Included 4.0% CHL NOS and 2.8% UC HL. LSGJP= Lymphoma Study Group of Japanese Pathologists.

The above developments have been summarized by Farrell and Jarrett [12] in the following lines: microdissection coupled with analysis of immunoglobulin genes revealed that HRS cells are usually clonal B-cells. HRS cells, from nearly all CHL cases, and LP cells have detectable rearrangements of Ig heavy and/or light chain genes, confirming a B-cell origin and, in any given case, the rearrangements are identical, proving the clonal nature of the disease. Furthermore, the Ig variable (IgV) gene regions show evidence of somatic hypermutation, revealing a germinal centre (GC) or post-GC origin. In LP cells intraclonal IgV gene diversity is observed, indicating ongoing somatic hypermutation, whereas HRS cells show identical somatic hypermutation consistent with a later stage of B-cell differentiation, 'crippling' mutations, resulting in non-functioal Ig genes, are observed in around 25% of CHL cases. Rarely (<2%), HRS cells harbor rearranged T cell receptor genes, suggesting a T-cell origin in a small minority of cases.

Nature of Hodgkin's Lymphoma

Two findings, in particular, make HL a unique malignant hematopoietic disease: first, the malignant mononucleated Hodgkin- and the multinucleated Reed-Sternberg (HRS) cells represent only a small fraction of cells (about 1% cells in tumor tissue) in the affected lymph nodes and are embedded in an infiltrate of reactive hematopoietic cells, composed of B- and T-lymphocytes, eosinophils, and plasma cells among others, and second, the HRS cells do not display a phenotype that can be assigned to a defined hematopoietic cell type. [123] One of the earliest reports on Hodgkin's lymphoma involving immunohistochemical parameters was undertaken by Aisenberg and Wilkes [124] to study the lymphocyte population in Hodgkin's disease (HD) and reactive hyperplasia (RH) using a panel of 10 monoclonal antibodies and rosetting techniques; in both Hodgkin's disease and hyperplasia, 60%-70% of the cells were T lymphocytes and approximately 80% of these were inducer/helper subset and 20% cytotoxic/suppressor subset. The most prominent difference between HD and RH was explained by greater affinity of the sheep cell receptor on the surface of T lymphocyte of HD as compared to RH. Facchetti et al. [125] observed that plasmacytoid monocytes (so called plasmacytoid T-cells) were one of the monocyte-derived cells that contributed to the cellular reaction in HD (LP, NS and MC); they occurred at the periphery of lymphoid aggregates which mimicked the composite nodules of reactive lymph node but contained RS-cell and its variants.

In the past, various possibilities put forth regarding nature of Hodgkin's disease. Before 1950s the nature of Hodgkin's disease was thought to be inflammatory, [4, 5, 126]neoplastic [127-129]and an intermediate state between the two. [3, 130] A fourth possibility was put forth by Kaplan and Smithers, [131]who suggested that Hodgkin's disease might represent an autoimmune process. During late 1960s and 1970s, evidence in favor of neoplastic nature of Hodgkin's disease emerged. Studies involving incorporation of tritiated thymidine into DNA proved that Hodgkin cells and Reed-Sternberg cells were the proliferating cells. [132-134] Kaplan and Gartner [103]not only demonstrated incorporation of tritiated thymidine in DNA of Hodgkin cells and R-S cells but also observed binucleated mitotic figures, which proved that R-S cells arise by nuclear replication rather than by cell fusion. Aneuploidy of Hodgkin's cells was demonstrated [135, 136] and their clonal derivation was described, thus fulfilling two of the most fundamental attributes of neoplasia. According to Gruss and Kadin, [1] the neoplastic nature of HD is based on aggressive clinical progression, presence of the proliferating and atypical H-RS cells, aneuploidy and cellular clonality; the histopathological presentation and characteristic histopathological features of HD correlates with the unbalanced production of multiple cytoknes and thus, HD is defined as a tumor of cytokine-producing cells in which the proportion of malignant H-RS cells to reactive cellular components and fibrosis is dependent on the production of particular cytokines and this allows sub-typing of HD cases.

WHO Classification of Hodgkin's Lymphoma

New discoveries on nature of Hodgkin's disease and its pathognomonic neoplastic cells led to formulation of new classifications of Hodgkin's disease under auspices REAL/WHO. [137] As discussed earlier Hodgkin's disease was renamed Hodgkin's lymphoma and classified under WHO classification of hematopoietic neoplasms [9, 58] into two broad categories, viz., nodular lymphocytic predominance Hodgkin's lymphoma (NLPHL) and classical Hodgkin's lymphoma (CHL); CHL in turn under WHO classification, was classified into four subtypes: lymphocyte-rich (LRCHL), nodular sclerosis (NSCHL), mixed cellularity (MCCHL) and lymphocyte depletion (LDCHL), with a wide geographical variation in frequency (Table 3). [38, 42, 47, 48, 52, 53, 115, 138-147] However, unlike the Rye classification, no definite geographical trend was observed in distribution of subtypes, which may be due to smaller number of studies. The range and median values for frequency of various subtypes were as follows: NLPHL (0.0% to 10.2%, 4.2%), LRCHL (1.0% to 12.5%, 3.4%), NSCHL (17.4% to 69.5%, 46.0%), MCCHL (4.8% to 72.7%, 36.4%), LDCHL (0.0%-12.1%, 3.4%) and UCCHL (0.0% to 14.3%, 4.5%), respectively. Although the frequency of reports having >50%NSCHL was more, and >5% NLPHL, >5% LRCHL, >30% MCCHL, >5% LDCHL was less in the Far-East countries as compared to rest of the world, the difference was not significant (p=0.28006 to =1.00000).

Nodular Lymphocytic Predominant Hodgkin's Lymphoma (NLPHL)

NLPHL is a distinct HL subtype composed of few neoplastic lymphocyte predominant (LP) cells in a background of reactive small B and T cells. [148] Initial description of NLPHL was one characterized by a nodular, or nodular and diffuse proliferation of scattered and large neoplastic cells (lymphocytic and/or histiocytic [L&H] cells or "popcorn" cells) in large spherical mesh-works of follicular dendritic cells (FDCs) filled with non-neoplastic small lymphocytes, mainly of B-cell type. [149] At present the term lymphocytic predominant (LP) cell has replaced the "L&H" or "popcorn" cell. The recent description of NLPHL by Mani and Jaffe [150] is as follows: The LP cell has a polylobated nucleus with finely dispersed chromatin and small, usually basophilic nucleoli, and relatively sparse cytoplasm, which is immunohistochemially CD15-, CD30- (rare weak+), CD20+, CD79a+, CD45+, J-chain+, OCT+, BOB1+, PU1+, PAX+, and EBV-. Background shows small lymphocytes in a nodular or nodular and diffuse pattern (with focal presence of nodular pattern at least). The small lymphocytes in the background are small B-cells with a mantle cell phenotype (IgD+, IgM-). There are expanded mesh-works of FDC, as seen by CD21 immunostain. Epithelioid histiocytes are present in varying numbers.

Classical Hodgkin's Lymphoma (CHL)

The HRS cells of CHL possess single to multilobated nuclei with peripherally condensed chromatin, large and often eosinophilic nucleoli and abundant cytoplasm; the HRS cells are CD15+ (membrane and/or Golgi region), CD30+ (membrane and/or Golgi region), CD20 variable + (positive in 30-40% cases), CD79a- to variable weak+, CD45-, J-chain-, OCT-2- (often), BOB1- (often), PU1-, PAX5+ (weak), and EBV+ (variable). [150] The histopathological features of four subtypes of CHL are as follows:

- LRCHL: By definition, lymphocyte-rich CHL is a diffuse tumor with relatively infrequently R-S cells, which are of classic type, However, a nodular or follicular variant occurs, in which classical HRS cells are few in number and can be seen in marginal/mantle zone around regressed GCs with dense FDC meshwork. Aggregates of epithelioid histiocytes may be present, but eosinophils and neutrophils are rare.
- NSCHL: Capsular fibrosis and broad collagen bands, which are often perivascular, characterize this subtype; lacunar cells (a special type of HRS cells) and mummified cells are important features. Grade I and II differ in number of HRS cells and necrosis is a feature of grade II.
- MCCHL: There is diffuse lymph node effacement with numerous HRS cells and a mixed inflammatory background with lymphocytes, eosinophils, plasma cells and histiocytes. Granulomas may be present.
- LDCHL: Whereas diffuse fibrosis variant has a hypo-cellular background, abundant disorderly arranged non-birefringent fibrosis, abundant histiocytes but fewer lymphocytes; the reticular variant shows numerous HRS cells with bizarre cytological features.

Lymphocyte depleted classical Hodgkin lymphoma (LDCHL) is a vanishing category of classical. Hodgkin lymphoma, accounts for approximately <1% of all cases in the most modern series. [151]

Difference between NLPHL and CHL

Pinkus and Said [152] observed that the L&H variant of R-S cells detected in LPHL, nodular were strongly immunoreactive for leukocyte common antigen and B-cell-specific antigens but uniformly non-reactive to Leu-1, granulocyte-related antigen; on the other hand the other types of R-S cells detected in NS, MC, and LD subtypes were strongly reactive for Leu-1 but non-reactive or rarely positive for LCA and negative for pan-B-cell monoclonal antibodies. According to these authors, [152] the L&H variants of RS-cells represent a distinct type of transformed cells, possibly of B-cell origin, and do not share a common lineage with other type of R-S cells; therefore LPHL, nodular may represent a distinct entity. Subsequently this distinct entity was named nodular lymphocytic predominant Hodgkin's disease (NLPHD). In all cases of NLPHD, the L&H cells were L26 positive. Other variants of RS cells, e.g., lacunar, mononuclear and diagnostic forms, which were present in NS, MC and LD subtypes, L26 positivity was noticed in <5% cells in 87% cases and in the remaining cases a larger proportion of these cells expressed L26. [153] Poppema [154] reported on the immunophenotype of nonneoplastic, small lymphocytes associated with HL; the T-cells in NLPHL, nodular sclerosing Hodgkin's lymphoma (NSHL) and mixed cellular Hodgkin's lymphoma (MCHL) displayed an activated CD4+ immunophenotype. However, the T-lymphocytes in NLPHL differed from NSHL and MCHL in that they showed reactivity for Leu 7 (CD57). Moreover, T-cells were found surrounding the R-S cells and variants in all three forms of HL but in only NLPHL these T-cells demonstrated CD57 reactivity. Poppema [154] suggested that CD57 immunoreactivity may be a helpful criterion for diagnosis of NLPHL. In an attempt to test the above hypothesis, Kamel et al. [155] used an image analysis system and found that the average of CD57 reactivity was 18.9% of small lymphocytes in NLPHL, 3.9% in NSHL, 4.3% in TCRBCL and 2.1% in follicular lymphoma. Further, the CD57+ lymphocytes showed a distinctive pattern in NLPHL, forming a ring of cells around the large L&H cells. According to Montes-Moreno, [156]the characteristic lymphocyte-predominant (LP) cells of NLPHL exhibit a germinal center (GC) phenotype profile with expression of GC markers such as BCL6, GCET1 and LMO2, together with expression of transcriptional factors related to a sustained B cell program such as OCT2 and BOB1. Interestingly, the GC-related profile is seen not only in LP cells but also in the surrounding T cells, which characteristically create a rosette-like pattern typical of NLPHL. These rosetting T-cells have a follicular T-cell phenotype with expression of CD3/CD4/CD57, bcl6, PD1 and, interestingly, CXCL13, a chemokine that is known to induce B-cell homing to lymphoid follicles and that plays a role in the T cell-dependent B cell affinity maturation process. These observations suggest that NLPHL is characterized by a GC phenotype in both LP and surrounding T-cells. This combination is not found in classical HL (CHL), with the exception of lymphocyte-rich CHL, which has a profile intermediate between NLPHL and CHL with overexpression of B-cell transcription program markers and the presence of follicular T-cell background in a substantial proportion of cases. This is not the case of other types of CHL in which the B cell program and the germinal center microenvironment is lost.

As it stands today, the NLPHL can be distinguished from CHL based on clinical, morphological, immunophenotypical and genetic features. The growth pattern in NLPHL is at least in part nodular mostly and diffuse pattern is very rare; the neoplastic cells are LP cells (L&H cells or popcorn cells) with nuclei resemble those of centroblasts having polylobular profile, finely dispersed chromatin and small nucleoli adjacent to nuclear membrane. The immunophenotype of the neoplastic cells in NLPHL are CD45+, CD20+, CD22+, CD79a+, J chain±, EMA±, CD15- and CD30- or weak+. The lymph node in CHL is largely effaced although remnants of follicle can be detected in some cases. In CHL, the typical Hodgkin's and Reed-Sternberg cells can be easily detected and can be associated with peculiar variants and the immunophenotype of H&RS cells is CD30+ (98%), CD15+ (80%), CD45-, EMA-, CD20+ (30%-40%) and CD79a (even less frequently); one or more T-cell markers are seen in a minority of H&RS cells in some cases. More specifically, the nodular lymphocyte-rich variant of classical Hodgkin lymphoma (CHL), can be differentiated NLPHL from based on immunophenotype. In contrast to CHL, tumor cells of NLPHL do not express CD30 and

CD15, but they are positive for B-cell markers (CD20, CD79a), immunoglobulins, J chain, and EMA. [149] The B-cell phenotype and genetic features of NLPHL, exhibiting clonally rearranged immunoglobulin genes with ongoing mutations, [157, 158] indicate its close relationship to B-cell non-Hodgkin lymphomas. [9, 159]

Differential Diagnosis of Hodgkin's Lymphoma

When the Rye classification on Hodgkin's disease was formulated in 1966, [10] it was regarded by many as a formidable classification since the diagnostic criteria for Hodgkin's disease were very sound, which could not be challenged easily. During 1970s, understanding of the nature of cells in the formation of non-Hodgkin's lymphoma (NHL) led to the emergence of a number of classifications and a wide range of controversies was associated with it. Unlike non-Hodgkin's lymphoma, the fortress of Hodgkin's lymphoma seemed invincible in seventies through eighties into early nineties. However, as seen in table 1, 1.2% to 5.2% cases were unclassified as lymphomas other than HL and NHL with a median of 3.8% in six studies. [19, 22, 37, 42, 46, 51] When Hodgkin's disease were classified as per Rye classification, in 12 of the 33 studies (Table 2), 0.7% to 26.8% HL cases were also unclassified. [16, 69-73, 75, 77, 78, 82, 85]This is again highlighted in WHO classification (Table 3), wherein 12 out of 17 studies had 1.8% to 14.3% cases were unclassified HL. [38, 42,47, 115, 138, 139, 141-144, 146,147] These findings indicate that there were cases in which decision between NHL and HL was difficult or not possible, and also cases in which classifying HL into subtypes based not only on morphological features but even with all ancillary parameters was difficult. In earlier reports, the so called pathognomonic HRS cells or HRS-like cells were reported not only in benign lymphoproliferative conditions like reactive lymphoid hyperplasia and infectious mononucleosis, but some of nonHodgkin lymphoma subtypes, e.g., chronic lymphocytic leukemia, mycosis fungoides, Burkitt's lymphoma, lymphoepithelioid lymphoma and immunoblastic lymphoma, and non-lymphoid malignancies like metastatic carcinoma, melanoma, sarcoma and germ cell tumors revealed presence of RS-like cells. [160-162] The application of T-cell and B-cell lymphoid markers for immunophenotyping and/or genetic probe methods have further confirmed the suspicion of pathologists that morphologic similarities do exist between HD, and some pleomorphic T-cell lymphomas, [163]T-cell-rich B-cell lymphoma (TCRBCL) [164] and anaplastic large cell lymphoma (ALCL). [165]Review of HL cases in some of the studies yielded NHL ranging from 1.9% to 14.3% with a median of 10.4%.[69, 72, 166, 167].

According to Harris, [168] the immunophenotype and genetic features are useful in the classification of HL and in distinguishing HL from two recently described, aggressive lymphomas that were in the past often diagnosed as HL, i.e., anaplastic large-cell lymphoma, T-cell type, and T-cell/histiocyte-rich large B-cell lymphoma. Elgin et al. [169] felt that immunoperoxidase markers are useful and often essential in distinguishing among lymphocytic predominant Hodgkin's lymphoma, T-cell-rich B-cell lymphoma, and lymphocyte-rich classical Hodgkin's lymphoma; however, it is becoming increasingly clear that these "entities" are closely related clonal B-lineage neoplasms that may inter-transform and/or coexist. Das et al. [170] reported that ALCL and TCRBCL are the most common NHL subtypes to be confused with HL but other entities like pleomorphic T-cell lymphomas and some large B-cell lymphomas may give rise to the diagnostic difficulties. This will be apparent from the few other reported studies in yester years. In a study of 2 NPHL and 43 CHL cases by Liu et al., [170] the NLPHL cases were CD20+, CD15-, CD30-; CD57+ cells and small B-lymphocytes were predominant cells in the background infiltration; diagnostic RS cells and other tumor cells in 43 CHL cases were positive for CD30 (100%), CD15 (81%), and CD20 (7%). Whereas six TCRBCL cases were negative for CD15 and CD30, two ALCL cases were CD30+, ALK1+, CD3+, CD15- and CD20-. The reactive inflammatory cell infiltration present in CHL cases were rich in TIA1+ cytotoxic lymphocytes but CD57+ cells were rarely encountered. The comparative genomic hybridization (CGH) profiles of THCRBCL and NLPHL showed some common and several distinct features, in particular with respect to the number of genomic imbalances (average of 4.7 in T/HRBCL versus 10.8 in LPHL) and their distribution (usually 1 to 5 in T/HRBCL versus 6 to 22 in LPHL). [171]Thus, T/HRBCL constitutes a separate lymphoma entity, possibly originating from the same precursor cell as LPHL. In a cyto-histologic study of 15 ALCL and 48 HL cases, Mourad et al. [172] observed an immunohistochemical profile of CD15+, CD30+ and CD45- pattern in HL, and CD15-, CD30+ and CD45+ in ALCL cases; immunostaining with ALK antibody revealed positive reaction in 3 of 8 ALCL cases. As per a review of literature by Marafioti et al., [173] the neoplastic cells of TCRBCL were LSP-1 positive and PU.1 negative, whereas the L&H cells of lymphocyte predominance HL were mostly LSP-1 negative, with variable PU.1 expression; however, the two markers did not distinguish between TCRBCL and lymphocyte-rich classical HL. The transcription factor PU.1 is down-regulated in TCRBCL compared with lymphocyte predominant HL; PU.1 regulates the transcription of genes relevant to the development of B-cells, macrophages and myeloid cells. Leukocyte-specific phosphoprotein (LSP1) is present in the neoplastic cells of most large B-cell lymphomas, but usually absent in lymphocyte-predominant HL.

Etiology of HL: Role of Epstein Barr Virus (EBV) and Other Viral Agents

EBV plays an important role in several neoplasms, in particular, African endemic Burkitt's lymphoma and Chinese nasopharyngeal carcinoma in south-east Asia; other diseases such as Hodgkin's disease, some NHL, gastric cancer and esophageal cancer have some relationship with EBV. [85, 174] According to Jarrett, [175] EBV is an extremely efficient transforming agent and when EBV infects B-cells in vitro, six EBNA (EBNA-6) proteins (EBNA 1, 2, 3a, 3b, 3c and LP) are expressed alongside three membrane proteins (LMP1, LMP2A and LMP2B). Recent molecular studies provide support for the idea that EBV is involved in the pathogenesis of HD. EBV genomes are consistently found in a proportion of tumor biopsies, EBV infected cells are clonal; not only the EBV genomes have been localized to Reed Sternberg cells, EBV latent gene products are expressed in R-S cells. [176] Furthermore, since majority of samples from patients aged greater than 50 years and less than 15 years are fund to be EBV positive, it is suggested that EBV plays a role in HD in children and older adults but that other agents, possibly other viruses, are involved in young adults. [176]In the Chinese population, tumor cells of 39% of CHL patients were EBV+ and this was significantly associated with male sex, mixed cellular subtype, young age (<20y). [177] A review by Chang et al. [74] showed that patients with HD have abnormally high levels of antibodies against EBV antigens and EBV-associated infectious mononucleosis patients have an increased risk of HD over control populations. A review by Makar et al. [139]of 14 studies from Arabian Gulf and Middle East region, Asia, North America and Western Europe and Africa and South America revealed EBV positivity in 382/776 (49.2%) cases; the positivity in LP, NS, MC, LD and unclassifiable cases was 10/57 (17.5%), 168/447 (37.6%), 201/276 (72.8%), 22/32 (68.8%), and 3/8 (37.5%), respectively. Testing of EBV within the RS and Hodgkin cells was carried out in childhood Hodgkin's lymphoma in 10 different countries. The proportion of LMP1 positive cases varied significantly, being 50% of cases from UK, South Africa, Egypt, and Jordan, 60% from UAE, 70% from Australia, 81% from Costa Rica, 88% from Iran, 90% from Greece, and 100% of the 56 cases from Kenya. [178] Peh et al. [78] found that in younger (<15 years) patients, 93% were positive for EBV and in older patients 52% were positive. According to Liu et al., [79] the association of EBV with HL is intimately related to socioeconomic status with high prevalence in developing countries and low prevalence in developed countries; in a study of 70 HL cases from Taiwan overall EBV positivity was 44 (62.9%). A comparative study of 33 HD cases from Kenya and 31 cases from Nagasaki, Japan revealed EBER positivity by ISH in 79% in Kenya and 59% in Nagasaki. [174] The frequency of EBV positivity by LMP-1 by IHC and EBER by ISH from 14 different studies (11 on Rye classification and 3 based on WHO classification of HL) has been depicted in table 4. [74, 78-83, 85-87, 115, 139, 143, 144] Overall EBV positivity ranged from 26.1%to 93.8%, with a median 46.8%. Under Rye classification, the range and median of EBV positivity for the subtypes were as follows: LP (0%-100%, 0%), NS (15%-100%, 29.6%), MC (38.1%-100%, 74.2%) and LD (14%-100%, 50.0%), respectively. [74, 78-83, 85-87, 143] In WHO classification, the range and median of EBV positivity in various subtypes were as follows: NLPHL (0%-2%, 2%), LRCHL (25%-100%, 50%), NSCHL (27.3%-478%, 34.2%), MCCHL (52.9%-100%, 79.2%) and LDCHL (50%-100%, 75%), respectively. [115, 139, 144]

Benharroch et al. [179] in a cohort of 154 HD patients detected positive immunostaining for at least two anti-measles antibodies in 82 (54.3%); while immunostaining for EBV LMP-1 protein was positive in 46 (31.1%); reverse transcriptase-PCR and ISH for measles RNA were positive in 7 and 10 of 28 patients, respectively. In setting of high prevalence HIV infection in South Africa, 2225 new cases of lymphoproliferative disorders were diagnosed during 2007-2009 as compared with 1897 cases diagnosed during 2004-2006; [180] a significant increase in both high-grade B-cell lymphomas and Hodgkin's lymphoma was documented during 2007-2009 and this was associated with a statistically significant increase in HIV prevalence in those tested (from 44.3% in 2004-2006 to 62.0% in 2007-2009).

Phenotypic, Genomic and Molecular Defects in HRS Cells: The Significance

Hodgkin's lymphomas belong to the most curable neoplasti diseases in adults; about 80% of patients in all anatomical stages and of all histological subtypes can be cured with modern treatment strategies. [181] It has been observed since long that patients with lymphocyte depletion, NOS, and mixed cellularity subtype of HL have a significantly worse prognoses compared to patients who had nodular sclerosis, whereas patients who had lymphocytic predominance had the best prognosis. [182] Using three marker (CD15, CD20 and CD30) in 1751 classical (non-lymphocytic predominant) HD cases Von Wasielewsky et al. [183] found 83% with classical phenotype (CD15+, CD30+, CD20-); 12% lacked CD15 positivity (CD15-, CD30+, CD20-) and 5% showed other combinations. According to these authors, [183] clinical follow-up of 1286 cases revealed significant difference for freedom from treatment failure (p=0.0022) and overall survival (p=0.0001) between cases with classical immunophenotype and those with CD15- (CD30+, CD20-); multivariate Cox regression analysis showed that lack of CD15 expression in classical HD is an independent negative prognostic factor for relapse (p=0.022) and survival (p= 0.0035). In a study 110 HD patients by Smolewski et al., [184] 69 obtained complete remission (CR) after first-line treatment and 41 did not respond. Evaluating apoptosis by TUNEL technique (TdT-mediated dUTP nick end labeling), these authors [184] found positive TUNEL reaction in 43 patients with apoptotic index (AI) varying between 10% and 60%; in the remaining 57 patients AI of H-RS cells was <10%; the mean AI in non-responding patients was significantly higher than in CR group (p=0.015); the high frequency of AI was also negatively correlated with the progression free survival time (p=0.031) and the overall survival (p=0.042).

Quite a few immunophenotypic and molecular studies on the prognosis of HL are based on Epstein Barr virus (EBV). Two pathogenic mechanisms are probably influenced by the presence of EBV in the H-RS cells: resistance of the H-RS cells to apoptosis; and escape of H-RS cells from a cytotoxic T lymphocyte immune response; [185] latent membrane protein-1 (LMP-1) is most likely the EBV-encoded protein responsible for this putative EBV-mediated pathogenic effect. Oudejans et al. [185] found that with the use of conventional therapy regimens, the presence of EBV bears little influence on clinical presentation and treatment outcome of HD. However, the difference in regulation of both apoptosis and immune escape mechanisms between EBV+ and EBV- cases may be important determinants of the success of immune therapy to treat Hodgkin's disease. Krugmann et al., [86] observed that patients with EBV-associated classical HL were predominantly mixed cellular type; were more frequent in male patients, in those above 45 years of age, in Stage III and IV disease, and in patients with B-symptoms; showed a significantly longer mean time of first relapse of 99 months as compared with 49 months for EBV-negative cases (p<0.02). However, overall survival did not correlate with EBV-association. Thus, the presence of EBV has a beneficial effect on the length of failure-free survival despite the higher frequency of risk factors such as higher tumor stage or advanced age. According to Keegan et al., [186] EBV in HL cells has been considered a prognostic marker for this heterogeneous disease, but studies have yielded mixed findings, likely because of selected patients series and failure to acknowledge the effect of age. In a study by these authors, [186] EBV presence in children less than 15 years old was suggestively associated with favorable survival (p=0.07); in adults aged 15 to 44 years, EBV did not affect HL outcome, although a protective effect was suggested; in older adults (45 to 96 years), EBV presence nearly doubled the risk of overall and HL-specific mortality but only with nodular sclerosis subtype. Thus, EBV tumor presence is associated with better survival in young patients in HL and poorer survival in older patients with NS HL.

Table 4. Epstein-Barr virus (EBV) studies in Hodgkin's disease/lymphoma as per Rye and WHO classification [74, 78-83, 85-87, 115, 139, 143, 144]

Author and year	Country	No of cases studied		+vity in %	EBV +vity in subtypes of HL in percentages					
		Ove-rall	LMP1(L) /EBER (E)		NLP	LP/ LR*	NS	MC	LD	UC
Chang et al., 1993 [74]	Peru		LMP: 25	78.1		0	77.3	90.0	25.0	-
			EBER: 30	93.8		100	100	100	50.0	-
Peh et al., 1997 [78]	Malaysia	81		50.6		0	22.2	86.4	50.0	100
Monterosso et al., 1998 [80]	Costa Rica		LMP: 40	40.0		0	15.0	85.7	100	-
Liu et al., 1998 [79]	Taiwan	70		62.9		16.7	63.9	69.2	100	-
Mourad et al., 1998 [81]	Saudi Arabia	62		46.8		0	46.7	88.9	-	
Enblad et al., 1999 [82]	Sweden	117		27.4		20.	23.0	38.1	100	0
Macák et al., 2000 [83]	Czech Republic	142		33.1		38.5	25.0	38.7	66.7	-
De Oliveira et al., 2002 [85]	Brazil	96		63.5		0	29.6	83.9	25.0	100
Krugmann et al., 2003 [86]	Austria		LMP: 119	26.1		0	21.4	38.5	33.3	-
			EBER: 107	29.0		0	23.4	44.1	33.3	-
Almasri and Khalidi, 2004 [87]	Jordan	64		46.9		0	28.6	64.7	-	-
Keresztes et al., 2006 [143]	Hungary	109		43.1		-	34.8	49.3	-	-
Makar et al., 2003 [139]	Kuwait	107*		56.1	2	50.0	34.2	79.2	100	33.3
Al-Salam et al., 2008 [144]	UAE	45*		37.8	0	100	27.3	52.9	50.0	-
Chang et al., 2009 [115]	Taiwan	34*	LMP: 13	38.2						
			EBER: 18	52.9	0	25.0	47.8	100	-	100

* These studies were based on WHO classification and LP subtype of Rye classification was replaced with lymphocyte-rich (LR) subtype and nodular lymphocyte predominant (NLP) HL was a separate entity from CHL.

Significance of Microenvironment in HL

In a study by Von Wasielewski et al., [187] prominent eosinophilia was detected 38% of HL cases overall, which differed among histologic subtypes: LP (0%), LRCHL (14%), NS1CHL (40%), NS2CHL (55%), MCCHL (43%) and LDCHL (54%). In a multivariate analysis, tissue eosinophilia proved to be the strongest prognostic factor (indicating poor prognosis) for freedom of treatment failure (P<0.001) and overall survival (P<0.001), and this effect was most significant among NSCHL, especially NS1CHL cases, however, in MCCHL no significant effect of eosinophilia on survival could be demonstrated. [187] Eosinophils secrete CD30 ligand that is capable of binding to CD30 positive HRS cells, which in turn leads to activation of TRAF2, followed by NF-κB and thereby neoplastic proliferation and apoptosis protection of HRS cells. With the possibility that eosinophils are only passive indicators of unknown prognostic determinants, it may be concluded that the positive clinical outcome of eosinophilia-negative NSCHL cases could be due to lower NF-κB activity. Applying a cutoff score of >0.82% CD68+ tumor macrophages, Tzankov et al. [147] observed worse overall survival in increased number of CHL cases (mean 185 months, median 192 months) compared to cases with lower number (mean 285 months, median not reached); eleven of 62 CHL patients with ≤0.82% tumor macrophages died, compared to 19 of 43 with >0.82% (p<0.001). Expression of markers for various tumor associated macrophages (TAMs), viz., CD68, HLA-DR, CD163, HLA-DR/CD68 (M1) and CD163/CD68 (M2) were immunohistochemically studied by Zaki et al. [188] in classical HL. Number of CD163+ cells and M2+ cells was significantly correlated with shorter overall survival (p<0.05), while it was marginally significant for CD68+ cells (p=0.0827). While confined to MC subtype, number of M1+ cells correlated with favorable prognosis (p<0.05), while M2 did not (p=0.7). At multivariate analysis, number of CD63+ cells, M2+ cells, and age were independent factors for poor overall survival (p=0.03, =0.02, and =0.01, respectively). Thus, CD163+ cells and M2+ cells might work as tumor promoter cells in CHL and M1+ cells might be tumor suppressive in MC subtype. Sohani et al. [148] observed 11 NLPHL in which, in addition to typical B-cell-rich nodules containing LP cells (areas of NLPHL) there were areas of atypical T-cells. 9 of these contained sheets of atypical T-cells surrounding primary and secondary follicles in a pattern mimicking the T-zone lymphoma of PTCL-NOS; the remaining 2 cases contained atypical T-cells presented as large clusters at the periphery of B-cell-rich nodules. The atypical T-cells showed no pan-T-cell antigen loss or aberrant T-cell antigen expression in any case, and PCR or Southern blot analysis showed no evidence of T-cell clonality in 6 cases tested. In comparision with control patients, NLPHL patients with atypical T-cells were more likely to develop recurrent NLPHL (71.4% vs. 13.6%, p=0.008) and to have a shorter time to relapse (p=0.04).

In CHL, together with genetic lesions affecting the neoplastic population, the malignant component is tightly regulated by interactions with the microenvironment. [156] Of particular interest is the presence of biased T-cell populations in HL cases, evidence for a dis-regulation of T cell immune function. In this sense, a considerable fraction of infiltrating CD4+ T cells are regulatory (Treg) cells which have been shown to display immunosuppressive activity on HL Th2 cells. The monocyte/macrophages prove to be a major determinant of prognostic outcome, the higher the content of CD68+ macrophages in diagnostic biopsy samples, the greater the risk of progression after primary treatment and relapse, following autologous stem cell transplantation. On the other hand, patients with limited-stage disease and without elevated numbers of CD68+ cell have a long-term disease-free survival of 100% using current treatment strategies.

Despite significant advances in the treatment of HL, considerable long term toxicity of conventional therapies requires the development of new non-genotoxic therapeutic strategies. The insight into the molecular pathogenesis of HL is likely to help in development of these new strategies. [189]

Pathogenesis of Hodgkin's Lymphoma

Whereas Kaplan and Smithers [131] hypothesized that Hodgkin disease might represent an autoimmune process, DeVita [190] called it a lymphocyte civil war. Kay, [191] in a scanning electron microscopic study of Hodgkin's tissue, found that T-cells cause cytolysis of R-S cells in a definite sequential manner and defined the pathogenesis of Hodgkin's disease on the basis of "a war between T-lymphocytes and transformed macrophages". According to him, [191] the various histopathological subtypes of HD and their prognosis depend upon the relative strength of both the forces, i.e., T-lymphocytes versus HR-S cells, and the outcome of the war, respectively. The R-S cell/lymphocyte interaction was further defined by Payne et al., [97, 192] who observed an antigen dependent lymphocyte/ macrophage contact and proposed the involvement of a unique receptor system for this interaction.

The pathogenesis of HL is still largely unresolved, but only over the last 15 years significant advances regarding its molecular pathogenesis has been achieved; [189] the reason behind this delay being the lack of a specific lineage profile in combination with the low number of malignant mononuclear Hodgkin- and multinucleated Reed-Stenberg-(HRS-) cells in the affected lymph nodes that prevented for a long time both the identification of its cell of origin and of genomic and molecular defects. The HRS cells harbor genetic lesions that contribute to or cause increase in the activity of transcription factors of the NF-kappaB and STAT families. [122] This aberrant activation of several signaling pathways (such as the NFkappaB pathway) is of key importance for HRS cell survival [121] because they protect HRS cells from apoptotic cell death. [189, 193] According to Schmitz et al., [122] HRS cells are found within a mixed reactive cellular infiltrate and interact with these non-malignant cells in a complex fashion that appears to be essential for HRS cell survival and proliferation; less is known about the pathogenesis of L&H cells in NLPHL, but an increase in the activity of receptor tyrosine kinase, NF-kappaB, and JAK/STAT has also been detected. NF-kappaB triggers proliferation and provides a molecular basis of cells' aberrant growth and cytokine gene expression. In HL pathogenesis associated with Epstein-Barr virus (EBV) infection, the activation of NF-kappaB is induced by viral latent protein 1 (LMP1); CD99 is down-regulated by LMP1 through NK-kappaB signaling pathway, which leads to the generation of cells with H-RS phenotypes related to the clinical and histologic characteristics of HL. [193]A biological link between 2 characteristic features of H-RS cells: CD30 overexpression and constitutive NF-kappaB activation has been observed; ligand-independent signaling by over expressed CD30 was shown to be a common mechanism that induced constitutive NF-kappaB activation in these cells, which suggest the self-growth-promoting potential of H-RS cells and redefine the biology of HL composed of H-RS cells and lymphocytes. [194]

With the above mentioned background information the molecular pathogenesis of Hodgkin's lymphoma can be explained as follows: There is compelling evidence that HRS cells are clonal B-cells that have lost their B-cell phenotype. [12] In other words, with the description of clonally rearranged immunoglobulin (Ig) genes with a high frequency of somatic mutations it has become clear that HRS cells are in most cases derived from germinal center (GC) or post GC B-cells, and despite their B-cell origin, HRS cells have, in most cases, lost the B-cell-specific gene expression program. [123] According to Yurchenko and Sidarenko, [195] due to reprogramming of gene expression, these lymphoma cells have lost the expression of most B-cell specific genes and acquired expression of multiple genes that are typical for other hematopoietic cells. According to Janz and Mathas, [123] the genomic alterations in HRS cells include activation of the transcription factor kappa B (NF-κB), activator protein 1 (AP-1), members of the STAT signaling pathway and deregulated NOTCH1 signaling; the NF-κB and AP1 transcription factors are thought to synergistically regulate not only genes involved in apoptosis protection and proliferation but also the abundant number of cytokines and chemokines produced by HRS cells. Furthermore, the AP1 and NOTCH1 signaling pathways have been shown to be involved in the loss of B-cell phenotype, characteristic of the HRS cells. Normally mature GC B-cells lacking functional B-cell receptors (BCR) complex would die by apoptosis, and therefore, the survival of HRS cells in the face of apoptotic triggers is considered central to CHL oncogenesis. The escape from apoptosis and transcriptional reprogramming of HRS cells are interlinked and appear central to the pathogenesis of Hodgkin lymphoma [12]: Epstein-Barr virus (EBV) is present in the HRS cells of a proportion of cases and express genes with plausible oncogenic function. It is likely that EBV plays a role in reprogramming and survival through dysregulation of several signaling networks and transcription factors, including nuclear factor (NF)-κB. Activation of NF-κB is a feature of all HRS cells and mutations affecting this pathway appear common in EBV-negative HL. The HRS cell furthers its own survival by attracting a supportive microenvironment of immune and stromal cells, and suppressing local immune responsiveness. The stromal background of HL include non-malignant T and B lymphocytes, plasma cells, histiocytes/macrophages, granulocytes, eosinophils, mast cells, interdigitating reticulum cells and fibroblast cells in collagen bands. [196] HRS cells can express and secrete a variety of cytokines, including IL-1, IL-2—IL-10, IL-13, IL-15, IL-21, ganulocyte-macrophage-colony-stimulating factor (GMCF), lymphotoxin-alpha (LF-α), transforming growth factor–beta (TGFβ), members of CCsubfamily of chemokines: CC chemokine ligand 5 (CCL5/RANTES), CCL17/TARC, CCL20, CCL22: and also a number of tumor necrosis factor (TNF) family cytokines (TNFα, BAFF, APRIL, RANKL, NGF). [196, 197] According to their functional role, cytokine in HL may be grouped in (1) attracting cells into microenvironment, (2) suppressing immune cells and (3) autocrine and/or paracrine regulators of HRS survival.

References

[1] Gruss HJ, Kadin ME. Pathophysiology of Hodgkin's disease: functional and molecular aspects. *Baillieres Clin Hematol* 1996; 9: 417-446.

[2] Hodgkin T. On some morbid appearances of the absorbent glands and spleen. *Med Chir Trans* 1832; 17:69-97.
[3] Wilks S. Cases of enlargement of the lymphatic glands and spleen (or Hodgkin's disease), with remarks. *Guy's Hosp Rep* 1865; 11:56-67.
[4] Sternberg C. Uber eine eigenartige unter dem Bilde der Pseudoleukamic verlaufende Tuberculose des lymphatischen Apparates. *Ztschr Heilk* 1898; 19:21-30.
[5] Reed DM. On the pathological changes in Hodgkin's disease, with special reference to its relation to tuberculosis. *Johns Hopkins Hospital Reports.* 1902; 10:133-136.
[6] Olu-Eddo AN, Omoti CE. Hodgkin lymphoma: Clinicopathologic features in Benin City, Nigeria and update on its biology and classification. *Nigerian J Clin Pract* 2011; 14:440-444.
[7] Cozen W, Katz J, Mack TM. Risk patterns of Hodgkin's disease in Los Angeles vary by cell type. *Cancer Epidemiol Biomarkers Prev* 1992; 1:261-268.
[8] Foss HD, Marafioti T, Stein H. Hodgkin lymphoma. Classification and pathogenesis. *Pathologe* 2000; 21: 113-123.
[9] Jaffe ES, Harris NL, Stein H, Vardiman JW, editors. World Health Organization classification of tumors. *Pathology and genetics of tumors of hematopoietic and lymphoid tissues.* Lyon: IARC Press; 2001.
[10] Lukes RJ, Craver LF, Hall TC, Rappaport H, Ruben P. Report of the nomenclature committee. *Cancer Res* 1966; 26:1311.
[11] Hartge P, Devesa SS, Fraumeni JF Jr. Hodgkin's and non-Hodgkin's lymphomas. *Cancer Surv* 1994; 19-20:423-453.
[12] Farrell K, Jarrett RF. The molecular pathogenesis of Hodgkin lymphoma. *Histopathology* 2011; 58:15-25.
[13] Landgren O, Caporaso NE. New aspects in descriptive, etiologic, and molecular epidemiology of Hodgkin's lymphoma. *Hematol Oncol Clin North Am.* 2007;21:825-840.
[14] Morton LM, Wang SS, Devesa SS, Hartge P, Weisenburger DD, Linet MS. Lymphoma incidence patterns by WHO subtype in the United States, 1992-2001. *Blood* 2006; 107:265-276.
[15] Eichenauer DA, Engert A, Dreyling M. Hodgkin's lymphoma: ESMO Clinical Practice Guidelines for diagnosis, treatment and follow-up. *Ann Oncol* 2011; 22 (S): vi55-58.
[16] Wu S-J, Chen C-Y, Su I-J, Tang J-L, Ko B-S, Huang S-Y, Yao M, Tsay W, Chen C-H, Tien H-F. Cliical characteristics and treatment response of Hodgkin's lymphoma in Taiwan. *J Formos Med Assos* 2008; 107: 4-12.
[17] Bastien H, Teisseyre A, Dusserre P, Michiels R, Cayot F, Lamy M, Cabanne F. Malignant lymphomas in Burgundy, France (1976--1977): a new approach using computerized pathological diagnoses. *Bull Cancer* 1979; 66:287-292.
[18] Radaszkiewicz T. Malignant and benign lymphomas: histologic classification and immunomorphologic studies. Results of 838 cases. *Wien Klin Wochenschr* 1980; 92:819-833.
[19] Kelényi G, Várbiró M. Malignant lymphoma reference centre—Hungary, 1978. *Virchows Arch A Pathol Anat Histol* 1980; 388:213-219.
[20] Shimizu M, Miura M, Kitahara M, Katayama I. Non-Hodgkin's lymphomas. Analysis of 109 Japanese cases with the use of LSGJ classification. *Am J Pathol* 1982; 106:30-39.

[21] Ho FC, Todd D, Loke SL, Ng RP, Khoo RK. Clinico-pathological features of malignant lymphomas in 294 Hong Kong Chinese patients, retrospective study covering eight-year period. *Int J Cancer* 1984; 34:143-148.

[22] Su IJ, Shih LY, Kadin ME, Dun P, Hsu SM. Pathologic and immunologic characterization of malignant lymphoma in Taiwan. With special reference to retrovirus-associated adult T-cell lymphoma/leukemia. *Am J Clin Pathol* 1985; 84:715-723.

[23] Calderon B, Villalon A, Augustion B, Jaier B, Zamuco J, Mori S Malignant lymphoma in Manila—a clinicopathologic study at the University of Philippines-Philippines General Hospital Medical Center. *Jpn J Clin Oncol* 1986; 16:21-27.

[24] Burla M, Egli F, Rhyner K. malignant lymphoma: a study of an outpatient cohort. *Schweiz Rundsch Med Prax* 1990; 79:101-110.

[25] Okpala IE, Akang EE, Okpala UJ. Lymphomas in University College Hospital, Ibadan, Nigeria. *Cancer* 1991; 68:1356-1360.

[26] Walter PR, Koltz F, Alfy-Gattas T, Minko-Mi-Etoua D, Nguembi-Mbina C. Malignant lymphomas in Gabon (equatorial Africa): a morphologic study of 72 cases. *Hum Pathol* 1991; 22:1040-1043.

[27] Ramani A, Kumar KA, Rao KK, Vidyasagar MS, Kundaje GN. Clinico-pathological profile of lymphomas in south India: a prospective rural hospital study of 103 cases. *J Assos Physicians India.* 1991; 39:322-325.

[28] Obafunwa JO, Akinsete I. Malignant lymphomas in Jos, Nigeria: a ten-year study. *Cent Afr J Med* 1992; 38:17-25.

[29] Ngendahayo P, Schmauz R. Pattern of malignant lymphoma in Rwanda. Bull Cancer 1992; 79:1087-1096.

[30] Ji X, Li W. Malignant lymphoma in Beijing. *J Environ Pathol Toxicol Oncol* 1992; 11:327-329.

[31] Yang K. A histopathologic and immunopathologic sudy of 209 malignant lymphoma cases from four regions of China: Suzhou, Nanjing, Qindao and Shenyang. *Zhonghua Zhong Liu Za Zhi* 1993; 15:86-90.

[32] Dasgupta A, Mukherjee C, Ghosh RN, Sengupta J. Malignant lymphoma—a 15-year study report. *J Indian Med Assos* 1993; 91:35-37.

[33] Cool CD, Bitter MA. The malignant lymphomas of Kenya: morphology, immunophenotype, and frequency of Epstein-Barr virus in 73 cases. *Hum Pathol* 1997; 28:1026-1033.

[34] Chai SP, Peh SC, Kim LH, Lim LY, Gudum HR. The pattern of lymphoma in east Malaysian patients as experienced in the University Hospital, Kuala Lumpur. *Malays J Pathol* 1999; 21:45-50.

[35] Chuang SS, Lin CN, Li C. Malignant lymphoma in southern Taiwan according to the revised European-American classification of lymphoid neoplasms. *Cancer* 2000; 89:1586-1592.

[36] Castella A, Joshi S, Raaschou T, Mason N. Pattern of malignant lymphoma in the United Arab Emirates—a histopathologic and immunologic study in 208 native patients. *Acta Oncol* 2001; 40:660-664.

[37] Getachew A. Malignant lymphoma in western Ethiopia. *East Afr Med J.* 2001; 78:402-404.

[38] Naresh KN, Agarwal B, Sangal BC, Basu DD, Kothari AS, Soman CS. Regional variation in the distribution of subtypes of lymphoid neoplasms in India. *Leuk Lymphoma.* 2002; 43:1939-1943.

[39] He S, Zhang JB, Zhang JG, Yang SY, Han F. The WHO (1997) classification of 370 cases of malignant lymphomas. *Zhonghua Xue Ye Xue Za Zhi* 2003; 24:519-522.

[40] Sukpanichnant S. Analysis of 1983 cases of malignant lymphoma in Thailand according to the World Health Organization classification. *Hum Pathol* 2004; 35:224-230.

[41] Haddadin WJ. Malignant lymphoma in Jordan: a retrospective analysis of 347 cases according to World Health Organization classification. *Ann Saudi Med* 2005; 25:398-403.

[42] Shivarov V, Dimitrov J, Guenova M. Lymphoid neoplasms in Bulgaria according to the WHO classification (2001). The experience of the National Center of Haematology. *Hematol J* 2005; 90:74-75.

[43] Wang JF, Wang YZ, Chen ZW, Taylor RC. Prevalence of lymphoma subtypes in Shaxi according to latest WHO classification. *Zhonghua Bing Li Xue Za Zhi* 2006; 35:218-223.

[44] Hashemi-Bahremani M, Parwaresch M-R, Tabrizchi H, Gupta RK, Raffii MR. Lymphomas in Iran. *Arch Iranian Med* 2007; 10:343-348.

[45] Jeong SY, Chang YH, Lee JK, Hong J, Hong SI, Lee SS. Incidence and histologic patterns of bone marrow involvement of malignant lymphoma based on the World Health Organization classification: a single institution study. *Korean J Lab Med* 2007; 27:383-387.

[46] Akhtar SS, Haque IU, Wafa SM, El-Saka H, Saroor AM, Nadrah HM. Malignant lymphoma in Al-Qassim, Saudi Arabia, reclassified according to the WHO classification. *Saudi Med* J 2009; 30:677-681.

[47] Yoon SO, Suh C, Lee DH, Chi H-S, Park CJ, Jang S-S, Shin H-R, Park B-H, Huh J. Distribution of lymphoid neoplasms in the Republic of Korea: Analysis of 5318 cases according to the World Health Organiztion classification. *Am J Hematol* 2010; 85:760-764.

[48] Mwakigonja AR, Kaaya EE, Heiden T, Wannhoff G, Castro J, PK F, Porwit A, Biberfed P. Tanzanian malignant lymphomas: WHO classification, presentation, ploidy, proliferation and HIV/EBV. *BMC Cancer* 2010; 10:344.

[49] Chen W-L, Tsai W-C, Chao T-Y, Sheu L-F, Chou J-M, Kao W-Y, Chen Y-C, Ho C-L. The clinicopathological analysis of 303 cases with malignant lymphoma classified according to the World Health Organization classification system in a single institute of Taiwan. *Ann Hematol* 2010; 89:553-562.

[50] Chakrabarti S, Sarkar S, Goswami BK, Mondal S, Roy A, Das S. Hodgkin's and non-Hodgkin's lymphoma in an rural medical institution: Comparative clinicopathologic analysis. *Asian Pac J Cancer Prev* 2010; 11:1605-1608.

[51] Jayasekara H, Karahalios A, Juneja S, Thursfield V, Farrugia H, English DR, Giles GG. Incidence and survival of lymphohematopoietic neoplasms according to the World Health Organization classification: a population-based study from the Victorian Cancer Registry in Australia. *Leuk Lymphoma* 2010; 51:456-468.

[52] Yago RT, Hughson MD, Sulayvani FK, Al-Allawi NA. Malignant lymphoma in northern Iraq: A retrospective analysis of 270 cases according to the World Health Organization classification. *Indian J Cancer* 2011; 48:446-451.

[53] Yang Q-P, Zhang W-Y, Yu J-B, Zhao S, Xu H, Wang W-Y, Bi C-F, Zou Z, Wang X-Q, Huang J, Dai L, Liu W-P. Subtype distribution of lymphomas in Southwest China: Analysis of 6,382 cases using WHO classification in a single institution. *Diagn Pathol* 2011; 6:77.

[54] Matteo E, Barón AV, Chabay P, Porta J, Dragosky M, Preciado MV. Comparision of Epstein-Barr virus presence in Hodgkin lymphoma in Pediatric versus adult Argentine patients. *Arch Pathol Lab Med* 2003; 127:1325-1329.

[55] Jackson Jr H, Parker Jr F. Hodgkin's disease. *II Pathology New Eng J Med* 1944; 231:35-44.

[56] Lukes RJ, Butler JJ. The pathology and nomenclature of Hodgkin's disease. *Cancer Res* 1966; 26:1063-1083.

[57] Harris NL, Jaffe ES, Stein H, Banks PM, Chan JK, Cleary ML, Delsol G, De Wolf-Peeters C, Falini B, Gatter KC, et al. A revised European-American classification of lymphoid neoplasms: a proposal from the international lymphoma study group. *Blood* 1994; 84:1361-1392.

[58] Swerdlow SH, Campo E, Harris NL, Jaffe ES, Pileri S, Stein H, Thiele J, Vardiman JW. *WHO Classification of Tumours of the Haematopoietic and Lymphoid Tissues.* Lyon, France: IARC Press; 2008 : 312-316.

[59] Das DK, Gupta SK, Datta BN, Sharma SC. Fine needle aspiration cytodiagnosis of Hodgkin's disease and its subtypes. I: Scope and limitations. *Acta Cytol* 1990; 34:329-336.

[60] Das DK, Gupta SK. Fine needle aspiration cytodiagnosis of Hodgkin's disease and its subtypes. II: Subtyping by differential cell counts. *Acta Cytol* 1990; 34:337-341.

[61] Fuggle WJ, Crocker J, Smith PJ. A quantitative study of eosinophil polymorphs in Hodgkin's disease. *J Clin Pathol* 1984; 37:267-271.

[62] Crocker J, Jones EL, Curran RC. A quantitative study of α-naphthyl acetate esterase-positive cells in Hodgkin's disease. *J Clin Pathol* 1982; 35:1301-1306.

[63] Kadin ME, Gladstein E, Dorfman RF. Clinicopathologic studies in 117 untreated patients subjected to laparotomy for staging of Hodgkin's disease. *Cancer* 1971; 27:1277-1294.

[64] Gough J. Hodgkin's disease. A correlation of histopathology with survival. *Int J Cancer* 1970; 5:273-281.

[65] Farrer-Brown G, Bennet MHarrison CV, Millet Y, Jellife AM. The pathological findings following laparotomy in Hodgkin's disease. *Br J Cancer* 1971; 25:449-457.

[66] Wright DH. Lymphoreticular neoplasms: In *Tumors of a tropical country. A survey of Uganda* (1964-68). AC Templeton Ed. RRCR 1973; 41:270.

[67] Mehrotra RML, Wahal KM, Kushwaha MRS, Bagchi M, SarkarB. Hodgkin's disease: A clinicopathological study of 300 cases. *Indian J Cancer* 1977; 14:249-255.

[68] Das DK. *Cytomorphological, cytochemical and immunological characterization of lymphomas.* Doctoral thesis. Postgraduate Institute of Medical Education and Research, Chandigarh, India. 1983.

[69] Petrella T, Michiels JF, Michiels R, Collin F, Nabholtz JM, Friedman S, Fargeot P. CD15 antigen in Hodgkin's disease. *Pathol Res Pract* 1989; 185:886-890.

[70] Liang R, Choi P, Todd D, Chan TK, Choy D, Ho F. Hodgkin's disease in Hong Kong Chinese. *Hematol Oncol* 1989; 7:395-403.
[71] Soriano Rosas J, Lazos Ochao M, Rojo Medina J, Manrique JJ, Herrera Verdugo D. Hodgkin's disease in the Hospital General de México, Study of 309 cases. *Sangre (Barc)* 1990; 35:447-450.
[72] Carde P. Hodgkin's disease-I: identification and classification. *Br Med J* 1992; 305:99-102.
[73] Bernhards J, Fischer R, Hübner K, Schwarze EW Georgil A. Histological classification of Hodgkin's lymphoma. Results from the reference pathology of the German Hodgkin Trial. *Ann Oncol* 1992; S4:31-33.
[74] Chang KL, Albújar PF, Chen Y-Y, Johnson RM, Weiss LM. High prevalence of Ebstein-barr virus in the Reed-Sternberg cells of Hodgkin's disease occurring in Peru. *Blood* 1993; 81:496-501.
[75] Medeiros LJ, Greiner TC. Hodgkin's disease. *Cancer* 1995; 75:357-369.
[76] Rana R, Chopra R, Masih K, Zachariah A, Prabhakar BR, Mahajan MK. Hodgkin's disease: a clinicopathologic study. *Indian J Pathol Microbiol* 1995; 38:245-249.
[77] De Souza CA, Vassallo J, Lorand-Metze I. Hogkin's disease in Brazil: a clinicopathologic study. *Haematologica* 1997; 82:127-128.
[78] Peh SC, Looi LM, Pallesen G. Epstein-Barr virus (EBV) and Hodgkin's disease in a multi-ethnic population in Malaysia. *Histopathology* 1997; 30:227-233.
[79] Liu SM, Chow KC, Chiu CF, Tzeng CH. Expression of Epstein-Barr virus in patients with Hodgkin's disease in Taiwan. *Cancer* 1998; 83:367-371.
[80] Monterroso V, Zhou Y, Koo S, Glackin C, Bujan W, Medeiros LJ. Hodgkin's disease in Costa Rica: a report of 40 cases analyzed for Epstein-Barr virus. *Am J Clin Pathol* 1998; 109:618-624.
[81] Mourad W, Alsohaibani MO, Saddik M, Bazerbashi S. Epstein-Barr virus expression in Hodgkin's disease: Correlation with histologic subtypes and T and B lymphocyte distribution. *Ann Saudi Med* 1998; 18:296-300.
[82] Enblad G, Sandvej K, Sundström C, Pallesen G, Glimelius B. Epstein-Barr virus distribution in Hodgkin's disease in an unselected Swedish population. *Acta Oncol* 1999; 38:425-429.
[83] Macák J, Habanec B, Fabián P. Detection of Epstein-Barr virus in Hodgkin's lymphoma (patients in the Czech Republic). *Neoplasma* 2000; 47:156-161.
[84] Glavina-Durdov M, Jakic-Razumovic J, Capkun V, Murray P. Epstein–Barr virus encoded latent membrane protein-1expression in Hodgkin's disease. *British Journal of Cancer,* 2001; 84:1227–1234.
[85] De Oliveira DE, Bacchi MM, Abreu ES, Niero-Melo L, Bacchi CE. Hodgkin disease in adult and juvenile groups from two different geographic regions in Brazil. *Am J Clin Pathol* 2002; 118:25-30.
[86] Krugmann J, Tzankov A, Gschwendtner A, Fischhofer M, Greil R, Fend F, Dirnhofer S. Longer failure-free survival interval of Epstein-Barr virus-associated classical Hodgkin's lymphoma: a single-institution study. *Mod Pathol* 2003; 16: 566-573.
[87] Almasri NM, Khalidi HS. Epstein-Barr virus expression in Hodgkin's disease in Jordan. *Saudi Med* J 2004; 25:770-775.

[88] Vassalo J, Pinto Paes F, Augusto Soares F, Menezes Y, Aldred V, de Cássia Braga Ribeiro K, Correa Alves A. Histological classification of 1,025 cases of Hodgkin's lymphoma from the state of São Paulo, Brazil. *Sao Paulo Med J* 2005; 123:134-136.

[89] Steidl C, Connors JM, Gascoyne RD. Molecular pathogenesis of Hodgkin's lymphoma: increasing evidence of the importance of the microenvironment. *J Clin Oncol* 2011; 29:1812-1826.

[90] Hoffman GT, Rottino A. Phase microscopy studies of Hodgkins disease lymph nodes in relation to histogenesis of Sternberg-Reed cell. *Blood* 1950; 5: 74-78.

[91] Seif GSF, Spriggs AI. Chromosome changes in Hodgkin's disease. *J Natl Cancer Inst.* 1967; 39: 557-570.

[92] Rappaport H. *Tumors of the hematopoietic system. Atlas of tumor pathology.* Section III. Fascicle 8. Armed Forces Institute of Pathology, Washington DC, 1966.

[93] Dorfman RF. Enzyme histochemistry of cells in Hodgkin's disease and allied disordes. *Nature* 1961; 190: 925-926.

[94] Order S, Hellman S. Pathogenesis of Hodgkin's disease. *Lancet* 1972; I: 571-572.

[95] Biniaminov M, Ramos B. Possible T-lymphocyte origin of Reed-Sternberg cells. *Lancet* 1974; I; 368.

[96] Herva E, Ryhanen P, Banco G, Jarvenppa K, Helin H, Alavaiko M. Acid alpha-naphthyl aetate esterase (ANAE) activity and DNA synthesis of lymph node cells in Hodgkin's disease. *Scand J Haematol* 1979; 23: 277- 284.

[97] Payne SV, Jones DB, Wright DH. Reed-Sternberg cells/lymphocyte interaction. *Lancet* 1977; II: 768-769.

[98] Leech J. *Immunoglobulin positive Reed-Sternberg cells in Hodgkin's disease.* 1973; II: 265-266.

[99] Taylor CR. An immunohistological study of follicular lymphoma, reticulum cell sarcoma and Hodgkin's disease. *Eur J Cancer* 1976; 12: 61- 75.

[100] Berneau D, Fildmann G, Vorhauer W. Hodgkin's disease. Ultrastructural localisation of intracytoplasmic immunoglobulins within malignant cells. *Br J Haematol* 1978; 40: 51-57.

[101] Papadimitrou CS, Stein H, Lennert K. The complexity of immunohistochemical staining pattern of Hodgkin and Sternberg-Reed cells: demonstration of immunoglobulin, albumin, alpha 1-antichymotrypsin and lysozyme. *Int J Cancer* 1978; 21: 531-541.

[102] Kadin ME, Stites DP, Levy R, Warnke R. Exogeneous immunoglobulin and the macrophage origin of Reed-Sternberg cells in Hodgkin's disease. *N Engl J Med* 1978; 299: 1208-1214.

[103] Kaplan HS, Gartner S. "Sternberg Reed" giant cells of Hodgkin's disease. Cultivation in vitro, heterotransplantation and characterization as neoplastic macrophages. *Int J Cancer* 1977; 19: 511-525.

[104] Long JC, Zamecnik PC, Aisenberg AC, Atkins L. Tissue culture studies in Hodgkin's disease. *J Exp Med* 1977; 145: 1484-1500.

[105] Kaplan HS. Hodgkin's disease: Unfolding concepts concerning its nature, management and prognosis. 1980; 45: 2439-2474.

[106] Poppema S, Elema JD, Haile MR. The significance of intracytoplasmic proteins in Reed-Sternberg cells. *Cancer* 1978; 42: 1973-1803.

[107] Maksem JA, Hassan MO, Carter JR. The ultrastrutural heterogeneity of the Reed-Sternberg cell and its resemblance to monocyte-macrophage differentiation in vivo. *Ultrastruct Pathol* 1983; 4:379-389.

[108] Diehl V, Burrichter H, Schaadt M, Kirchnner HH, Fonatsch C, Stein H, Gerdes J, Heit W, Ziegler A. Hodgkin's cell lines: characteristics and possible pathogenetic implications. *Hematol Oncol* 1983; 1:139-147.

[109] Drexler HG, Gignac SM, Hoffbrand AV, Minowada J. Formation of multinucleated cells in a Hodgkin's-disease-derived cell line. *Int J Cancer* 1989; 43:1983-1090.

[110] Marafioti T, Hummel M, Foss HD, Laumen H, Korbjuhn P, Anagnostopoulos I, Lammert H, Demel G, Theil J, Wirth T, Stein H. Hodgkin and Reed-Sternberg cells represent an expansion of a single clone originating from a germinal center B-cell with functional immunoglobulin gene rearrangements but defective immunoglobulin gene transcription. *Blood* 2000; 95: 1443-1450.

[111] Drexler HG. Recent results on the biology of Hodgkin and Reed-Sternberg cells. I. Biopsy material. *Leuk Lymphoma* 1992; 8: 283-313.

[112] Wachi E, Nakamura N, Abe M, Wasaka H. Hodgkin's disease with CD20 (B1) positive Reed-Sternberg cells—an immunohistochemical and immunoelectron microscopic study. *Fukushima J Med Sci* 1989; 35:69-77.

[113] Schmid C, Pan L, Diss T, Isaacson PG. Expression of B-cell antigens by Hodgkin's and Reed-Sternberg cells. *Am J Pathol* 1991; 139:701-707.

[114] Zukerberg LR, Collins AB, Ferry JA, Harris NL. Coexpression of 223. CD15 and CD20 by Reed-Sternberg cells in Hodgkin's disease. *Am J Pathol* 1991; 139: 475-483.

[115] Chang KC, Chang Y, Jones D, Su IJ. Aberrant expression of cyclin A correlates with morphogenesis of Reed-Sternberg cells in Hodgkin's lymphoma. *Am J Clin Pathol* 2009; 132: 50-59.

[116] Bai MC, Jiwa NM, Horstman A, Vos W, Kluin PH, Van der Valk P, Mulink H, Walboomers JM, Meijer CJ. Decreased expression of cellular markers in Epstein-Barr virus positive Hodgkin's disease. *J Pathol* 1994; 174: 49-55.

[117] Siebert JD, McClure SP, Banks PM, Gulley ML. Hodgkin's disease, mixed cellularity type, with B-cell immunophenotype. Report of a case and review of literature. *Arch Pathol Lab Med* 1995; 119: 474-479.

[118] Stein H, Hummel M. Cellular origin and clonality of classic Hodgkin's lymphoma: immunophenotypic and molecular studies. *Semin Hematol* 1999; 36: 233-241.

[119] Küppers R, Rajewsky K. The origin of Hodgkin and Reed/Sternberg cells in Hodgkin's disease. *Annu Rev Immunol* 1998; 16: 471-493.

[120] Küppers R. Identifying the precursors of Hodgkin and Reed-Sternberg cells in Hodgkin's disease: role of the germinal center B-cell lymphomagenesis. *J Acquir Immune Defic Syndr* 1999; 21 Suppl: S74-S79.

[121] Küppers R, Hansmann ML. The Hodgkin and Reed-Sternberg cell. *Int J Biochem Cell Biol* 2005; 37: 511-517.

[122] Schmitz R, Stanelle J, Hansmann ML, Küppers R. Pathogenesis of classical and lymphocyte-predominant Hodgkin lymphoma. *Annu Rev Pathol* 2009; 4: 151-174.

[123] Janz M, Mathas S. The pathogenesis of classical Hodgkin's lymphoma: What can we learn from analyses of genomic alterations in Hodgkin and Reed-Sternberg cells? *Hematologica* 2008; 93:1292-1295.

[124] Aisenberg AC, Wilkes BM. Lymph node T cells in Hodgkin's disease: analysis of suspensions with monoclonal antibody and resetting techniques. *Blood* 1982; 59:522-527.

[125] Facchetti F, De Wolf-Peeters C, van den Oord JJ, Desmet VJ. Plasmacytoid monocytes (so called plasmacytoid T cells) I Hodgkin's disease. *J Pathol* 1989; 158:57-65.

[126] Wise NB, Poston MA. Co-existence of brucella infection and Hodgkin's disease: clinical, bacteriologic and immunologic study. *JAMA* 1940; 155:1976-1984.

[127] Benda C. *Zur histology der pseudoleukamischen: Verhandl deut-pathology-Gessel.* 1904; 7:123-131.

[128] Warthin AS. Genetic neoplastic relationships of Hodgkin's disease, aleukemic and leukemic lymphoblastoma and mycosis fungoides. *Am Surg* 1931; 93:153-161.

[129] Gall EA, Mallory TB. Malignant lymphoma. A clinicopathologic survey of 618 cases. *Am J Pathol* 1942; 18:381-429.

[130] Chevalier P, Bernard J. *La Maladie de Hodgkin. Pans*, Messon.

[131] Kaplan HS, Smithers DW. Aut0immunity in man and homologous disease in mice in relation to the malignant lymphoma. *Lancet* 1959; 2:1-4.

[132] Peckham MJ. Quantitative cytology and cytochemistry of Hodgkin's tissue labelled in vivo with tritiated thymidine. *Br J Cancer* 1973; 28: 332-339.

[133] Schiffer LM. Proliferation of cells in Hodgkin's disease. *Natl Cancer Inst Monogr* 1973; 36: 191-194.

[134] Kadin ME, Ausberg AK. Long term cultures of Hodgkin's tissue: A morphologic and radioautographic study. *Lab Invest* 1973; 28:181-184.

[135] Whitelaw DM. Chromosome complement of lymph node cells in Hodgkin's disease. *Can Med Assos J.* 1969; 101: 74-81.

[136] Olinici CD. Cytogenetic observation in different cell lines in Hodgkin's disease. *Acta Cytol (Basel)* 1972; 48: 283-287.

[137] Harris NL, Jaffe ES, Diebold J, Flandrin G, Muller-Hermelink HK, Vardiman J. Lymmphoma classification—from controversy to consensus: The REA and WHO classification of lymphoid neoplasms. *Ann Oncol* 2000; 11 (Suppl 1):3-10.

[138] Lymphoma Study Group of Japanese Pathologists (No name listed). The World Health Organization classification of malignant lymphomas in Japan: Incidence of recently recognized entities. *Pathol Int* 2000; 50:696-702.

[139] Makar RR, Saji T, Junaid TA. Epsein-Barr virus expression in Hodgkin's lymphoma in Kuwait. *Pathol Oncol Res* 2003; 9:159-165.

[140] De Matteo E, Barón AV, Chabay P, Porta J, Dragosky M, Preciado MV. Comparision of Epstein-Barr virus presence in Hodgkin's lymphomain pediatric versus adult Argentine patients. *Arch Pathol Lab Med* 2003; 127:1325-1329.

[141] Zhang J-R, Raza AS, Greaves TS, Cobb CJ. Fine-needle aspiration diagnosis of Hodgkin lymphoma using current WHO classification-Re-evaluation of cases from 1999-2004 with new proposals. *Diagn Cytopathol* 2006; 34:397-402.

[142] Lee M-Y, Tan T-D, Feng A-C, Liu M-C. Clinicopathological analysis of 598 malignant lymphomas in Taiwan: Seven-year experience in a single institution. *A J Hematol* 2006; 81:568-575.

[143] Keresztes K, Miltenyi Z, Bessenyei B, Beck Z, Szollosi Z, Nemes Z, Olah E, Illes A. Association between the Epstein-Barr virus and Hodgkin's lymphoma in the North-

Eastern part of HungaryL Effects on therapy and survival. *Acta Haematol* 2006; 116:101-107.

[144] Al-Salam S, John A, Daoud S, Chong SM, Castella A. Expression of Epstein-Barr virus n Hodgkin's lymphoma in a population of United Arab Emirates nationals. *Leuk Lymphoma* 2008; 49:169-1777.

[145] Hundall SD, Betancourt E, Barnhart E, Patel J. Comparative flow immunophenotypic features of the inflammatory infiltrates of Hodgkin lymphoma and lymphoid hyperplasia. *Cytometry Part B* (Clin Cytometry) 2008; 74B:1-8.

[146] Fong D, Steurer M, Greil R, Gunsilius E, Spizzo G, Gastl G, Tzankov A. Hodgkin lymphoma in Tyrol--a population-based study. *Ann Hematol* 2009; 88:449-456.

[147] Tzankov A, Matter MS, Dirnhofer S. Refined prognostic role of CD68-positive tumor macrophages in the context of the cellular micromileu of classical Hodgkin lymphoma. *Pathobiology* 2010; 77:301-308.

[148] Sohani AR, Jaffe ES, Harris NL, Ferry JA, Pittaluga S, Hasserjian RP. Nodular lymphocyte predominant Hodgkin lymphoma with atypical T cells: a morphologic variant mimicking peripheral T-cell lymphoma. *Am J Surg Pathol* 2011; 35:1666-1678.

[149] Anagnostopoulos I, Hansmann ML, Franssila K, Harris M, harris NL, Jaffe ES, Han T, van Krieken JM, Poppema S, Marafioti T, Franklin J, Sextro M, Diehl V, Stein H. European Task Force on Lymphoma project on lymphocyte predominance Hodgkin disease: histological and immunohistological analysis of submitted cases reveals 2 types of Hodgkin disease with a nodular pattern and abundant lymphocytes. *Blood.* 2000; 96: 1889- 1899.

[150] Mani H, Jaffe ES. Hodgkin lymphoma: An update on it biology with newer insights into classification. *Clin Lymphoma Myeloma* 2009; 9:206-216.

[151] Slack GW, Ferry JA, Haserjian RP, Sohani AR, Longtine JA, Harris NL, Zukerberg LR. Lymphocyte depleted Hodgkin lymphoma: an evaluation with immunophenotyping and genetic analysis. *Leuk Lymphoma* 2009; 50:937-943.

[152] Pinkus GS, Said JW. Hodgkin's disease, lymphocyte predominance type, nodular—a distinct entity? Unique staining profile for L&H variants of Reed-Sternberg cells defined by monoclonal antibodies to leukocyte common antigen, granulocyte-specific antigen, and B-cell-specific antigen. *Am J Pathol* 1985; 118:1-6.

[153] Pinkus GS, Said JW. Hodgkin's disease, lymphocyte predominance type, nodular—further evidence for a B cell derivation. L&H variant of Reed-Sternberg cells express L26, a pan B cell marker. *Am J Pathol* 1988; 133:211-217.

[154] Poppema S. The nature of the lymphocytes surrounding Reed-Sternberg cells in nodular lymphocyte predominance and other types of Hodgkin's disease. *Am J Pathol.* 1989; 135: 351- 357.

[155] Kame OW, Gelb AB, Shibuya RB, Warnke RA. Leu 7 (CD57) reactivity distinguishes nodular lymphocyte predominance Hodgkin's disease from nodular sclerosing Hodgkin's disease, T cell-rich B cell lymphoma and follicular lymphoma. *Am. J. Pathol.* 1993.;142: 541-546.

[156] Montes-Moreno S. Hodgkin's lymphoma: A tumor recognized by its micro-environment. *Adv Hematol* 2011; doi:10.1155/2011/142395.

[157] Marafioti T, Hummel M, Anagnostopoulos I, Foss HD, Falini B, Delsol G, Isaacson PG, Pileri S, Stein H. Origin of nodular lymphocyte-predominant Hodgkin's disease

from a clonal expansion of highly mutated germinal-center B cells. *N Engl J Med.* 1997; 337:453-458.

[158] Braeuninger A, Küppers R, Strickler J, Wacker HH, Rajewsky K, Hansmann ML. Hodgkin and Reed-Sternberg cells in lymphocyte predominant Hodgkin disease represent clonal populations of germinal centre-derived tumor cells. *Proc Natl Acad Sci U S A* 1997; 94:9337-9342.

[159] Rüdiger T, Jaffe ES, Delsol G, de Wolf Peeters C, Gascovne ED, Georgii A, Harris NL, Kadin ME, ac Lennan KA, Poppema S, Stein H, Weiss LE, Müller-Hermelink HK. Workshop report on Hodgkin's lymphoma and related disease ('grey zone'lymphoma). *Ann Oncol* 1998; 9 (S):s31-s38.

[160] Das DK, Gupta SK, Pathak IC, Sharma SC, Datta BN. Burkitt-type lymphoma: diagnosis by fine needle aspiration cytology. Acta Cytol 1987; 31:1-7.

[161] Yazdi HM, Burns BF. Fine-needle aspiration biopsy of Ki-1-positive large-cell anaplastic lymphoma. *Acta Cytol* 1991; 35: 306- 310.

[162] Caraway NP. Strategies to diagnose lymphoproliferative disorders by fine-needle aspiration using ancillary studies. *Cancer (Cytopathol)* 2005; 105: 432- 442.

[163] Banks PM. The distinction of Hodgkin's disease from T-cell lymphoma. *Seminar Diagn Pathol.* 1992; 9: 279-283.

[164] Tani E, Jahansson B, Skoog L. T-cell-rich B-cell lymphoma: Fine-needle aspiration cytology and immunocytochemistry. *Diagn Cytopathol.* 1998; 18: 1-4.

[165] Frizzera G. The distinction of Hodgkin's disease from anaplastic large cell lymphoma. *Seminar Diagn Pathol* 1992; 9:291- 296.

[166] Woodruff RD. Reviewing histologic diagnosis of lymphoma: comparision of original and review diagnoses in 269 cases. *Arch Pathol Lab Med* 1981; 105:573-576.

[167] Liu Y, Zhuang H, Liao X, Luo D, Cai X. Immunophenotype and differential diagnosis of Hodgkin's lymphoma. *Zhonghua Xue Ye Xue Za Zhi* 2002; 23: 524-527.

[168] Harris NL. Hodgkin's disease: classification and differential diagnosis. *Mod Pathol* 1999; 12: 159-175.

[169] Elgin J, Phillips JG, Reddy VV, Gibbs PO, Listinsky CM. Hodgkin's and non-Hodgkin's lymphoma: spectrum of morphologic and immunophenotypic overlap. *Ann Diagn Pathol* 1999; 3: 263-275.

[170] Das DK, Francis IM, Sharma PN, Sathar SA, John B, George SS, Mallik MK, Sheikh ZA, Haji BE, Pathan SK, Madda JP, Mirza K, Ahmed MS, Junaid TA. Hodgkin's lymphoma: diagnostic difficulties in fine-needle aspiration cytology. *Diagn Cytopathol.* 2009; 37: 564-573.

[171] Franke S, Wlodarska I, Maes B, Vandenberghe P, Achten R, Hagemeijer A, De Wolf-Peeters C. Comparative genomic hybridization pattern distinguishes T-cell/histiocyte-rich B-cell lymphoma from nodular lymphocyte predominance Hodgkin's lymphoma. *Am J Pathol* 2002; 161:1861-1867.

[172] Mourad WA, Al Nazer M, Tulbah A. Cytomorphologic differentiation of Hodgkin's lymphoma and Ki-1+ anaplastic large cell lymphoma in fine needle aspirates. *Acta Cytol* 2003; 47: 744-748.

[173] Marafioti T, Mancini C, Ascani S, Sabattini E, Zinzani PL, Pozzobon M, Pulford K, Falini B, Jaffe ES, Müller-Hermelink HK, Mason DY, Pileri SA. Leukocyte-specific phosphoprotein-1 and PU.1: two useful markers for distinguishing T-cell-rich B-cell

lymphoma from lymphocyte predominant Hodgkin's disease. *Haematologica.* 2004; 89: 957- 964.

[174] Kusuda M, Toriyama K, Kamidigo NO, Itakura H. A comparision of epidemiologic, histologic, and virologic studies on Hodgkin's disease in Western Kenya and Nagasaki, Japan. *Am J Trop Med Hyg* 1998; 59:801-807.

[175] Jarrett RF. Viruses and Hodgkin's lymphoma. *Ann Oncol* 2002; 13:23-29.

[176] Jarrett RF. Hodgkin's disease. *Baillieres Clin Haematol* 1992; 5:57-79.

[177] Huang X, Nolte I, Gao Z, Vos H, Hepkema B, Poppema S, van den Berg A, Diepstra A. Epidemiology of classical Hodgkin lymphoma and its association with Epstein Barr virus in Nothern China. *PLOS One* 2011;6: e21152 [Epub].

[178] Weinreb M, Day PJ, Niggli F, Powell JE, Raafat F, Hesseling PB, Sceneider JW, Hartley PS, Tzortzatou-Stathopoulou F, Khalek ER, Mangoud A, El-Safi ER, Madanat F, Al Sheyyab M, Mpofu C, Revesz T, Rafii R, Tiedemann K, Waters KD, Barrantes JC, Nyongo A, Riyat MS, Mann JR. The role of Epstein-Barr virus in Hodgkin's disease from different geographical areas. *Arch Dis Child* 1996; 74:27-31.

[179] Benharroch D, Shemer-Avni Y, Myint YY, Levy A, Mejirovsky E, Suprun I, Shendler Y, Prinsloo I, Arad S, Rager-Zisman B, Sacks M, Gopas J. Measles virus: evidence of an association with Hodgkin's disease. *Br J Cancer* 2004; 91:572-579.

[180] Wiggill TM, Mantina H, Willem P, Perner Y, Stevens WS. Changing pattern of lymphoma subgroups at a tertiary academic complex in a high-prevalence HIV setting: a South African perspective. *Acquir Immune Defic Syndr* 2011; 56:460-466.

[181] Diehl V, Stein H, Hummel M, Zollinger R, Connors JM. Hodgkin's lymphoma: biology and treatment strategies for primary, refractory and relapsed cases. *Hematology Am Soc Hematol Educ Program* 2003; 225-247.

[182] Allemani C, Sant M, De Angelis R, Marcos-Gragera R, Coebergh JM, and the EUROCARE Working Group. Hodgkin's disease survival in Europe and the US: Prognostic significance of morphologic groups. *Cancer* 2006; 107:352-360.

[183] von Wasielewski R, Mengel M, Fischer R, Hansmann ML, Hübner F, Franklin J, Tesch H, Paulus U, Werener M, Diehl V, Geogii A. Classical Hodgkin's disease. Clinical impact of the immunophenotype. *Am J Pathol* 1997; 151: 1123-1130.

[184] Smolewski P, Niewiadomska H, Los E, Robak T. Spontaneous apoptosis of Reed-Sternberg and Hodgkin cells; clinical and pathological implications in patients with Hodgkin's disease. *Int J Oncol* 2000; 17: 603-609.

[185] Oudejans JJ, Jiwa NM, Meijer CJ. Epstein-Barr virus in Hodgkin's disease: more than just an innocent bystander. *J Pathol* 1997; 181: 353-356.

[186] Keegan TH, Glaser SL, Clarke CA, Gulley ML, Craig FE, Digiuseppe JA, Dorfman RF, Mann RB, Ambinder RF. Epstein-Barr virus as a marker of survival after Hodgkin's lymphoma: a population-based study. *J Clin Oncol* 2005; 23: 7604-7613.

[187] von Wasielewski R, Seth S, Franklin J, Fischer R, Hübner K, Hansmann ML, Diehl V, Georgii A. Tissue eosinophilia correlates strongly with poor prognosis in nodular sclerosing Hodgkin's disease, allowing for known prognostic factors. *Blood* 2000; 95:1207-1213.

[188] Zaki MAA, Wada N, Iked J, Shibayaa H, Hashimoto K, Yamagami T, Tatsumi Y, Tsukaguchi M, Take H, Tsudo M, Morii E, Aozasa K. Prognostic implication of type of tumor-associated macrophages in Hodgkin lymphoma. *Virchows Arch* 2011; 459:361-366.

[189] Mathas S, Dörken B, Janz M. The molecular pathogenesis of classical Hodgkin lymphoma. *Dtsch Med Wochenschr* 2009; 134: 1944-1948.
[190] De Vita VT. Lymphocyte reactivity in Hodgkin's disease: lymphocyte civil war. *N Engl J Med* 1973; 289: 801-802.
[191] Kay MMB. Hodgkin's disease: A war between T-lymphocytes and transformed macrophages. *Monographs on lymphocytes, macrophages and cancer.* RRCR1976; 56:111-121.
[192] Payne SV, Nowell DG, Jones DG, Wright DH. The Reed-Sternberg cell lymphocyte interaction: Ultrastructure and characteristic of binding. *Am J Pathol* 1980; 100: 7-24.
[193] Lee IS, Kim SH, Song HG, Park SH. The molecular basis for the generation of Hodgkin and Reed-Sternberg cells in Hodgkin's lymphoma. *Int J Hematol* 2003; 77: 330-335.
[194] Horie R, Higashihara M, Watanabe T. Hodgkin's lymphoma and CD30 signal transduction. *Int J Hematol* 2003; 77: 37-47.
[195] Yurchenko M, Sidorenko SP. Hodgkin lymphoma: The role of cell surface receptors in regulation of tumor cell fate. *Exp Oncol* 2010; 32:214-223.
[196] Aldinucci D, Gloghini A, Pinto A, De Filippe R, Carbone A. The classical Hodgkin's lymphoma microenvironment and its role in promoting tumor growth and immune escape. *J Pathol* 2010; 221:248-263.
[197] Skinnider BF, Mak TW. The role of cytokines in classical Hodgkin lymphoma. *Blood* 2002; 99:4283-4297.

Index

A

B

C

D

E

F

G

H

I

M

N

O

Q

R

S

T

U

V

W

X

Y

Z